Review and Resource Manual

Psychiatric-Mental Health Nurse Practitioner

5th Edition

By Allyson Matney Neal, DNP, PMHNP-BC, PMHCNS-BC, PNP

Published by the American Nurses Association and
the American Psychiatric Nurses Association

Completion of this or any other course(s)/material(s) does not imply eligibility for certification or successful performance on any certification examination, nor is it a requirement to qualify for certification. The American Nurses Credentialing Center (ANCC) does not endorse any products or services.

About the American Nurses Association
The American Nurses Association (ANA) is the only full-service professional organization representing the interests of the nation's 4.2 million registered nurses through its constituent/state nurses associations and its organizational affiliates. ANA advances the nursing profession by fostering high standards of nursing practice, promoting the rights of nurses in the workplace, projecting a positive and realistic view of nursing, and by lobbying Congress and regulatory agencies on health care issues affecting nurses and the public.

American Nurses Association
8403 Colesville Road,
Silver Spring, MD 20910

About the American Psychiatric Nurses Association
The American Psychiatric Nurses Association (APNA) is your resource for psychiatric-mental health nursing. A professional organization with more than 15,500 members, APNA provides leadership to promote psychiatric-mental health (PMH) nurses; improve mental health care for culturally diverse individuals, families, groups, and communities; and shape health policy for the delivery of mental health services. To facilitate professional advancement, APNA provides quality psychiatric-mental health nursing continuing education; a wealth of resources for established, emerging, and prospective PMH nurses; and a community of dynamic collaboration. APNA champions psychiatric-mental health nursing and mental health care through the development of positions on key issues; the dissemination of current knowledge and developments in PMH nursing; and collaboration with stakeholders to promote advances in recovery-focused assessment, diagnosis, treatment, and evaluation of persons with mental health and substance use conditions. For more information, go to www.apna.org.

Library of Congress Control Number: 2024944240

ISBNs
Print: 978-1-963052-03-9
KDP Print: 979-8-303517-68-4
ePDF: 978-1-963052-04-6
ePUB 978-1-963052-05-3
Mobi: 978-1-963052-06-0
SAN: 851-3481

CONTENTS

A NOTE ABOUT MEDICATION NAMES

Generic names of medications/drugs are utilized throughout this text. The recognized practice of not capitalizing the generic form is employed.

CHAPTER 1

PREPARING FOR THE CERTIFICATION EXAMINATION

BEFORE YOU BEGIN STUDYING

Confirm the eligibility criteria. The eligibility criteria will vary for each exam but may include things like clinical practice hours, degree and license required, etc. Please check the American Nurses Credentialing Center (ANCC) website for details on the particular eligibility criteria for your exam.

Review the ANCC Certification Handbook. The ANCC Certification Handbook can be found on ANCC's website under "Additional Information and Resources" (www.nursingworld.org/certification/certification-policies/). It provides information on how the exam is scored, policies, etc.

Take advantage of all of ANCC's resources:

1. Test content outline: The test content outline includes the number of questions for each domain of practice and identifies the areas that are included on the examination.
2. Test reference list: Review the test reference list for review resources. While the list is not all-inclusive, it will act as a guide to help you prepare.
3. Sample questions: In addition to the review questions at the back of this book, you can find sample questions that are similar to those on the actual examination on ANCC's website. For many exams there are also banks of practice questions available from the American Nurses Association's (ANA) website: www.nursingworld.org/continuing-education/ce-subcategories/certification-review/. Make sure to look at practice tests designed for the exam.
4. Readiness tests: Take a practice test in a simulated test environment either at a Prometric Testing Center or via Live Remote Proctoring to increase your comfort with the test environment and procedures. Find more details about readiness tests on ANCC's website: www.nursingworld.org/certification/readiness-tests/

Develop a personal study plan approximately 3 months before you plan to take your exam. This could include self-study, finding a study buddy or group, taking a review course, taking an online narrated review course, reviewing current textbooks and articles, or other methods. The key is to have a study plan that works for you and follow through on it.

Arrange for special testing accommodations. ANCC and its testing vendor make every effort to reasonably accommodate candidates with documented disabilities as defined by the Americans with Disabilities Act (ADA). If you have a disability as defined under the ADA, you must notify ANCC by submitting a report regarding your request from your physician or a qualified healthcare professional. The information must be on the physician's or other qualified healthcare professional's letterhead, as well as typed, dated, and signed by the healthcare professional. Refer to the ANCC Certification Handbook for more details.

TIPS FOR PREPARING FOR THE EXAM

STEP ONE: ASSESS CURRENT KNOWLEDGE

General Content

Examine the table of contents of this book and the test content outline, available at https://www.nursingworld.org/our-certifications/

- What content do you need to know?
- How well do you know these subjects?

Take a Review Course

- Taking a review course is an excellent way to assess your knowledge of the content that will be included in the exam.
- If you plan to take a review course, take it well before the exam so you will have plenty of time to master any areas of weakness the course uncovers.
- If some topics in the review course are new to you, concentrate on these in your studies.

STEP TWO: DEVELOP YOUR STUDY PLAN

- Write up a formal plan of study.
    - Include topics for study, a timetable, resources, and methods of study that work for you.
    - Decide whether you want to organize a study group or work alone.

    - ◊ Schedule regular times to study.
    - ◊ Avoid cramming; it is counterproductive. Try to schedule your study periods in 1-hour increments.
    - ◊ Gather your study resources (ANCC Certification Handbook, test content outline, test reference list, review manual, sample questions, etc.).
- You will need to know facts and be able to interpret and analyze this information utilizing critical thinking.

Personalize Your Study Plan

- How do you learn best? Choose study methods that fit your learning style.
- Have a specific place with good lighting set aside for studying. Find a place with no distractions. Assemble your study materials.
- Make sure to focus on the areas in which you are weakest and reassess periodically.

STEP THREE: IMPLEMENT YOUR STUDY PLAN

- Refer to your study plan regularly. Write it up or type it out and put it someplace you will see it regularly. Post it at your desk or even put it into your calendar.
- Stick to your schedule.
- Take breaks when you get tired.
- If you start procrastinating, get help from a friend or reorganize your study plan.
- It is not necessary to follow your plan rigidly. Adjust as you learn where you need to spend more time.
- Make sure you reference the test reference list and test content outline on ANCC's website for the latest updates and information about the exam.

Pace Your Studying

- Stop studying for the examination when you start to feel overwhelmed and take a break. If you need to, adjust your study plan:
    - ◊ Break overwhelming tasks into smaller tasks that you know you can do.
    - ◊ Try a new study method.

Work With Others

- Put together a study group.
  - Study groups can provide practice in analyzing cases, interpreting questions, and critical thinking.
  - You can discuss a topic and take turns presenting cases for the group to analyze.
  - Study groups can also provide moral support and help you stay on track.

STEP FOUR: FINAL PREPARATION

Use practice exams when studying to get accustomed to the exam format and time restrictions. The ANA has a bank of sample questions available online in many specialty areas.

Practice tests can help you learn to judge the time it should take you to complete the exam and are useful for gaining experience in analyzing questions. However, keep in mind that books of questions may not uncover the gaps in your knowledge that a more systematic content review text like this manual will reveal. If you feel that you don't know enough about a topic, refer to a text from the reference list to learn more. After you feel that you have learned the topic, practice questions are a wonderful tool to help improve your test-taking skills.

Know your test-taking style and be aware of your potential pitfalls. Do you rush through the exam without reading the questions thoroughly? Practice reading the question completely, including all four choices. Choice "a" may sound good at first glance, but "d" is actually correct. Do you get stuck and dwell on a question for a long time? Remember that computer-based exams allow you to mark questions you are unsure about and go back to them later. You should spend about 45 to 60 seconds per question and finish with time to review the questions you marked. There is also no penalty for guessing; you are encouraged to respond to every examination question.

THE NIGHT BEFORE THE EXAM

- Be prepared to get to the exam on time.
  - Know the test site location and how long it takes to get there.
  - Take a "dry run" beforehand to make sure you know how to get to the testing site, if necessary.
- Get a good night's sleep.
- Eat sensibly.
- Avoid alcohol the night before.

- Assemble the required material to be admitted to the exam. Make sure you have the required form of ID. Reference the ANCC Certification Handbook for information about what you'll need.
- Read over the exam room rules. Know what you can and cannot bring with you.

THE DAY OF THE EXAM

- Get there early. You must arrive to the test center at least 15 minutes before your scheduled appointment time. If you are late, you may not be admitted.
- You will be given a dry erase board, which will be collected at the end of the exam.
- Nothing else is allowed in the exam room. You will be required to put all personal items in a designated area such as a locker.
- Items such as eyewear, jewelry, etc. are subject to visual inspection.
- No water or food will be allowed. You may leave the testing room to use the restroom or get a drink of water, but you will need to sign out according to the instructions that will be explained at the test site. Your testing time will not be increased to accommodate a break.
- Think positively. You have studied hard and are well-prepared.
- Remember your anxiety reduction strategies.

TIPS FOR DEALING WITH ANXIETY

LEADING UP TO THE EXAM

Everyone experiences anxiety when faced with taking the certification exam.

- Taking a review course or setting up your own study plan will help you feel more confident about taking the exam. There is no substitute for being well-prepared.
- Take practice tests and time yourself to get used to the feeling of working on a timer. Remember that the total time for each test is usually 4 hours. Time is not meant to be a factor in the examination.
- Brush up on test-taking skills.
- Practice relaxation techniques. A few minutes of deep breathing, meditation, or even just listening to soothing music can help you calm down and focus.

- Don't put too much stock in what others tell you about their exam experience. Remember that everything they can tell you is based on their memory of a stressful situation; it may not be very accurate. People tend to remember those items with which they are less comfortable; for instance, those with a limited background in women's health may say that the exam was "all women's health." In fact, the test content outline ensures that the exam covers multiple content areas without overemphasizing any one topic.

EXAM DAY ANXIETY

Test anxiety is a specific type of anxiety. Symptoms include upset stomach, sweaty palms, tachycardia, trouble concentrating, and a feeling of dread. There are ways to cope with test anxiety.

- Avoid alcohol, excess caffeine, and any new medications that might sedate you, dull your senses, or make you feel agitated.
- Take a few deep breaths and concentrate on the task at hand.
- Use relaxation techniques such as breathing exercises, progressive muscle relaxation, or imagery and visualization.
- Go into the exam with a strategy in mind. Plan to take water and bathroom breaks at specific intervals and take that opportunity to stretch. Mark questions you're unsure of to come back to them later rather than spending too much time on one question.

INTERNET RESOURCES

- ANCC website: https://www.nursingworld.org/our-certifications/psychiatric-mental-health-nurse-practitioner/
  - Test content outline
  - Test reference list
  - Sample questions
  - Readiness tests
- ANCC Certification Handbook: https://www.nursingworld.org/globalassets/certification/ancc-certification-handbook.pdff
- ANA Bookstore: www.nursingworld.org/education-events/Books/
  - Nursing: Scope and Standards of Practice, 4th edition
  - Psychiatric-Mental Health Nursing: Scope and Standards of Practice, 3rd edition

- ◊ Code of Ethics for Nurses
- ◊ Other titles that may be listed on your test reference list

♦ ANA certification review resources: www.nursingworld.org/continuing-education/ce-subcategories/certification-review/

- ◊ Practice questions
- ◊ Webinars and review courses
- ◊ Strategies for Certification Exam Success

CHAPTER 2

PSYCHIATRIC-MENTAL HEALTH NURSE PRACTITIONER ROLE, SCOPE OF PRACTICE, AND REGULATORY PROCESS

Starting in the 1950s with the seminal work of two psychiatric nurses, June Mellow (1968) and Hildegard Peplau (1952), psychiatric nursing has been a well-established, well-recognized subspecialty of nursing. The emergence of the psychiatric-mental health nurse practitioner (PMHNP) role reflects the growth of the advanced practice role, the acceptance of a brain-based etiology of psychiatric disorders, and an awareness of the need to provide holistic nursing care that does not artificially separate mind and body (Stuart, 2013). The PMHNP role is built on fundamental, advanced practice core knowledge that is common to all nurse practitioners (NPs). This base of knowledge is expanded to include the specific knowledge of the subspecialty of psychiatry. This chapter reviews the role of the PMHNP, the scope of practice, and the regulatory process.

Advanced practice nurses specializing in psychiatry are educationally prepared at the master's or doctoral level, possess in-depth knowledge and skills in the specialty area, and provide primary psychiatric care to individuals or families at risk of or currently experiencing a psychiatric disorder.

NURSE PRACTITIONER ADVANCED PRACTICE CORE CONTENT

All NPs upon graduation are expected to meet a set of core competencies (National Organization of Nurse Practitioner Faculties [NONPF], 2022). NONPF revised the competencies to be in alignment with The Essentials: Core Competencies for Professional Nursing Education (American Association of Colleges of Nursing [AACN], 2021). Specialty competencies, such as the Psychiatric-Mental Health Nurse Practitioner Competencies (NONPF, 2013), are then built upon these core competencies.

AACN ESSENTIALS: CORE COMPETENCIES

- Domain 1: Knowledge of Nursing Practice
  - NONPF NP Domain 1: Knowledge of Practice
- Domain 2: Person-Centered Care
  - NONPF NP Domain 2: Person-Centered Care
- Domain 3: Population Health
  - NONPF NP Domain 3: Population Health
- Domain 4: Scholarship for Nursing Discipline
  - NONPF NP Domain 4: Practice Scholarship and Translational Science
- Domain 5: Quality and Safety
  - NONPF NP Domain 5: Quality and Safety
- Domain 6: Interprofessional Partnerships
  - NONPF NP Domain 6: Interprofessional Collaboration in Practice
- Domain 7: Systems-Based Practice
  - NONPF NP Domain 7: Health Systems
- Domain 8: Informatics and Healthcare Technologies
  - NONPF NP Domain 8: Technology and Information Literacy
- Domain 9: Professionalism
  - NONPF NP Domain 9: Professional Acumen
- Domain 10: Personal, Professional, and Leadership Development
  - NONPF NP Domain 10: Personal and Professional Leadership

NURSE PRACTITIONER ADVANCED PRACTICE SPECIALIZED CONTENT

The specialty competencies are designed specifically for entry-level PMHNP. These specialty competencies are to be used with the Nurse Practitioner Role Competencies (NONPF, 2022). The specialty competencies address the life span PMHNP focus, including families and populations. As changes occur within the health care system, these competencies will also change.

LEADERSHIP COMPETENCIES

- Participates in community and population-focused programs that evaluate programs, promote mental health, and prevent or reduce risk of mental health problems
- Advocates for complex client and family medicolegal rights and issues
- Collaborates with interprofessional colleagues about advocacy, and policy to reduce health disparities and improve outcomes for populations

QUALITY COMPETENCIES

- Evaluates the appropriate uses of seclusion and restraints in the care process

POLICY COMPETENCIES

- Employs opportunities to influence health policy to reduce the impact of stigma on services for the prevention and treatment of mental health problems and psychiatric disorders

INDEPENDENT PRACTICE COMPETENCIES

- Develops individualized, age-appropriate treatment plans
- Includes differential diagnosis
- Assesses the impact of acute and chronic medical problems on psychiatric treatment
- Conducts individual, couples, group, and family psychotherapy
- Applies supportive psychodynamic, cognitive, behavioral, and other evidence-based psychotherapies to brief and long-term practice
- Applies recovery-oriented principles
- Demonstrates best practices of family care approaches
- Plans care to minimize the development of complications and promote function
- Treats acute and chronic psychiatric disorders and problems
- Ensures client safety through the appropriate prescription of pharmacologic and nonpharmacologic interventions

- Explains the risks, benefits, and alternatives of treatment to client and family
- Identifies the role of PMHNP in risk-mitigation strategies in areas of substance use and misuse
- Seeks consultation
- Uses self-reflection to improve care
- Provides consultation to health care providers and others to enhance quality and reduce cost
- Guides clients in evaluating the appropriate use of complementary and alternative treatment
- Uses individualized outcome measures to evaluate psychiatric care
- Manages psychiatric emergencies
- Refers clients appropriately
- Facilitates the transition of clients across levels of care
- Uses outcomes to evaluate care
- Attends to the client–NP relationship as a vehicle for change
- Maintains a therapeutic relationship over time with individuals and groups
- Therapeutically concludes the client–NP relationship
- Demonstrates an ability to address sexual and physical abuse, substance use, sexuality, and spiritual conflicts
- Applies therapeutic relationship strategies based on theory and research
- Applies principles of self-efficacy, empowerment, and others to effect change
- Identifies and maintains professional boundaries
- Teaches clients, families, and groups
- Provides psychoeducation
- Modifies the treatment approach based on client readiness
- Considers motivation and readiness to improve self-care
- Demonstrates knowledge of the appropriate use of seclusion and restraint
- Documents the appropriate use of seclusion and restraints

HISTORY OF THE NP ROLE

The NP role was introduced in 1965 by Loretta C. Ford, EdD, and Henry K. Silver, MD, at the University of Colorado (Mirr Jansen & Zwygart-Stauffacher, 2006). They identified new roles in which experienced registered nurses (RNs) with advanced education and skills were performing clinical duties traditionally reserved for physicians. Universities were slow to implement NP programs at the master's level. However, RNs embraced the new role and rushed into continuing education programs of varying length, quality, and focus to accomplish the necessary educational preparation for this new role.

In 2008, the License, Accreditation, Certification, and Education (LACE) consensus model was finalized and adopted by many nursing organizations. The consensus model identified four Advanced Practice Registered Nurse (APRN) roles: Certified Registered Nurse Anesthetist (CRNA), Certified Nurse Midwife (CNM), Clinical Nurse Specialist (CNS), and Certified Nurse Practitioner (CNP). As part of the LACE model, psychiatric-mental health was identified as a population focus. The APNA and International Society of Psychiatric-Mental Health Nurses (ISPN) recommendation was for PMHNPs to be prepared across the life span (American Psychiatric Nurses Association [APNA], 2011). In 2015, APRN in psychiatric-mental health nursing moved to certification examination, PMHNP–Life Span, with the American Nurses Credentialing Center (ANCC).

Proven competence brought an acceptance of the NP role in the health care system, with acceptance and recognition of the title and role by consumers and other health care professionals. NP programs are accredited by one of two organizations to achieve standardization and control over quality: the Commission on Collegiate Nursing Education (CCNE, 2023) and the Accreditation Commission for Education in Nursing (ACEN, 2023). NPs are recognized providers under many third-party insurance coverage plans (e.g., Medicare, Medicaid, Civilian Health and Medical Program of the Uniformed Services, federal programs funding school-based clinics, U.S. military, Veterans Administration).

GROWTH OF THE NP ROLE

- Facilitating factors for growth
  - Consumer demand for services
  - Acceptance of the advanced practice nursing role
  - Emergence of the PMHNP role
  - Decreasing stigmatization
  - Emphasis on integrated health care services

- Constraining factors for growth
  - Growing competition in the job market in general for NPs
  - Reimbursement struggles with Medicare and private insurance companies
  - Overlapping scope of practice with other NPs
  - Increased concerns over reimbursement fraud and abuse (e.g., issues of coding and billing for services)
  - Scope of practice and need for formal supervisory or collaborative relationships with physicians

REGULATORY AND STATUTORY DIMENSIONS OF THE NP ROLE

- State legislative statutes
  - Grant legal authority for NP practice
  - The Nurse Practice Act of every state
    - Provides title protection (who may be called an NP)
    - Defines advanced practice
    - Prevailing state laws that define scope of practice (what NPs may do)
    - Places restrictions on practice
    - Sets NP credentialing requirements (e.g., educational requirements, certification)
    - States grounds for disciplinary action
      - Practicing without valid license
      - Falsification of records
      - Medicare fraud
      - Failure to use appropriate nursing judgment
      - Failure to follow accepted nursing standards
      - Failure to complete accurate nursing documentation
    - May specifically require that an NP develop a collaborative agreement with a physician
      - Collaborative agreement: Also known as a protocol that describes what types of drugs might be prescribed and defines some form of oversight for NP practice
- Statutory law
  - Rules and regulations differ for each state

    - May further define scope of practice and practice requirements
    - May provide restrictions in practice that are unique to a specific state
- Licensure
    - A process by which an agency of state government grants permission to persons to engage in the practice of that profession
    - Also prohibits all others from legally doing protected practice
- Credentialing
    - A process used to protect the public by ensuring a minimum level of professional competence
- Certification
    - A credential that provides title protection
    - Determines scope of practice (i.e., who NPs can see and what NPs can treat)
    - The process by which a professional organization or association certifies that a person licensed to practice as a professional has met certain predetermined standards specified by that profession for specialty practice
    - Assures the public that a person has mastery of a specified body of knowledge
    - Ensures that the person has acquired the skills necessary to function in a particular specialty
    - ANCC, a subsidiary of the American Nurses Association (ANA), Is the only certifying body for advanced practice psychiatric nursing.
- Certification offered as a PMHNP–Life Span (ANCC, 2023)
- Scope of practice
    - Defines NP roles and actions
    - Identifies competencies assumed to be held by all NPs who function in a particular role
    - Varies broadly from state to state
    - Advanced practice PMHNP standards are identified in Psychiatric-Mental Health Nursing: Scope and Standards of Practice (ANA, APNA, & ISPN, 2022).
- Standards of practice
    - Authoritative statements that describe the quality and type of practice that should be provided
    - Provide a way to judge the nature of care provided
    - Reflect the expectation for the care that should be provided to clients with various illnesses
    - Reflect professional agreement focused on the minimum levels of acceptable performance

- ◊ Can be used to legally describe the standard of care that must be met by a provider
- ◊ May be precise protocols that must be followed or more general guidelines that recommend actions

PROFESSIONAL ROLE RESPONSIBILITIES

- Confidentiality
  - ◊ The client's right to assume that information given to the health care provider will not be disclosed
  - ◊ Protected under federal statute through the Medical Records Confidentiality Act of 1995 (S.1360)
  - ◊ Pertains to verbal and written client information
  - ◊ Requires that the provider discuss confidentiality issues with clients, establish consent, and clarify any questions about disclosure of information
  - ◊ Requires that the provider obtain a signed medical authorization and consent form to release medical records and information when requested by the client or another health care provider
- Health Insurance Portability and Accountability Act (HIPAA)
  - ◊ The first national comprehensive privacy protection act
  - ◊ Guarantees clients four fundamental rights
    - To be educated about HIPAA privacy protection
    - To have access to their own medical records
    - To request amendment of their health information to which they object
    - To require their permission for disclosure of their personal information
- The Health Information Technology for Economic and Clinical Health Act (HITECH) of 2009 (U.S. Department of Health and Human Services [HHS], 2017)
  - ◊ Provides incentive payments for sharing specific electronic health record (EHR) data
  - ◊ Provides meaningful-use incentives
  - ◊ EHRs can improve both individual and population-based health outcomes (Friedman et al., 2013).
  - ◊ EHRs can improve quality, safety, efficiency, effectiveness, and outcomes (HHS, Office for Civil Rights, 2013).
- E-prescribing
- Computerized physician order sets

- Tracking care and avoiding duplication of services
- Telehealth
  - The use of electronic information and telecommunication technologies to support long-distance clinical health care (Health Resources and Services Administration [HRSA], 2022). It is often used for those who may otherwise not be able to access care.
  - Must follow the same standards as care delivered in person
  - Must be practiced in accordance with international, federal, and state regulatory agency standards
  - Must include provisions for emergency care of the client
  - The PMHNP must ensure that HIPAA regulations regarding confidentiality and maintenance of the health record are followed.
- Exceptions to guaranteed confidentiality
  - When appropriate persons or organizations determine that the need for information outweighs the principle of confidentiality
  - If a client reveals an intent to harm self or others
  - Information given to attorneys involved in litigation
  - Releasing records to insurance companies
  - Answering court orders, subpoenas, or summonses
  - Meeting state requirements for mandatory reporting of diseases or conditions
  - Tarasoff principle (Tarasoff v. Regents of the University of California, 1976): Duty to warn potential victim of imminent danger of homicidal clients
  - In cases of child or elder abuse
- Informed consent
  - The communication process between the provider and the client that results in the client's acceptance or rejection of the proposed treatment
  - An explanation of relevant information that enables the client to make an appropriate and informed decision
  - The rights of all competent adults or emancipated minors
    - Emancipated minors: Persons younger than 18 years who are married, are parents, or are self-sufficiently living away from the family domicile
  - Elements of informed consent
    - Nature and purpose of proposed treatment or procedure
    - Risks or discomforts and benefits of treatment
    - Risks and benefits of not undergoing treatment
    - Alternative procedures or treatments

- Diagnosis and prognosis
  - The provider must document in the medical record that informed consent has been obtained from the client.
  - The PMHNP is responsible for ensuring that the client is cognitively capable of giving informed consent.
    - Capacity is the ability to use information given related to the diagnosis and treatment to make decisions regarding the plan of care.
    - Capacity is not fixed and must be assessed throughout treatment
      - Disorders and conditions that may affect cognition and, therefore, capacity include:
        - Neurocognitive disorders
        - Mental health disorders
          - Schizophrenia
          - Depression
          - Substance use
        - Traumatic brain injury
        - Hospitalized adults
        - End of life
      - Elements of decision-making capacity
        - Understanding: is able to state the diagnosis, risks, benefits, options
        - Expressing a choice: is able to clearly state the decision
        - Appreciation: expresses how the information applies
        - Reasoning: is able to compare the information given and possible consequences
  - A person is described as having adequate, marginal, or inadequate decision-making capacity
- Ethics
  - Important aspect of the NP role that deals with moral duties, obligations, and responsibilities
  - What is right versus what is wrong
  - Bioethical principles provide the foundation and direction in clinical decision-making:
    - Justice: Doing what is fair; fairness in all aspects of care
    - Beneficence: Promoting well-being and doing good
    - Nonmaleficence: Doing no harm

- Fidelity: Being true and loyal
- Autonomy: Doing for self
- Veracity: Telling the truth
- Respect: Treating everyone with equal respect

◊ In 2015, ANA published the Code of Ethics for Nurses with Interpretive Statements (ANA, 2015). Its nine provisions are:

1. The nurse practices with compassion and respect for the inherent dignity, worth, and unique attributes of every person.
2. The nurse's primary commitment is to the client, whether an individual, family, group, community, or population.
3. The nurse promotes, advocates for, and protects the rights, health, and safety of the client.
4. The nurse has the authority, accountability, and responsibility for nursing practice; makes decisions; and takes action consistent with the obligation to promote health and provide optimal care.
5. The nurse owes the same duties to self as to others, including the responsibility to promote health and safety, preserve wholeness of character and integrity, maintain competence, and continue personal and professional growth.
6. The nurse, through individual and collective effort, establishes, maintains, and improves the ethical environment of the work setting and conditions of employment that are conducive to safe, quality health care.
7. The nurse, in all roles and settings, advances the profession through research and scholarly inquiry, professional standards development, and the generation of both nursing and health policy.
8. The nurse collaborates with other health professionals and the public to protect human rights, promote health diplomacy, and reduce health disparities.
9. The profession of nursing, collectively through its professional organizations, must articulate nursing values, maintain the integrity of the profession, and integrate principles of social justice into nursing and health policy.

◊ Important ethical principles in psychiatry

- Clients must be involved in decision-making to the full extent of their capacity (shared decision-making).
- Clients have a right to treatment in the least-restrictive setting.
- Clients have a right to refuse treatment unless a legal process resulting in a mandatory court order for treatment has been obtained.

◊ Ethical dilemma

- Occurs in a situation in which there are two or more justifiable alternatives
- Occurs when the choice is made to promote good

- Which option sacrifices the fewest high-priority values (a harm-reduction approach)?

◊ Theoretical approaches to ethical decision-making

- Deontological theory: An action is judged as good or bad based on the act itself regardless of the consequences.
- Teleological theory: An action is judged as good or bad based on the consequence or outcome.
- Virtue ethics: Actions are chosen based on moral virtues (e.g., honesty, courage, compassion, wisdom, gratitude, self-respect) or the character of the person making the decision.

ETHICS OF DISCLOSURE BY PROVIDERS

- Clients have a right to know what is happening during the course of their treatment.
- Providers have an ethical responsibility to disclose medical errors, accidents, injuries, and negative results to clients.
- As a result of the disclosure, a client may have a legal right to compensation for harm suffered due to medical misadventures (Sadock et al., 2017).

RISK VERSUS BENEFITS OF DISCLOSURE OF DISABILITY REGARDING EMPLOYMENT

- The Americans with Disabilities Act (ADA) works to prevent discrimination by employers with 15 or more employees against qualified persons in hiring, firing, advancement, job training, compensation, and workplace conditions (Buppert, 2021).
- The ADA is federal legislation granting Americans who have disabilities, including mental illness, the opportunity for employment on an equal basis with the nondisabled.
- Employers are required to make reasonable accommodations for qualified applicants or employees with a disability.

Risk of Disclosure

- Employers may find ways to avoid hiring persons known to have a disability.
- Coworkers may harass or discriminate against persons with psychiatric illnesses.
- It may be unfairly assumed that persons with psychiatric illnesses may be less productive.

- May limit an employee's chance for advancement in career.
- Feedback for improvement may not be given to the employee because others may attribute the employee's behavior to the psychiatric illness.
- Labeling oneself as "disabled" may affect one's beliefs or self-image.

Benefits of Disclosure

- Ability to request reasonable accommodations
- Opportunity to have a job coach come to the worksite and communicate directly with employer
- Employee can involve an employment service provider, employee assistance program, or other third party in the development of accommodations
- Easier for employee to come to work during an exacerbation of symptoms
- May help with the recovery process
- Allows coworkers to offer personal support
- May empower another employee to disclose

LEGAL CONSIDERATIONS

- Malpractice insurance
    - Provides financial protection against claims of malpractice
    - Provides coverage for negligent professional acts
    - Provides coverage for highly technical or professional skills required by health care professionals, including NPs
    - Is recommended universally for all NPs
    - Does not protect NPs from charges of practicing outside their legal scope of practice
    - Provides NPs with their own legal representation to advocate for them even if their agency also carries malpractice liability insurance protection
    - Four elements of negligence that must be established to prove malpractice
        1. Duty: The NP had a duty to exercise reasonable care when undertaking and providing treatment to the client.
        2. Breach of duty: The NP violated the applicable standard of care in treating the client's condition.

3. Proximate cause: There is a causal relationship between the breach in the standard of care and the client's injuries.
4. Damages: The client experiences permanent and substantial damages as a result of the breach in the standard of care.

COMPETENCY

- A legal, not a medical, concept
- A determination that a client can make reasonable judgments and decisions regarding treatment and other health concerns
- A person is considered competent until a court rules the person to be incompetent.
- If a person is deemed incompetent, a court-appointed guardian will make health-related decisions for that person.

COMMITMENT

- The process of forcing a person to receive involuntarily evaluation or treatment
- The process may differ from state to state.
- Basic criteria
  - Person has a diagnosed psychiatric disorder
  - Person is harmful to self or others as a consequence of the disorder
  - Person is unaware of or unwilling to accept the nature and severity of the disorder
  - Treatment is likely to improve functioning
- Involuntary admission
  - Admission to a hospital or other treatment facility against the person's will
  - Clients maintain all civil liberties except the ability to come and go as they please.
  - Amount of time clients can be kept against their wishes varies by state.
- Voluntary admission
  - Admission to a hospital or other treatment facility that a person desires or agrees to
  - Client maintains all civil liberties
  - Client consents to potential confinement within the structure of a hospital setting

ROLES OF THE PMHNP

SCHOLARLY ACTIVITIES

- It is important for NPs to engage in the following scholarly activities:
  - Publishing
  - Lecturing or presenting
  - Precepting PMHNP students continuing education

MENTORING (APNA, 2022)

- Mentoring implies a knowledge or competence gradient, in which the teaching–learning process contributes to a sharing of advice or expertise, role development, and formal and informal support to influence the career of the protégé (Jakubik et al., 2016)
- A mutually agreed upon relationship with goals and methods for accountability
- A process in which a more experienced NP agrees to guide and support a junior colleague in the role, competencies, and skills
- Requires mutual respect and an interactive process of learning
- Most mentoring relationships are long term and end when mutually agreed to do so.

CLIENT ADVOCACY

- Means to stand up for clients' rights and empower them to become their own advocates
- Reduces the stigma of mental illness
- Helps clients receive available services
- Promotes mental health by participating in one or more of these professional organizations:
  - American Nurses Association (ANA)
  - American Psychiatric Nurses Association (APNA)
  - International Society of Psychiatric Nurses (ISPN)

HEALTH POLICY

- Advanced practice nurses have a legal and ethical responsibility to be client advocates.
  - Participation in local, state, national, and international health policy activities (Buppert, 2021)
  - Involvement: Testify at a public meeting, lobby, or work with the media to bring awareness to an issue
  - Phases of policy-making: Formulation, implementation, and evaluation (Abood, 2007)

CASE MANAGEMENT

- A system of controlled oversight and authorization of services and benefits provided to clients
- Consists of coordinating care, ensuring quality outcomes, monitoring plan of care, and doing advocacy
- Overall goal is to promote quality, cost-effective outcomes

Risk Assessment

- Continuous monitoring for high-risk situations
- Assessing persons for nonhealthy behaviors

Risk Management

- Activities or systems designed to recognize and intervene to reduce the risk of injury to clients
- Appropriate interventions implemented to reduce unhealthy behaviors in clients and high-risk situations
- Recognition and intervention to reduce subsequent claims against health care providers

ADVANCE DIRECTIVES

- Durable power of attorney for health care, also known as health care proxy
  - Legally binding in all 50 states

- ◊ Designates, in writing, an agent to act on behalf of a person should they become unable to make health care decisions
- ◊ Not limited to terminal illness; also covers other aspects of illness, such as making financial decisions during a person's illness
- ◊ Should be considered as an aspect of relapse planning for clients with chronic psychiatric disorders

- ♦ Living will: Document prepared while client is mentally competent to designate preferences for care if client becomes incompetent or terminally ill
    - ◊ Not legally binding in all states

CULTURALLY COMPETENT CARE AND SPECIAL POPULATIONS

- ♦ Treating clients from diverse cultures, viewing each client as a unique person, and noting a potential relationship between clients' cultural experiences and their symptom presentation and perceptions
- ♦ Assumes that if the NP becomes more sensitive to cultural issues influencing the client's symptoms and treatment, more comprehensive health care can be provided
- ♦ Culture: The learned beliefs and behaviors or the socially inherited characteristics that are common among all members of a group; may be a racial, social, ethnic, or religious grouping
- ♦ Culture-bound syndromes: Specific behaviors related to a person's culture and not linked to a psychiatric disorder
    - ◊ Be cognizant of inaccurately judging a client's behavior as psychopathology when it is really related to their culture.

BARRIERS TO CULTURAL AND SPIRITUAL COMPETENCES

- ♦ It is the responsibility of the provider to recognize and address barriers on an ongoing basis. Barriers have been identified as the following:
    - ◊ Lack of diverse providers and organizational leadership
    - ◊ Limited awareness of differences
    - ◊ Lack of training
    - ◊ Ethnocentrism
    - ◊ Unrecognized prejudice

CULTURAL INFLUENCES AND DETERMINANTS OF HEALTH

- Family: A group of adults and children who are usually related and whose adults participate in carrying out the essential functions of providing food, clothing, shelter, safety, and education of children
  - Concept broadened beyond the traditional husband–wife–children pattern
  - Family initially teaches the belief patterns, religion, culture, and mores of a society
- Ethnicity: Self-identified race, tribe, or nation with which a person or group identifies and that greatly influences beliefs and behavior
- Community: A group of individuals linked together due to their common characteristics or interests
- Social determinants of health:
  - Economic stability
  - Educational access and quality
  - Health care access and quality
  - Neighborhood and built environment
  - Social and community context

BEING UNHOUSED

Being unhoused is an enormous problem affecting the United States and the world. It can have devastating effects on individuals' and families' emotional and physical health. Substance use, violence, and severe mental illnesses are just a few major issues faced by persons who are unhoused. The practitioner must be aware of the challenges faced by this vulnerable population. Possessing appropriate communication skills and knowledge of available resources is invaluable.

- Unhoused person
  - Someone who does not have stable or consistent nighttime housing or who maintains permanent residence at shelters, hotels, transitional housing, or public places not appropriate for human beings to live in; someone intended to be institutionalized who is in an institution for transitory residence
  - Men, women, and children make up the unhoused population. The number of unhoused families is on the rise.
- The majority of unhoused families are headed by a single parent, usually a woman.
  - Female-headed households are at high risk for becoming unhoused if the head of household has limited education or employment skills, low-paying employment with little or no benefits, and limited access to affordable housing.

    - Teen mothers are at high risk due to lack of education and incomes that older parents possess.
- Reasons for becoming unhoused
    - Mental illness
    - Substance use disorders
    - Poverty
    - Unemployment
    - Inadequate public assistance
    - Domestic violence
    - Lifestyle choice
- Mental illness and substance use disorders in the unhoused population
    - Approximately 50% of people who are unhoused have co-occurring substance use disorders and serious mental illness, including bipolar disorder, schizophrenia, and depression.
    - Severe mental illness accounts for 25% to 30% of the U.S. unhoused population (Padgett, 2020; Sadock et al., 2017).
    - Symptoms are often active and untreated.
    - Untreated serious mental illness results in symptoms such as paranoia, hallucinations, mania, anxiety, and depression, making it difficult for people to maintain employment, relationships, and activities of daily living.
    - People who are unhoused with co-occurring disorders are at a greater risk for violence, medication nonadherence, and treatment resistance.

Strategies for Reducing Rates of Unhoused Individuals

- Outreach: Introducing services to persons who are unhoused with serious mental illness in various settings; building an empathetic, consistent, and caring relationship to provide treatment
- Integrated care: Treatment combining mental health and medical care to improve overall functioning in the community; may also include access to dental care and pharmacy services
- Co-location: Providing mental health and primary care services at a single site
- Supporting services to persons in housing: Effective in moving persons who are unhoused with serious mental illness directly to independent housing with support and intensive attention
- Prevention: Beginning with discharge planning in inpatient settings, provide resources for mental health care, housing, transitioning service, and follow-up

MIGRANT AND SEASONAL FARM WORKERS

- Migrant: Persons who leave their permanent residences to take agricultural jobs in different locations
- Seasonal: Workers who travel from their permanent residences seasonally for agricultural employment
- Includes men, women, and children of all cultures
- It is estimated that more than 3 million migrant and seasonal farm workers work in the United States (National Center for Farmworker Health, 2023).
  - Hard to get an accurate census because families and workers move a great deal
- Working conditions; problems with the process of acculturation, isolation, discrimination; and impaired access to health care play a role in a high prevalence of mental illness among migrant and seasonal farm workers.
- Very high incidence of depression, anxiety, and substance use
- Physical and emotional abuse of women is harder to address because of frequent changes of location.
- Meeting the mental health needs of this vulnerable population can pose a challenge because of the ways specific cultures perceive mental illness. Displaying an empathic, understanding, and culturally sensitive attitude is imperative when promoting care to this population.

SEXUAL ORIENTATION AND GENDER IDENTITY

Possessing a thorough understanding of sexuality is of great importance when communicating with clients of different sexual orientations. The practitioner must possess an open, supportive, sensitive, and empathetic attitude toward the client. Understanding the client's viewpoint and what they are seeking will help facilitate an effective psychiatric evaluation. In addition, an awareness of the factors that the client may have faced because of their sexuality is crucial (Sadock et al., 2017).

- Gender identity: A person's identity along a continuum between normative constructs of masculinity and femininity. Note that some clients may identify with genders outside of these normative constructs (e.g., nonbinary, genderfluid)
  - Influences on gender identity may consist of biological and social factors.
  - Biological factors may include pre- and postnatal hormone levels and gene expression.

    - ◊ Social factors may include gender messages from family, mass media, and cultural attitudes.

- Gender dysphoria: The formal diagnosis to describe a marked incongruence between one's experienced and expressed gender, and the gender assigned at birth
- Sexual orientation: The direction of sexual attraction; preferred over "sexual preference" or "lifestyle," which imply choice, whereas "orientation" does not; some prefer "sexual identity" because it allows people to determine their own identities. Sexual orientation does not always relate to gender identity.
- Asexual: Does not experience sexual attraction to others
- Bisexual: Attracted to both sexes
- Pansexual: Attraction to others not limited by sex, current gender identification, or gender expression
- Heterosexual: Attracted to the opposite sex
- Homosexual: Attracted to the same sex
- Transgender: Umbrella term describing persons whose gender identity does not conform to gender norms associated with the gender they were assigned at birth; does not imply a particular sexual orientation
- Transsexualism: This is an outdated term and could be offensive to some clients. It should be avoided unless a client specifically requests to use this term. Persons who identify as the opposite gender from the one they were assigned at birth; some change their bodies hormonally and surgically to conform to their gender identity
- LGBTQIA+: Lesbian, gay, bisexual, transgender, queer or questioning, asexual, and intersex
- Many clients seek treatment from a provider of the same orientation
- Sexual behavior: The manner in which humans experience and express their sexuality; includes attracting partners, sexual interactions, and social interactions

Caring for Clients in the LGBTQIA+ Population

People with gender identity and sexual orientation outside of the perceived societal norms

- Have increased rates of mental illness
- Have increased high-risk behaviors
- Have increased attempts to end their own life

- Have increased lack of stable housing, especially youth
- Have less access to care because of provider or clinic bias

Because of the preceding, this population is often medically and psychiatrically underserved. The following are mental health statistics for the LGBTQIA+ population (National Alliance on Mental Illness [NAMI], 2023):

- LGBTQIA+ adults are more than twice as likely as heterosexual adults to experience a mental health condition.
- LGBTQIA+ people are at a higher risk than the general population for suicidal thoughts and attempts to end their own life.
- Youths who identify as lesbian, gay, or bisexual are almost four times as likely to attempt to end their own life compared to their heterosexual peers.
- 48% of all transgender adults report that they have considered suicide in the past 12 months, compared to 4% of the overall U.S. population.

Equity, diversity, and inclusion include the following ideals:

- Patient-perspective care values the viewpoint and preference of the individual (Carey, 2016).
- Intentionally create a welcoming environment that embraces diverse people, perspectives, and experiences.
- Clients, families, and communities are equal partners in promoting well-being.

Best practices are as follows:

- Allow people to self-identify
    - Pronouns or identified pronouns
        - Avoid using the term "preferred pronouns" as it insinuates that gender identity is a choice
        - Use requested names and pronouns
- Accept parents outside the mother–father dyad (e.g., two mothers can come into the ICU)
- Be respectful
- Ask about their lives and what is important in their care; accept the answers

The following are ways to navigate documentation and legal issues:

- Have a way to document in the EHR the requested name and gender if it does not match official documentation.

- Documented names and genders are needed only for legal items such as consents or prescriptions.
- It is acceptable to use preferred name and gender in notes if there is notation of this elsewhere in the chart.

Unique Medical Needs of Transgender Clients

There is no standard stage of physical transition. It is highly variable due to time since transition, various ages when transition starts, ability to have surgery or take hormones, and client preference. It is impossible to tell by visual exam.

Document the medications and hormones that the client is taking, plus a list of surgical procedures and an "organ list" that the client has presented. This will inform what preventive care and routine screenings are needed.

Examples include transgender men with breasts and traditionally female genitalia and sexual organs or transgender women with prostates and testicles.

The PMHNP needs to be aware of the policies and regulations impacting gender affirming care, which can vary by state.

The following are guidelines for medical or surgical transitioning (Coleman et al., 2022; World Professional Association for Transgender Health, n.d.):

- The diagnosis of gender dysphoria or gender incongruence is made by a mental health professional prior to surgical or medical treatment by an endocrinologist.
- A mental health professional needs to be involved in the diagnosis and treatment of gender dysphoria or gender incongruence in adolescents.
- The adolescent client has reached the Tanner stage 2 of puberty prior to the initiation of pubertal suppression.
- Gender affirming surgery is considered only after a minimum of 12 months of gender affirming hormone therapy.
- Mental health care is recommended due to the risk of side effects from the medications used and the stresses of transitioning.

Gender-Affirming Medical Treatment—Hormone Therapy (Unger, 2016)

Testosterone ("T"): Used as a monotherapy (US Food and Drug Administration [FDA] off-label use)

- Provided as intramuscular < subcutaneous (IM < SubQ) and topical formulations

- Risk of cardiovascular events, hyperlipidemia, and increased blood pressure when using testosterone; increased monitoring required
- Risk of increased depression and suicidal ideation
- Can interact with oral hypoglycemic agents with increased lowering of blood sugar

Leuprolide

- Hormonal suppression for male-to-female transition in combination with estrogen; off-label use
- Given as a depot shot, 1-month and 3-month formulations
- Increased risk of hyperglycemia and cardiac events when used with transgender women
- Possible psychiatric side effects include emotional lability, irritability, anger, and aggression

Estrogen

- Used to reduce the male secondary sexual characteristics
- Formulations transdermal or oral
- Concerns with prolonged use include breast cancer and decrease in bone density

Spironolactone

- A potassium-sparing diuretic; is also a mineralocorticoid receptor antagonist
- Given orally
- Commonly used in the United States as an aldosterone blocker in combination with estrogen due to higher cost and IM dosing of leuprorelin
- Potassium levels need to be monitored

FORENSICS AND CORRECTIONS

Deinstitutionalization began in the 1970s, leaving many with a mental illness or intellectual disability in need of housing in the community. One of the places that persons with a mental illness are overrepresented is in the criminal justice system (Kennedy-Hendricks et al., 2016, p. 1077). Persons in the prison system have higher rates of serious mental illnesses as compared to those in the community (Prins, 2014).

According to the Prison Policy Initiative (2023)

- 43% of the state prison population have a diagnosed mental health disorder

- 44% of those incarcerated in local jails are diagnosed with a mental health disorder
- 1 in 4 report experiencing serious psychological distress in jail
- 66% of federal and 74% of state inmates received no mental health treatment while incarcerated
- 27% of those incarcerated 3 or more times in 1 year reported a moderate or severe mental illness
- Mental health effects of being incarcerated
    - Posttraumatic stress disorder
    - Anxiety
    - Impaired decision-making
- 27% of police shootings in 2015 involved a mental health crisis

Unfortunately, lack of synchronized care among criminal justice, mental health, and public health systems results in repeat incarcerations (Baillargeon et al., 2010; Kushel et al., 2005). It is essential to remain neutral, calm, and objective and to be skilled in self-reflective techniques as well as acknowledging one's own emotional response and biases when providing care for imprisoned clients. Lyons (2009) recommends that the practitioner compartmentalize emotional responses and biases temporarily and debrief afterward.

- Forensic: The application of scientific knowledge to legal problems and legal proceedings, for example, in forensic anthropology, forensic dentistry, forensic medicine (legal medicine), forensic psychology, and forensic science
- Forensic science: The application of a broad range of sciences to answer questions of interest to the legal system; a high-technology field using electron microscopes, lasers, ultraviolet and infrared light, advanced analytical techniques, and computerized databanks to analyze and research evidence
- Forensic nursing: The practice of nursing when health and legal systems intersect; the forensic nurse provides direct services to individual clients; consultation services to nursing, medical, and legal agencies; and expert court testimony in areas dealing with trauma or investigations of questioned deaths, adequacy of services delivery, and specialized diagnoses of specific conditions as related to nursing

FORENSIC VERSUS CORRECTIONAL

- Forensic: Nurse–client relationship based on crime committed and investigational aspect of the interaction

- Correctional: Nurse–client relationship based on offender's current mental health and medical conditions
- Locations: Emergency departments, prisons (high-, medium-, and low-security units), courts, and police stations (Lyons, 2009)

Forensic Knowledge Base

- Relies on evidence-based practice as well as past clinical experience
- Incorporates both criminal justice and mental health systems
- The forensic PMHNP should possess theoretical and practical knowledge of the criminal justice and mental health systems.
    - Function of the court
    - Litigation procedures
    - Workings of the criminal justice system
    - Relevant case law and health litigation
    - Understanding of mental health, distorted thinking patterns, and impaired cognition
    - Areas of competence and skill: safety, security, management, and assessment of risk; management of aggression and violence; therapeutic relationship; offending behavior knowledge; prison culture; documentation; medical knowledge; psychopharmacology; and crisis de-escalation (Lyons, 2009)

Forensic Risk Assessment Versus Risk Assessment

- Forensic risk assessment: "Aims to assess whether a patient is a risk to themselves or others in terms of serious violence, dangerousness, absconding, and recidivism now or in the future" (Lyons, 2009, p. 53)
- Risk assessment:
    - Utilized throughout the process of interaction between the PMHNP and the client
    - May be initially performed in emergency department
    - Often implemented based on the need to keep the client safe and to protect healthcare workers
    - Should be continuous part of PMHNP's decision-making process to "predict and manage crises as they arise, control freedom of movement, and maintain safe levels of supervision and observation" (Lyons, 2009, p. 53)

CASE STUDY 1

A newly graduated PMHNP who worked as a psychiatric nurse before going to graduate school is considering a position at a community mental health center. The client population would consist of mainly adults with serious, chronic, and persistent mental illness; occasional children; clients in crisis; and emergent medical needs such as management of diabetes, hypertension, and chronic pain.

What does the PMHNP need to consider before accepting this position?

1. Is the PMHNP legally authorized to treat both children and adults?
2. What regulation, rule, or standard should be consulted to determine if the PMHNP is legally allowed to treat both children and adults?
3. What regulation, rule, or standard should be consulted to determine if the PMHNP is legally allowed to treat both physical and psychiatric disorders?
4. What is the role of professional psychiatric nursing organizations in assisting PMHNPs to determine the scope of practice that is appropriate for a new graduate?

The PMHNP decides not to take that job and instead has been working for about a year as a PMHNP in a nurse-managed primary mental health clinic. One day the PMHNP is asked to assess a client who is talking to people not present in the room, is anxious that other people want to harm them, and is expressing verbal threats against many persons at another clinical practice in town who had "malpracticed" them. The client is adamant that they do not wish any treatment and that they are not ill. To care for this client, the PMHNP must consider these questions:

5. Is the PMHNP able to treat the client if they do not consent to care?
6. What legal standards must be met to treat this client without his consent?

About 5 weeks later the previously mentioned client returns to the clinic for follow-up care. The client is clinically stable, on medication, and showing no active symptoms, and is interested in developing a relapse prevention plan and asks the PMHNP to assist them in this process. The PMHNP must consider thse additional questions:

7. Is the inclusion of a durable power of attorney an appropriate strategy in relapse planning for this client?
8. What quality indicators should be considered in planning the client's care with them?
9. What risk management and liability issues should be considered?

CASE STUDY 2

A PMHNP working in a rural mental health clinic is asked by a primary care provider to evaluate a 35-year-old client. The client insists they are not "depressed," but rather that they have been feeling understandably distressed after being fired from their job for excessive absenteeism related to "head, neck, and back pain." The client has difficulty falling and staying asleep, wakes up feeling tearful, and does not want to get out of bed. The client has become socially isolative and spends hours sitting in front of the television. For the past 6 months, the client has been taking 50 mg of amitriptyline that was prescribed by the primary care provider. After evaluating the client, the PMHNP decides that the criteria for major depression have been met and increases the dose of amitriptyline.

1. How should the PMHNP explain to the client their rationale for increasing the dose of the amitriptyline?
2. Because amitriptyline is a tricyclic antidepressant, is it reasonable for the PMHNP to continue and even adjust the dose of this medication—in other words, is this treatment within the scope of the PMHNP's practice?

ANSWERS TO CASE STUDY DISCUSSION QUESTIONS

CASE STUDY 1

1. The key word here is "legally." Professional standards and scope of practice documents suggest what is reasonable and prudent practice. Professional nursing organizations will provide information on what is seen as acceptable educational preparation for practice. However, the individual legislative regulations of each state determine what constitutes legal practice for each individual PMHNP.
2. The Nurse Practice Act and related legislation of the state in which the PMHNP practices will delineate the legal boundaries of their practice.
3. Professional standards and scope-of-practice documents suggest what is reasonable and prudent practice. The individual legislative regulations of each state determine what constitutes legal practice for each individual PMHNP.
4. Professional nursing organizations provide information through a scope and standards document about what is seen as an acceptable practice role for PMHNPs, but the PMHNP's practice is ultimately guided by the individual state's nurse practice act.
5. Any client, including a psychiatric client, has the right to refuse treatment. The PMHNP is legally and ethically bound to honor the client's rights.
6. The legal standard must be met in the state where the PMHNP practices to treat a client against their wishes. This usually entails performing the legal task of committing a client, and in most states, ensuring that the following criteria are met:
   - ◊ The person has a diagnosed psychiatric disorder.
   - ◊ The person is unaware of or unwilling to accept the nature and severity of disorder.
   - ◊ As a result of a mental disorder, a person is harmful to self or others.
   - ◊ As a result of a mental disorder, a person cannot take care of their basic needs of food, clothing, and shelter.
7. A durable power of attorney allows a person in a state of health to choose another person to act on their behalf should they become unable to make their own health care decisions. Chronic mental illness has the potential to render a person unable to make health care decisions, and a durable power of attorney document should be part of relapse planning.
8. Standardized client assessment and rating scales, evidence-based standards of care, and measures of quality, including client and family satisfaction, should be considered.
9. The PMHNP should adhere to standards and scope of practice and identify factors specific to this client that increase liability exposure.

CASE STUDY 2

1. The PMHNP must discuss the treatment plan in the context of the client's psychiatric symptoms. Without trying to convince the client that they have major depression, the PMHNP can discuss how chronic pain may have led to the distress that is currently being experienced and that the medication may address many of the distressing symptoms. The provider will also need to address the potential side effects from this tricyclic antidepressant and the usual course of treatment in terms of dosing and timeline.
2. Yes, if the PMHNP is using the medication to target the client's depressive symptoms and if it is believed that the benefit-to-risk ratio is reasonable in this instance, it is reasonable for the PMHNP to continue the medication and adjust the dose. The PMHNP must do all the relevant medical tests to prescribe this medication.

REFERENCES AND RESOURCES

Abood, S. (2007). Influencing health care in the legislative arena. Online Journal of Issues in Nursing, 12(1). https://doi.org/10.3912/OJIN.Vol12No01Man02

Accreditation Commission for Education in Nursing. (2023). Accreditation manual. www.acenursing.org/acen-accreditation-manual/

American Association of Colleges of Nursing. (2013). CCNE: Commission on Collegiate Nursing Education. www.aacn.nche.edu/ccne-accreditation/why-accreditation

American Association of Colleges of Nursing. (2021). The Essentials: Core Competencies for Professional Nursing Education. www.aacnnursing.org/Portals/42/AcademicNursing/pdf/Essentials-2021.pdf

American Nurses Association. (2000). Medicare and "incidental to" payment: Coverage of nursing services in hospital outpatient clinics and emergency departments. www.acenursing.org/accreditation-manual/

American Nurses Association. (2015). Code of ethics for nurses with interpretive statements (2nd ed.).

American Nurses Association, American Psychiatric Nurses Association & International Society of Psychiatric-Mental Health Nurses. (2022). Psychiatric-mental health nursing: Scope and standards of practice (3rd ed.).

American Nurses Credentialing Center. (2023). Psychiatric-mental health nurse practitioner (across the lifespan) certification (PMHNP-BC). www.nursingworld.org/our-certifications/psychiatric-mental-health-nurse-practitioner/

American Psychiatric Association. (2022). Diagnostic and statistical manual of mental disorders (5th ed., Text rev.).

American Psychiatric Nurses Association. (2011). APNA Board of Directors endorses APNA/ISPN Joint Task Force recommendation on the implementation of the 'Consensus model for APRN regulation: Licensure, accreditation, certification & education.' ww1.prweb.com/prfiles/2011/03/07/8187513/LACE.pdf

American Psychiatric Nurses Association. (2022). APNA Guidance regarding precepting and mentorship. www.apna.org/resources/apna-guidance-regarding-precepting-and-mentorship/

Baillargeon, J., Penn, J. V., Knight, K., Harzke, A. J., Baillargeon, G., & Becker, E. A. (2010). Risk of reincarceration among prisoners with co-occurring severe mental illness and substance use disorders. Administrative Policy in Mental Health, 37(4), 367–74. https://doi.org/10.1007/s10488-009-0252-9.

Brownson, R. C., & Petitti, D. (2006). Applied epidemiology: Theory to practice (2nd ed.). Oxford University Press.

Buppert, C. (2021). Nurse practitioner's business practice and legal guide (7th ed.). Jones & Bartlett Learning.

Burgess, A. W. (1998). Advanced practice psychiatric nursing. Appleton & Lange.

Carey, T. A. (2016). Beyond patient-centered care: Enhancing the patient experience in mental health services through patient-perspective care. Patient Experience Journal, 3(2), 46–49. https://doi.org/10.35680/2372-0247.1139

Coleman, E., Radix, A. E., Bouman, W. P., Brown, G. R., de Vries, A. L. C., Deutsch, M. B., Ettner, R., . . . Arcelus, J. (2022). Standards of care for the health of transgender and gender diverse people, Version 8. International Journal of Transgender Health, 23(sup1), S1–S259. https://doi.org/10.1080/26895269.2022.2100644

Commission on Collegiate Nursing Education. (2023). CCNE accreditation. https://www.aacnnursing.org/ccne-accreditation

Cotroneo, M., Kurlowicz, L. H., Outlaw, F. H., Burgess, A. W., & Evans, L. K. (2001). Psychiatric-mental health nursing at the interface: Revisioning education for the specialty. Issues in Mental Health Nursing, 22, 549–569.

Delaney, K., Chisholm, M., Clement, J., & Merwin, E. (1999). Trends in psychiatric mental health education. Archives of Psychiatric Nursing, 13(2), 67–73.

Donabedian, A. (1988). The quality of care. How can it be assessed? JAMA, 260(12), 1743–1748.

Edmunds, M. W., Horan, N. M., & Mayhew, M. S. (2000). Adult nurse practitioner review manual. American Nurses Association.

Farnam, C., Zipple, A. M., Tyrell, W., & Chittiinanda, P. (1999). Health status risk factors of people with severe and persistent mental illness. Journal of Psychosocial Nursing, 37, 16–19.

Fineout-Overholt, E., Melnyk, B. M., & Schultz, A. (2005). Transforming health care from the inside out: Advancing evidence-based practice in the 21st century. Journal of Professional Nursing, 21(6), 335–344.

Friedman, D. J., Parrish, G., & Ross, D. A. (2013). Electronic health records and US public health: Current realities and future promise. American Journal of Public Health, 103(9), 1560–1567.

Friedman, M. (2002). Family nursing: Research, theory, and practice (5th ed.). Appleton & Lange.

Ford, L. C. (1992). Advancing nursing practice: Future of the nurse practitioner. In L. H. Aiken & C. M. Fagin (Eds.), Charting nursing's future: Agenda for the 1990s. J. B. Lippincott.

Harris, E., & Barraclough, B. (1999). Excess mortality of mental disorder. British Journal of Psychiatry, 173, 476–481.

Health Resources and Service Administration. (2022). What is telehealth. www.hrsa.gov/telehealth/what-is-telehealth

Institute for the Future. (2000). Health and health care 2010: The forecast, the challenge. Jossey-Bass.

Institute of Medicine. (2010). The future of nursing: Leading change, advancing health. https://pubmed.ncbi.nlm.nih.gov/24983041/

Institute of Medicine, Board on the Health of Special Populations. (2011). The health of lesbian, gay, bisexual, and transgender people: Building a foundation for better understanding. National Academies Press.

Jakubik, L. D., Eliades, A. B., & Weese, M. M. (2016). Part 1: An overview of mentoring practices and mentoring benefits. Pediatric Nursing, 42(1), 37.

Johnson, M., Maas, M., & Moorhead, S. (Eds.). (2003). Nursing outcomes classification (3rd ed.). Mosby.

Karlawish, J. (2021). Assessment of decision-making capacity in adults. UpToDate. https://www.uptodate.com/contents/assessment-of-decision-making-capacity-in-adults

Kennedy-Hendricks, A., Huskamp, H.A., Rutkow, L. & Berry, C. L. (2016). Improving access to care and reducing involvement in the criminal justice system for people with mental illness. Health Affairs, 35(6), 1076–1083.

King, M., Semlyen, J., Tai, S. S., Killaspy, H., Osborn, D., Popelyuk, D., & Nazareth, I. (2008). A systematic review of mental disorder, suicide, and deliberate self-harm in lesbian, gay and bisexual people. BMC Psychiatry,8(70). https://bmcpsychiatry.biomedcentral.com/articles/10.1186/1471-244X-8-70

Kruks, G. (2010). Gay and lesbian homeless/street youth: Special issues and concerns. Journal of Adolescent Health, 12(7), 515–518.

Kushel, M. B., Hahn, J. A., Evans, J. L., Bangsberg, D. R., & Moss, A. R. (2005). Revolving doors: imprisonment among the homeless and marginally housed population. American Journal of Public Health, 95(10), 1747–1752.

Lyons, T. (2009). Role of the forensic psychiatric nurse. Journal of Forensic Nursing, 5, 53–57.

Macnee, C., & McCabe, S. (2000). Micro stressors: The impact of hassles and uplifts. In V. H. Rice (Ed.), Handbook of stress and coping: Implications for nursing research, theory, and practice. Sage.

Matlow, A. G., Wright, J. G., & Zimmerman, B. (2006). How can the principles of complexity science be applied to improve the coordination of care for complex pediatric patients? Quality and Safety in Health Care, 15, 85–88.

McBride, A., & Austin, J. (1996). Psychiatric-mental health nursing: Integrating the behavioral and biological sciences. W. B. Saunders.

McCabe, S. (2000). Bringing psychiatric nursing into the twenty-first century. Archives of Psychiatric Nursing, 14(3), 109–116.

McCabe, S. (2002). The nature of psychiatric nursing: The intersection of paradigm, evolution, and history. Archives of Psychiatric Nursing, 16(2), 51–60.

McCabe, S., & Macnee, C. L. (2002). Weaving a new safety net of mental health care in rural America: A model of integrated practice. Issues in Mental Health Nursing, 23, 263–278.

McCloskey, J. C., & Bulechek, G. M. (Eds.). (2000). Nursing interventions classification (3rd ed.). Mosby.

Medical Record Confidentiality Act of 1995, S. 1360, 104th Cong. (1995). https://www.gpo.gov/fdsys/pkg/BILLS-104s1360is/content-detail.html

Mellow, J. (1968). Nursing therapy. American Journal of Nursing, 68, 2365–2369.

Melnyk, B. M., Fineout-Overholt, E., Stillwell, S. B., & Williamson, K. (2010). The seven steps of evidence-based practice. American Journal of Nursing, 110(1), 51–53.

Mirr Jansen, M., & Zwygart-Stauffacher, M. (2006). Advanced practice nursing: Core concepts for professional role development. (3rd ed.). Springer Publishing.

Nagle, M., & Krainovich-Miller, B. (2001). Shaping the advanced practice psychiatric nursing role: A futuristic model. Issues in Mental Health Nursing, 22, 461–482.

National Alliance on Mental Illness. (2023). LGBTQ+. https://www.nami.org/Your-Journey/Identity-and-Cultural-Dimensions/LGBTQ.

National Center for Farmworker Health. (2023). Migrant and seasonal farmworker demographics. https://www.ncfh.org/naws-fact-sheet.html

National Organization of Nurse Practitioner Faculties. (2013). Psychiatric-mental health nurse practitioner competencies. National Panel for Nurse Practitioner Faculties.

National Organization of Nurse Practitioner Faculties. (2022). Nurse practitioner role competencies. National Panel for Nurse Practitioner Faculties. https://www.nonpf.org/page/NP_Role_Core_Competencies

Nettina, S. M., & Knudtson, M. (2001). The family nurse practitioner review manual. American Nurses Credentialing Center.

New York City Health and Hospitals. (2011). To treat me you have to know who I am. [Video]. YouTube. https://www.youtube.com/watch?v=NUhvJgxgAac

North American Nursing Diagnosis Association. (2000). Nursing diagnosis: Definitions and classifications 1999–2000.

Northouse, P. G. (2007). Leadership theory and practice (4th ed.). Sage Publications.

Padgett, D. (2020). Homelessness, housing instability and mental health: Making the connection. BJPsych Bulletin, 44(5), 197–201. https://doi.org/10.1192/bjb.2020.49

Peplau, H. (1952). Interpersonal relations in nursing. GP Putnam's Sons.

Perese, E. F. (2012). Psychiatric advanced practice nursing: A biopsychosocial foundation for practice. F. A. Davis.

Prins, S. J. (2014). The prevalence of mental illness in U.S. state prisons: A systematic review. Psychiatric Services, 65(7), 862–872.

Prison Policy Initiative. (2023). Mental health. www.prisonpolicy.org/research/mental_health

Reinhardt, A. C., & Ray, L. N. (2003). Differentiating quality improvement from research. Applied Nursing Research, 16(1), 2–8.

Richardson, K. A., Cilliers, P., & Lissack, M. (2001). Complexity science: A "gray" science for the "stuff in between." Emergence, Complexity and Organization, 3(2), 6–18.

Richardson, W. S., Wilson, M. C., Nishikawa, J., & Hayward, R. S. (1995). The well-built clinical question: A key to evidence-based decisions. ACP Journal Club, 123(3), A12–A13.

Sadock, B., Sadock, V., & Ruiz, P. (2017). Kaplan and Sadock's comprehensive textbook of psychiatry (10th ed.). Wolters Kluwer.

Shea, C. A., Pelletier, L., Poster, E. C., Stuart, G. W., & Verhey, M. P. (1999). Advanced practice nursing in psychiatric and mental health care. Mosby.

Sherwood, G. D., & Horton-Deutsch, S. (2012). Reflective practice transforming education and improving outcomes. Sigma Theta Tau International.

Stuart, G. W. (2013). Principles and practice of psychiatric nursing (10th ed.). Mosby.

Substance Abuse and Mental Health Services Administration. (2023, June 13). Lesbian, gay, and bisexual behavioral health: Results from the 2021 and 2022 national surveys on drug use and health. U.S. Department of Health and Human Services. https://www.samhsa.gov/newsroom/press-announcements/20230613/samhsa-releases-new-data-lesbian-gay-bisexual-behavioral-health

Tarasoff v. Regents at the University of California, 17 Cal. 3d 425, 551 P. 2d 334, 131 Cal. Rptr. 14 (Cal. 1976). www.ojp.gov/ncjrs/virtual-library/abstracts/tarasoff-vs-regents-university-california-et-al-mental-health Retrieved August 1, 2023

Unger C. A. (2016). Hormone therapy for transgender patients. Translational andrology and urology, 5(6), 877–884. https://doi.org/10.21037/tau.2016.09.04

U.S. Department of Health and Human Services. (2005). Healthy People 2010. Office of Disease Prevention and Health Promotion. https://wayback.archive-it.org/5774/20220415230712/https://www.healthypeople.gov/2010/

U.S. Department of Health and Human Services. Mental health: A report of the Surgeon General. Substance Abuse and Mental Health Service Administration, National Institute of Mental Health. https://www.loc.gov/item/2002495357/

U.S. Department of Health and Human Services. (2017). HITECH Act Enforcement Interim Final Rule.

U.S. Department of Health and Human Services. (2019). Healthy People 2020: Lesbian, Gay, Bisexual and Transgender Health. https://www.healthypeople.gov/2020/topics-objectives/topic/lesbian-gay-bisexual-and-transgender-health.

U.S. Department of Health and Human Services, Office for Civil Rights. (2013). Modifications to the HIPAA privacy, security, enforcement, and breach notification rules under the Health Information Technology for Economic and Clinical Health Act and the Genetic Information Nondiscrimination Act; other modifications to the HIPAA rules. Federal Register, 78(17). https://www.gpo.gov/fdsys/pkg/FR-2013-01-25/pdf/2013-01073.pdf

U.S. Institute of Medicine Committee on Lesbian, Gay, Bisexual, and Transgender Health Issues and Research Gaps and Opportunities. (2011). The Health of Lesbian, Gay, Bisexual, and Transgender People: Building a Foundation for Better Understanding. National Academies Press. https://doi.org/10.17226/13128

U.S. Department of Health, Education, and Welfare. (1979). The Belmont report. https://www.hhs.gov/ohrp/regulations-and-policy/belmont-report/index.html

Ward, B.W., Dahlhamer, J. M., Galinsky, A. M., Joesti, S. S. (2014). Sexual orientation and health among U.S. adults: National Health Interview Survey, 2013. National Center for Health Statistics. https://www.cdc.gov/nchs/data/nhsr/nhsr077.pdf

World Health Organization. (2023). International Statistical Classification of Diseases and Related Health Problems (ICD). https://www.who.int/standards/classifications/classification-of-diseases

World Professional Association for Transgender Health. (n.d.). Standards of care version 8. https://wpath.org/publications/soc8/

CHAPTER 3

THEORETICAL BASIS OF CARE

Although the psychiatric-mental health nurse practitioner (PMHNP) role is relatively new, psychiatric-mental health nursing has a long, well-established, and cherished tradition of advanced practice. As with all other specialty areas of nursing, advanced practice psychiatric nursing is theoretically grounded, and a wide array of theories form the basis for the PMHNP role. These theories help identify the foundational, core concepts of advanced practice psychiatric nursing. The scope of practice for the PMHNP is based on an understanding of foundational core concepts and theories (Alligood, 2022).

This chapter reviews the concepts of biopsychosocial theories that underpin PMHNP practice, which starts with the initial psychiatric interview and mental status exam (MSE).

- Psychiatric interview
  - Purpose
    - Establish rapport
    - Develop therapeutic relationship
    - Client's narrative
      - Chief complaint
      - History of the present problem
      - Precipitating factors
      - Developmental history
      - Allergies
      - Medications (current and past)
      - Past medical history
      - Past psychiatric history
      - Family background and medical and psychiatric history
      - Social and behavioral history
      - MSE
      - General physical and neurological exam (see Chapter 6)
      - Safety assessment
  - A well-developed interview and MSE lead to an accurate diagnosis and plan of care.

BIOPSYCHOSOCIAL FRAMEWORK OF CARE

RECOVERY

- Recovery is the single most important goal in the transformation of mental health care of the past 2 decades. Four major dimensions of recovery include health, home, purpose, and community (U.S. Department of Health and Human Services [HHS], Substance and Mental Health Services Administration [SMHSA], 2023).
- PMHNP interventions follow evidence-based practice guidelines, are always client goal–directed, and take into account the client's ethnicity and culture.
- PMHNPs help clients to recognize strengths, set attainable goals, and have hope for their future.
- A key part of the PMHNP's work is to use empirical evidence in educating their clients, clients' families, and the community about mental health, psychiatric illness, and effective management of illness.
- The PMHNP oversees and guides the psychiatric-mental health nurse in designing evidence-based health information and educational programs that are geared to client learning needs, ability, and readiness to learn.
- PMHNPs care for people with co-occurring medical and psychiatric disorders.
- Principles of mental health recovery are integrated into all levels of mental health care (American Nurses Association [ANA], American Psychiatric Nurses Association [APNA], & International Society of Psychiatric-Mental Health Nurses [ISPN], 2022).

CLASSIFICATION OF PSYCHIATRIC DISORDERS: DSM-5-TR

- Before the Diagnostic and Statistical Manual of Mental Disorders, Fifth Edition (DSM-5) became available in May 2013, psychiatric disorders were classified using standard criteria of the Diagnostic and Statistical Manual of Mental Disorders, Fourth Edition, Text Revision (DSM-IV-TR; American Psychiatric Association [APA], 2000). The Diagnostic and Statistical Manual of Mental Disorders, Fifth Edition, Text Revision (DSM-5-TR) became available in 2022 (APA).
- The DSM-5-TR updates include additional diagnostic entities, symptom codes, specifiers, and updated terminology (First, 2022).
  - New diagnostic entities
    - Prolonged grief disorder
      - Grief-related symptoms of emotional numbness, pain, and yearning that continue for at least 12 months resulting in impaired functioning

- Stimulant-induced mild neurocognitive disorder
  - Added to existing substance-induced mild cognitive disorders when neurocognitive symptoms are associated with stimulant use
- Unspecified mood disorder
  - When symptoms of mood do not meet the full criteria of depressive or bipolar disorder

◊ Other conditions that may be a focus of clinical attention

- Suicidal behavior and nonsuicidal self-injury disorder may be used independently and no longer require another diagnosis to monitor these behaviors.

◊ Diagnostic criteria

- The following diagnostic criteria were modified for clarity:
  - Autism spectrum disorder
  - Inclusion of gambling as a behavioral addiction
  - Substance/Medication-induced bipolar and related disorder
  - Major depressive disorder
  - Avoidant/Restrictive food intake disorder

◊ Specifiers

- Extensions added to a diagnosis that result in a more specific diagnosis.
- New specifiers:
  - Diagnosis: Bipolar I-current manic episode
    - Specifiers: Mild, moderate, severe
  - Diagnosis: Bipolar II-current episode
    - Specifiers: At least one manic and one major depressive episode are not better explained by another disorder
  - Diagnosis: Other specified obsessive–compulsive related disorder
    - Specifier: Olfactory reference disorder
  - Diagnosis: Persistent depressive disorder
    - Specifier: With anxious distress and atypical features remain

◊ Revised terminology

- Gender dysphoria: terminology changed to be more culturally sensitive and less stigmatizing
  - "Desired gender" changed to experienced gender
  - "Cross-sex medical procedure" changed to gender affirming medical procedure

    - "Cross-sex hormone treatment" changed to gender affirming hormone treatment
    - "Natal male" changed to individual assigned male at birth
    - "Natal female" changed to individual assigned female at birth
    - "Disorders of sex development" changed to differences in sex development
  - Racial and cultural considerations in presentations and prevalence, as well as racial and discrimination impact of experiences
  - "Neuroleptic medications" changed to antipsychotic medications or other dopamine-receptor blocking agents
  - "Intellectual disability" changed to intellectual developmental disorder
  - "Conversion disorder" changed to functional neurological syndrome

THERAPEUTIC RELATIONSHIP

- Assumes that the client and nurse enter into a mutual, interactive, interpersonal relationship specifically to focus on the identified needs of the client
- Therapeutic relationships are focused on the client's needs and are goal-directed, theory-based, and open to supervision.
- The following are a few characteristics of a therapeutic relationship:
  - Genuineness
  - Acceptance
  - Nonjudgment
  - Authenticity
  - Empathy
  - Respect
  - Professional boundaries
- The therapeutic relationship has specific and sequential phases (see Table 3–1).
- Transference and countertransference are key concepts in the nurse–client relationship.
  - Transference: Displacement of feelings for significant people in the client's past onto the PMHNP in the present relationship
  - Countertransference: The nurse's emotional reaction to the client based on the nurse's own past experiences
  - Signs indicating the presence of countertransference in the PMHNP include
    - Intense emotional reactions, positive or negative, on first contact with the client

- Recurrent anxiety or uneasiness while dealing with the client
- Uncharacteristic carelessness in interaction and follow-up with the client
- Difficulty empathizing
- Resistance to others treating or interacting with the client
- Preoccupation with or dreaming about the client
- Frequently running over time or cutting time short with client
- Depression or other strong emotions during or after interaction with client
- Feedback from others over involvement with client

◊ The PMHNP is expected to monitor their reaction to clients to constantly assess for the presence of countertransference.

TABLE 3–1.
PHASES OF A THERAPEUTIC NURSE–CLIENT RELATIONSHIP

PHASE	NURSING ACTION	COMMON CLIENT BEHAVIOR
Introduction (Orientation)	Creating a trusting environment Establishing professional boundaries Establishing the length of anticipated interaction Providing diagnostic evaluation Setting mutually agreed-upon treatment objectives	Initial hesitancy by the client to participate fully in assessment and treatment planning (approach avoidance)
Working (Identification and Exploitation)	Clarifying client expectations and mutually set goals Implementing treatment plan Monitoring health Undertaking preventative health care Measuring outcomes of care Evaluating outcomes of care Reprioritizing plan and objectives as indicated	Transference—client (countertransference—nurse) Client resistance to care practices Client resistance to change
Termination (Resolution)	Reviewing client's progress toward objectives Establishing long-term plan of care Focusing on self-management strategies Disengaging from relationship Referring client to other services as needed	Client resistance to termination Regression Reemergence of symptoms or problems

Note. Adapted from Wheeler, K. (2022). Psychotherapy for the advanced practice psychiatric nurse: A how-to guide for evidence-based practice (3rd ed.) Springer Publishing.

- ◇ If identified, countertransference is usually addressed through the supervisory process and in talking to coworkers about the issues.
    - Provided in peer–peer or peer–supervisor relationship
    - Examines interpersonal dynamics inherent in the PMHNP's relationship with clients

DEVELOPMENTAL THEORIES

- Growth, change, and development are a part of the dynamic, constant life process of being human.
- Humans develop uniquely from simple to complex.
- The health states of individuals and families can be viewed over a continuum of development.
- Developmental stages and the milestones or tasks that accompany them give insight into age-appropriate behaviors, measure levels of comprehension for client teaching, and provide a context within which to evaluate assessment data. Erikson believed crisis existed in each developmental stage; outcomes shape the individual (see Table 3–2).
- Example: The mental status finding of concrete thinking in a 9-year-old client would be normal and expected; however, the same finding in a 29-year-old client is nonnormative and suggestive of psychopathology (see Table 3–3 for typical age at onset for psychiatric disorders).

TABLE 3–2.
ERIK ERIKSON'S (1902–1994) STAGES OF HUMAN DEVELOPMENT

STAGE	AGE	OVERVIEW	SUCCESSFUL ATTAINMENT	LACK OF SUCCESSFUL ATTAINMENT
Trust vs. Mistrust	0–1 year	Infants develop trust when needs are met, while inattention leads to mistrust.	Able to form meaningful relationships, trust others, hope in the future	Poor relationships, suspiciousness, lack of hope
Autonomy vs. Shame and Doubt	1–3 years	Child asserts autonomy, uses "no"	Learns self-control	Lack of self-esteem, poor self-control, decreased independence
Initiative vs. Guilt	3–6 years	Child initiates motor and intellectual activity	Self-directed behavior, goal formation, sense of purpose	Lack of initiated behaviors and goal-directed behaviors

(Continued)

TABLE 3–2. (CONTINUED)

STAGE	AGE	OVERVIEW	SUCCESSFUL ATTAINMENT	LACK OF SUCCESSFUL ATTAINMENT
Industry vs. Inferiority	6–12 years	Child enters formal school and begins learning, works to acquire adult skills, learns to master tasks	Sense of achievement, feels competent	A sense of inferiority may lead to behavioral issues related to working and learning.
Identity vs. Role Confusion	12–20 years	Adolescent group identity and preoccupation with appearances; develop morals and ethics; sexual experimentation is common	Personal sense of identity	Struggle to develop identity, especially in group settings
Intimacy vs. Isolation	20–35 years*	Young adults establish intimate relations with friends and sexually intimate relationships.	Committed relationships	Emotional isolation, egocentrism
Generativity vs. Stagnation	35–65 years**	Adults come to terms with life in relation to accomplishments both professionally and personally.	Giving of time and talents to others, able to care for others	Self-absorbed, unable to grow, change, and care for others
Integrity vs. Despair	≥65 years	Older adults have a sense of satisfaction with one's life vs. despair over an inability to achieve one's goals.	Sense of fulfillment, an insightful, balanced perspective on life, willingness to face death	Despair over impending death, dissatisfaction with life, bitterness

*Intimacy vs. Isolation 21–40 years due to many young adults delaying marriage and committed relationships.

**Generativity vs. Stagnation 40–65 years due to delaying committed relationships.

Note. Adapted from Wheeler, K. (2022). Psychotherapy for the advanced practice psychiatric nurse: A how-to guide for evidence-based practice (3rd ed.) Springer Publishing.

TABLE 3–3.
EXAMPLES OF TYPICAL AGE AT ONSET FOR COMMON PSYCHIATRIC DISORDERS

DISORDER	AVERAGE AGE OF ONSET
Anxiety disorder	15–20 years—can occur at any age
Attention-deficit/Hyperactivity disorder	10–12 years
Bipolar disorder	12–24 years
Dementia	≥65 years—can occur earlier or later in life
Depressive disorder	30 years—can occur in childhood to older adult
Intellectual disability	Childhood to adolescence
Schizophrenia disorder	Approx. 25 years

Note. Adapted from Solmi, M., Radua, J., Olivola, M., Croce, E., Soardo, L., Salazar de Pablo, G., Il Shin, J., Kirkbride, J. B., Jones, P., Kim, J. H., Kim, J. Y., Carvalho, A. F., Seeman, M. V., Correll, C. U., & Fusar-Poli, P. (2022). Age at onset of mental disorders worldwide: large-scale meta-analysis of 192 epidemiological studies. Molecular Psychiatry, 27(1), 281–295. https://doi.org/10.1038/s41380-021-01161-7

- Piaget viewed human development related to knowledge acquisition (see Table 3–4). Intelligence is structured logically and a biological adaptation.

FOUNDATIONAL THEORIES SUPPORTING THE PMHNP ROLE

- Psychodynamic theory (also known as psychoanalytic theory) (Sigmund Freud, 1856–1939)
    - Focus is on concepts of intrapsychic conflict among the structures of the mind
    - Initially designed to explain neurosis and conditions of high anxiety such as phobias and hysteria
    - Theory later expanded to include normal and abnormal development and personality development
    - Basic tenets of psychodynamic theory
    - Psychoanalytical theory assumes that all behavior is purposeful and meaningful. All behavior has meaning.
- Principle of psychic determinism: Even apparently meaningless, random, or accidental behavior is actually motivated by underlying unconscious mental content.
    - Example: A person forgets where they parked the car because they really do not wish to go wherever it was that they were headed.
    - Most mental activity is unconscious—urges, feelings, and fantasies that would be unacceptable to the person's values if consciously experienced.

TABLE 3–4.
PIAGET

STAGE	AGE	OVERVIEW
Sensorimotor	0–2 years	Infant begins to acquire knowledge through sensory observation of their environment, begins to master motor function by exploring, and gains achievement through mastery. Object permanence is obtained in this stage.
Preoperational stage	2–7 years	Child views self as center of universe, believes that they are responsible for everything that occurs in their world, are egocentric, have animistic thinking, use symbols and language more.
Concrete operational stage	7–11 years	Child replaces operational thought with egocentricity, develops the ability to see things from another person's perspective.
Formal operations stage	≥11 years	Individual develops abstract thought; is able to reason deductively and think conceptually.

Note. Adapted from Wheeler, K. (2022). Psychotherapy for the advanced practice psychiatric nurse: A how-to guide for evidence-based practice (3rd ed.) Springer Publishing.

- ◊ Conscious behaviors and choices are affected by unconscious mental content.
- ◊ Childhood experiences shape adult personality.
- ◊ Instincts, urges, or fantasies function as drives that motivate thoughts, feelings, and behaviors.
    - Two types of normal drives: Sexual drives (libido) and aggressive drives
        - Drives affect behavior as an individual attempts to deal with the associated feelings and seeks gratification through release of the tension that the drives produce.
        - Normally, different actions or behaviors are used at different ages to discharge tension from drives and seek gratification.
        - Psychosexual stages of development have been identified to show the age-related behaviors commonly used for discharging drives and obtaining gratification (see Table 3–5).
- ◊ Three primary psychic structures make up the mind and personality and are responsible for mental functioning:
    1. The id
        - Contains primary drives or instincts, urges (hunger, sex, or aggression), or fantasies

TABLE 3–5.
FREUD'S PSYCHOSEXUAL STAGES OF DEVELOPMENT

STAGE	AGE	PRIMARY MEANS OF DISCHARGING DRIVES AND ACHIEVING GRATIFICATION	PSYCHIATRIC DISORDER LINKED TO FAILURE OF STAGE
Oral stage	0–18 months	Sucking, chewing, feeding, crying	Schizophrenia Substance use Paranoia
Anal stage	18 months–3 years	Sphincter control, activities of expulsion and retention	Depressive disorders
Phallic stage	3–6 years	Exhibitionism, masturbation with focus on Oedipal conflict, castration anxiety, and female fear of lost maternal love	Sexual identity disorders
Latency stage	6 years–puberty	Peer relationships, learning, motor skills development, socialization	Inability to form social relationships
Genital stage	Puberty forward	Integration and synthesis of behaviors from early stages, primary genital-based sexuality	Sexual perversion disorders

Note. Adapted from Wheeler, K. (2022). Psychotherapy for the advanced practice psychiatric nurse: A how-to guide for evidence-based practice (3rd ed.) Springer Publishing.

- Drives are largely unconscious, sexual, or aggressive in content, and infantile in nature
- Operates on the pleasure principle; seeks immediate satisfaction
- Is present at birth and motivates early infantile actions
- The id says, "I want"

2. The ego
   - Contains the concept of external reality
   - Rational mind; responsible for logical and abstract thinking
   - Functions in adaptation
   - Mediates between the demands of drives and environmental realities
   - Operates on the reality principle
   - Begins to develop at birth as infant struggles to deal with environment
   - Responsible for use of defense mechanisms
   - The ego says, "I think, I evaluate"

3. The superego
    - Is the ego-ideal
    - Contains sense of conscience or right versus wrong
    - Also contains aspirations, ideals, and moral values
    - Regulated by guilt and shame
    - Begins to fully develop around age six as a child comes into contact with external authority figures such as other parents, schoolteachers, coaches, or religious figures
    - The superego says "I should or ought"

- Psychic structures commonly come into conflict over what to do to achieve gratification.
- Although the exact nature of conflict is often unconscious, conflict is experienced consciously as anxiety.
- The function of anxiety is to alert the conscious mind to the presence of conflict.
- Conflict is normally dealt with through the use of defense mechanisms (see Table 3–6), which
    - Are a function of the ego,
    - Are unconsciously called into action,
    - Are used to reduce anxiety,
    - Become part of the personality,
    - Maintain a sense of safety,
    - Promote self-esteem and a sense of well-being,
    - May be used episodically or habitually, and
    - May be used constantly and become fixed, as seen in neurosis.

♦ Cognitive theory (Jean Piaget, 1896–1980)

◊ Piaget believed that human development evolves through cognition, learning, and comprehending.

◊ He believed that factors such as native endowment and biological and environmental factors set the course for a child's development.

◊ He described four stages of cognitive development:

1. Sensorimotor (birth–2 years): The critical achievement of this stage is object permanence—the ability to understand that objects have an existence independent of the child's involvement with them.
2. Preoperational (2–7 years): More extensive use of language and symbolism; magical thinking

TABLE 3–6.
DEFENSE MECHANISMS

DEFENSE MECHANISM	OVERVIEW
Immature Defenses	
Denial	Avoiding by ignoring painful/unpleasant realities
Projection	Unacceptable beliefs/feelings are attributed to others
Acting out	Impulsive actions used to avoid conscious experiences
Regression	Returning to an earlier stage of development to avoid a current conflict/stress
Hypochondria	Inflated illness resulting from feelings that are unacceptable
Introjection	Internalizing characteristics of others
Somatization	Bodily symptoms resulting from emotional states
Splitting	Inability to hold opposing feelings/thoughts
Neurotic Defenses	
Displacement	Transferring negative emotions from person/object to another
Dissociation	Disconnection between thoughts/feelings/self, resulting in an altered state of consciousness
Intellectualization	Intellect is used to avoid feelings/emotions that are distressing
Rationalization	Unacceptable behaviors are justified by using logical reasoning
Reaction formation	Expressed emotion is the opposite of the true feeling
Repression	Unconsciously blocking an unacceptable feeling/behavior
Mature Defenses	
Sublimation	Unacceptable impulses are directed toward acceptable activities
Suppression	Consciously not thinking about unpleasant thoughts/emotions
Altruism	Unselfish actions that provide benefit to others
Humor	Using humor to express feelings/thoughts that are uncomfortable

Note. Adapted from Wheeler, K. (2022). Psychotherapy for the advanced practice psychiatric nurse: A how-to guide for evidence-based practice (3rd ed.) Springer Publishing.

3. Concrete operations (7–12 years): Child begins to use logic; develops concepts of reversibility and conservation
    - Reversibility: The realization that one thing can turn into another and back again (e.g., water and ice)
    - Conservation: Ability to recognize that although the shape of an object may change, it will still maintain characteristics that enable it to be recognized as that object (e.g., clay)
4. Formal operations (12 years–adult): Ability to think abstractly; thinking operates in a formal, logical manner

- Interpersonal theory (Harry Stack Sullivan, 1892–1949)
    - Behavior occurs because of interpersonal dynamics.
    - Interpersonal relationships and experiences influence one's personality development, which is called the self-system (the total components of personality traits).
    - Understanding behavior requires understanding the relationships in the person's life.
    - There are two drives for behavior: the drive for satisfaction (basic human drives such as sleep, sex, and hunger) and the drive for security (conforming to social norms of a person's reference group).
    - When the person's need for satisfaction and security is interfered with by the self-system, mental illness occurs.
    - Humans experience anxiety, and behavior is directed toward relieving the anxiety, which then results in interpersonal security.
    - Sullivan also described stages of interpersonal development (see Table 3–7).

TABLE 3–7.
SULLIVAN'S STAGES OF INTERPERSONAL DEVELOPMENT

STAGE	TIME PERIOD	DEVELOPMENTAL TASK
Infancy	Birth–18 months	Oral gratification; anxiety occurs for the first time
Childhood	18 months–6 years	Delayed gratification
Juvenile	6–9 years	Forming of peer relationships
Pre-adolescence	9–12 years	Same-sex relationships
Early adolescence	12–14 years	Opposite-sex relationships
Late adolescence	14–21 years	Self-identity developed

Note. Adapted from Sadock, B. J., Sadock, V. A., & Ruiz, P. (2017). Kaplan and Sadock's comprehensive textbook of psychiatry (10th ed.).Wolters Kluwer

- Hierarchy of needs theory (Abraham Maslow, 1908–1970)
    - A health model rather than illness model
    - A hierarchical organization of needs
    - Hypothesizes that certain needs are more important than others
    - States that a person will attempt to meet more important needs first before satisfying other needs
    - Hierarchy of needs:
        1. Survival
            - Water
            - Air
            - Food
            - Sleep

2. Safety and security needs
    - Protection from harm, emotional and physical
3. Love and belonging
    - Affection, intimacy, and companionship
4. Self-esteem
    - Sense of worth
5. Self-actualization
    - Achieving one's potential
    - Being all that one can be

- ♦ Health belief model (Marshall Becker, 1940–1993)
    - ◊ Explains that healthy people do not always take advantage of screening or preventative programs because of the following certain variables:
        - Perception of susceptibility
        - Seriousness of illness
        - Perceived benefits of treatment
        - Perceived barriers to change
        - Expectations of efficacy
- ♦ Transtheoretical model of change
    - ◊ States that change such as in health behaviors occurs in five predictable stages (Prochaska et al., 1992):
        1. Precontemplation: The person has no intention to change.
        2. Contemplation: The person is thinking about changing; they are aware that there is a problem but not committed to changing.
        3. Preparation: The person has made the decision to change; they are ready for action.
        4. Action: The person is engaging in specific, overt actions to change.
        5. Maintenance: The person is engaging in behaviors to prevent relapse.
- ♦ Lewin's change theory
    - ◊ A three-stage change model of driving forces, restraining forces, and equilibrium (Petiprin, 2003)
        1. Unfreezing: Preparing for the change by letting go
        2. Change: Implementing the change
        3. Refreezing: Solidifying the change as it becomes the new habit
- ♦ Motivational interviewing (Wheeler, 2022)
    - ◊ Focused, goal-directive therapy
    - ◊ Builds on the transtheoretical model of change

  - Motivation is elicited from the client
  - Nonconfrontational, nonadversarial
- Self-efficacy and social learning theory (Albert Bandura, 1925–2021)
  - Behavior is the result of cognitive and environmental factors.
  - People learn by observing others, relying on role-modeling.
  - Self-efficacy is the perception of one's ability to perform a certain task at a certain level of accomplishment.
  - Behavioral change and maintenance are functions of outcome expectations and efficacy expectations.

NURSING THEORIES

- Theory of cultural care (Madeleine Leininger, 1925–2012)
  - Regardless of the culture, care is the unifying focus and the essence of nursing.
  - Health and well-being can be predicted through cultural care.
- Theory of self-care (Dorothy Orem, 1914–2007)
  - Self-care: Activities that maintain life, health, and well-being
- Therapeutic nurse–client relationship theory or interpersonal theory (Hildegard Peplau, 1909–1999)
  - First significant psychiatric nursing theory
  - Based in part on interpersonal theory (Sullivan, 1953)
  - Sees nursing as an interpersonal process in which all interventions occur within the context of the nurse–client relationship
  - The therapeutic nurse–client relationship is central to nursing
  - Includes phases of the nurse–client relationship (see Table 3–1):
    - Orientation phase
    - Working phase (identification, exploitation)
    - Termination phase (resolution)
  - Promoting adaptive responses is the goal of nursing
  - Behavior represents the person trying to adapt to internal or environmental forces
- Caring theory (Jean Watson, born 1940)
  - Caring is an essential component of nursing.
  - Carative factors guide the core of nursing and should be implemented in health care.
  - Carative factors are those aspects of care that potentiate therapeutic healing and relationships.

CASE STUDY 1

Thomas is a 19-year-old college freshman who uses the pronouns "he, him." During the second week of classes, he presented to his college's student health services clinic seeking help for "shyness." The PMHNP is responsible for assessment and care planning with this client.

As the PMHNP begins working with him, Thomas gives a chief complaint of feeling uncomfortable meeting new people and desiring to return home and drop out of school. The PMHNP has several issues to consider as they continue to work with Thomas.

1. Chronologically, what stage of development should Thomas be experiencing?
2. What are the tasks of this stage?
3. How would the PMHNP assess the actual developmental issues that Thomas is experiencing?
4. What factors does the PMHNP need to consider to determine whether Thomas is experiencing normative or nonnormative behaviors?
5. What characteristic does the PMHNP need to display to establish a therapeutic relationship with Thomas?

   Thomas reported that he has not been sleeping well, has experienced a decrease in appetite, and just wants to talk to someone about his problems in adjusting to school. In planning the follow-up care for Thomas, the PMHNP has many issues to consider.

6. What would be the goal of continued work with Thomas?
7. If the PMHNP were to start therapy with him, what kind of therapy would they consider?
8. According to DSM-5-TR, does Thomas have a mental illness?

CASE STUDY 2

J.T. is an 18-year-old, second-semester business major who presents to the university's mental health clinic because "my parents said I have to come here or they will pull me out of school. I don't think I need to be here." J.T. is on academic probation. The PMHNP learns that J.T.'s parents grew alarmed when, while home on holiday, J.T. was brought home by police after J.T and a friend were pulled over and friend was given a DUI. J.T. allows that perhaps "I partied too much" during the first semester at school but insists "I don't drink any more than anybody else." J.T. reluctantly agrees to see the PMHNP for an evaluation and for eight, weekly psychotherapy sessions "to please my parents."

1. What defense mechanism(s) is J.T. using?
2. How should the PMHNP approach working with this client?

ANSWERS TO CASE STUDY DISCUSSION QUESTIONS

CASE STUDY 1

1. Thomas' chronologic age should align with the developmental stage of adolescence.
2. According to Erikson, the developmental task of adolescence is identity versus role confusion.
3. The PMHNP should assess the degree of development of his personal sense of identity.
4. The PMHNP must have an awareness of the normal milestones of development and the behaviors that indicate failure of developmental stages. The client's history and behaviors are then matched to the known norm for comparison.
5. In order to develop a therapeutic relationship with Thomas, the PMHNP must display genuineness, acceptance, nonjudgmental attitude, authenticity, empathy, and respect for professional boundaries.
6. The goals of continued work with Thomas are assisting him to establish insight into behaviors and to increase range and maturity of coping behaviors.
7. Options for psychotherapy depend on factors such as a client's goals, motivation, past experiences with counseling, expectations for therapy, and resources.
8. Mental illness causes a disruption in the usual constitutions of mental health. Mental illness assumes an underlying psychopathology and can be defined as a clinically significant behavioral or psychological syndrome or pattern that occurs in a person that is associated with persistent distress or disability or with a significantly increased risk of death, pain, or an important loss of freedom. Thomas appears to be experiencing mental health concerns but based on available data does not meet the definition of mental illness.

CASE STUDY 2

1. J.T. is using denial and rationalization.
2. The PMHNP needs to work with J.T. to establish goals using the principles of the transtheoretical model of change and motivational interviewing.

REFERENCES AND RESOURCES

Alligood, M. R. (2022). Nursing theorists and their work (10th ed.). Elsevier.

American Nurses Association, American Psychiatric Nurses Association, & International Society of Psychiatric-Mental Health Nursing (2022). Psychiatric-mental health nursing: Scope and standards of practice (3rd ed.). American Nurses Association.

American Psychiatric Association. (2000). Diagnostic and statistical manual of mental disorders (4th ed., Text rev.).

American Psychiatric Association. (2022). Diagnostic and statistical manual of mental disorders (5th ed., Text rev.).

Burgess, A. W. (1998). Advanced practice psychiatric nursing. Appleton & Lange.

Erikson, E. H. (1963). Childhood and society. Basic Books.

First, M.B., Yousif, L.H., Clarke, D.E., Wang, P.S., Gogtay, N., & Appelbaum, P.S. (2022). DSM-5-TR: Overview of what's new and what's changed. World Psychiatry, 21(2), 218–219. https://doi.org/10.1002/wps.20989

Freud, S. (1923). The ego and the id. W. W. Norton & Company.

Freud, S. (1936). The problem of anxiety. Basic Books.

Haley, J. (1996). Learning and teaching therapy. Guilford Press.

Keltner, N., Schwecke, L. H., & Bostrom, C. E. (2006). Psychiatric nursing (5th ed.). Mosby.

Kerr, M. E., & Bowen, M. (1988). Family evaluation: An approach based on Bowen theory. W. W. Norton & Company.

Marsh, D. T. (1998). Serious mental illness and the family: The practitioner's guide. John Wiley & Sons.

Miller, W. R., & Rollnick, S. (2002). Motivational interviewing: Preparing people for change (2nd ed.). Guilford Press.

Minuchin, S., & Fishman, H. (1981). Family therapy techniques. Harvard University Press.

Mohr, W. (2000). Partnering with families. Journal of Psychosocial Nursing, 38, 15–19.

National Institute of Mental Health. (1990). Decade of the brain.

Peplau, H. (1952). Interpersonal relations in nursing. Putnam.

Petiprin, A. (2023). Lewin's change theory. Nursing Theory. https://www.nursing-theory.org/theories-and-models/lewin-change-theory.php

Prochaska, J., & DiClemente, C. (1984). The transtheoretical approach: Crossing traditional boundaries therapy. Dow Jones Irwin.

Prochaska, J., Norcross, J., & DiClemente, C. (1992). In search of how people change: Applications to addictive behaviors. American Psychologist, 47(9), 1102–1112. https://doi.org/10.1037//0003-066x.47.9.1102

Sadock, B., Sadock, V., & Ruiz, P. (2017). Kaplan and Sadock's comprehensive textbook of psychiatry (10th ed.). Wolters Kluwer.

Sherman, C. (2000). Assessment is good opportunity to change family dynamics. Clinical Psychiatric News, 3, 25–29.

Solmi, M., Radua, J., Olivola, M., Croce, E., Soardo, L., Salazar de Pablo, G., . . . Fusar-Poli, P. (2022). Age at onset of mental disorders worldwide: Large-scale meta-analysis of 192 epidemiological studies. Molecular psychiatry, 27(1), 281–295. https://doi.org/10.1038/s41380-021-01161-7

Stuart, G. W., & Laraia, M. (2004). Principles and practice of psychiatric nursing. Mosby.

Substance and Mental Health Services Administration. (2023). Recovery and recovery support. U.S. Department of Health and Human Services. https://www.samhsa.gov/find-help/recovery

Sullivan, H. S. (1953). Interpersonal theory of psychiatry. Basic Books.

Wheeler, K. (2022). Psychotherapy for the advanced practice psychiatric nurse: A how-to guide for evidence-based practice (3rd ed.). Springer Publishing.

Yalom, I., & Leszcz, M. (2020). The theory and practice of group psychotherapy (6th ed.). Basic Books.

CHAPTER 4

PSYCHIATRIC-MENTAL HEALTH NURSE PRACTITIONER PROFESSIONAL ROLE AND HEALTH POLICY

Leadership, Quality Improvement and Safety, Practice Inquiry, and Health Policy

LEADERSHIP

Nurses should be leaders and engage with health professionals to transform and redesign health care (Institute of Medicine [IOM], 2011).

- The nurse practitioner (NP) is educated to lead interdisciplinary treatment teams
  - Acts as full partner in health care
  - Designs, implements, evaluates, and advocates to redesign the U.S. health care system
  - Translates research into practice
- Team leadership model
  - Decision 1: Should the leader monitor the team or take action?
    - Seek out information to understand the team
    - Analyze information
    - Interpret the information and decide how to act
  - Decision 2: Should the leader intervene to meet the task or relational need?
    - Performance functions
    - Task functions
  - Decision 3: Should the leader intervene internally or externally?
    - Assess for conflicts between group members—action to maintain group performance
    - Assess for unclear goals
    - Assess for proper support (Northouse, 2007)

REFLECTIVE PRACTICE

- Reflection uses a model or framework for validation
- Process to tell a story about self and others to gain insight into practice
- Enhances critical thinking to problem-solve and enhance clinical reasoning and decision-making
- Link theory to practice

CONFLICT RESOLUTION, NEGOTIATION, MEDIATION, ARBITRATION, AND PROFESSIONAL CIVILITY

- Conflict: Occurs when a person believes their needs, interests, or values are incompatible with those of others
- Conflict resolution: Directed by a neutral third party who facilitates a "win–win" situation
- Negotiation: Discussion among two or more people with the goal of reaching an agreement
- Mediation: Voluntary and confidential process in which a third party facilitates discussion to reach an agreement
- Arbitration: Process in which a third party reviews evidence from both sides and makes a decision to settle the case
- Professional civility: Behavior that shows respect toward another person

CRITICAL THINKING

- Defined as the acquisition of knowledge with an attitude of deliberate inquiry
- Making clinical decisions based on evidence-based practice
    - Decreases the difficulty of choosing from conflicting or multiple recommendations when diagnosing and treating clients
- Develops self-awareness though a metacognitive process to gain new insights about self and in relation to others

RESEARCH

- Systematic inquiry or investigation to validate and refine existing knowledge and generate new knowledge
- Contribute to advancing knowledge that is generalizable
- Types of research
  - Quantitative: Collecting and analyzing numerical data to describe, predict, or control variables of interest (e.g., experimental, observational, descriptive)
  - Qualitative: Involves collecting and evaluating non-numerical data to understand concepts or subjective opinions (e.g., phenomenology, grounded theory, ethnography)
  - Mixed methods: Collecting, analyzing, and mixing quantitative and qualitative research and methods in a single study.
- Ethical considerations in research
  - The institutional review board (IRB) determines that the rights and welfare of human research participants are protected and has the authority to approve, require modifications, or disapprove of any research activities.

EVIDENCE-BASED PRACTICE

Evidence-based practice (EBP) is a problem-solving approach to the delivery of health care that integrates the best evidence from a body of research with a clinician's expertise and client's preferences and values to make the best decisions about client care (Melnyk & Fineout-Overholt, 2023). It is a seven step process:

1. Cultivate questioning attitude toward practice
2. Ask a formatted foreground question (i.e., P [patient)], I [intervention], C [comparison], O [outcome], T [time]; PICOT)
3. The systematic search for and collection of the most relevant evidence
4. Critically appraise the evidence (critical appraisal, evaluation, synthesis, and practice recommendations)
5. Integrate the evidence with one's clinical expertise and client preferences and values in making a practice decision or change
6. Evaluate outcomes
7. Disseminate the outcomes of the practice decision or change

Sources of Evidence

- External: Publications from research studies
- Internal: Local quality and outcome data
- Pre-appraised evidence: Systematic review is a synthesis of multiple research findings addressing a specific clinical question. Clinical practice guidelines contain practice recommendations based on systematic reviews of the evidence and the benefits and harms of interventions to optimize client care and outcomes.

Evidence Hierarchies

- Level of evidence based on research design is assigned according to established guidelines or frameworks, such as an evidence hierarchy pyramid, which ranks evidence from the highest level (e.g., systematic reviews and meta-analyses of randomized controlled trials) to the lowest level (e.g., expert opinion).
- Quality of evidence in research refers to the extent to which a study is conducted to ensure validity (truthfulness), reliability (clinical importance), and applicability (relevancy to the practice for my clients) of the results (Melnyk & Fineout-Overholt, 2023).

EBP Models

- Numerous models have been designed to help clinicians implement evidence-based change in practice. (i.e., Iowa model, Johns Hopkins Evidence-Based Practice model, Stetler model, other evidence-based practice quality improvement)
- Process models: Describe and or guide the process of translating research into practice
- Based on the EBP model, varying critical appraisal tools are available.

Quality Improvement

- Quintuple aim
  - Client experience
  - Population health
  - Reducing costs
  - Care team well-being
  - Health equity

The Model for Improvement: A framework to analyze the existing data within a local health care system to improve and standardize internal processes and outcomes (cost, productivity, quality, and safety).

- PDSA (Plan-Do-Study-Act) is an iterative process using tests of change that start on a small scale and scope toward meeting the health care system's specific aims.
    - Plan: Plan the test or observation, including a plan for collecting data.
    - Do: Execute the plan.
    - Study: Analyze the data and study the results.
    - Act: Refine the change based on what was learned from the test.
- Types of measures:
    - Outcome measures: How does the system impact clients' values, health, and well-being? What are the impacts on other stakeholders, such as payers, employees, or the community?
    - Process measures: Are the parts/steps in the system performing as planned? Are we on track in our efforts to improve the system?
    - Balancing measures: Are changes that are designed to improve one part of the system causing new problems in other parts of the system?
- Data are displayed graphically and plotted over time (run or control chart) to determine the common cause or special cause variation to establish the stability of the system's processes.
- Data-driven decisions (Institute for Healthcare Improvement [IHI], n.d.)

JUST CULTURE OF SAFETY

- "Position Statement: Just Culture" (American Nurses Association [ANA], 2010)
    - Supports collaboration efforts among state boards of nursing, professional organizations, client safety centers, and health care systems to develop Just Culture initiatives
    - Holds people accountable for their behaviors and investigates errors
    - Goal is to create an open and fair learning environment to design safe systems and manage choices
    - The mindset that affects the work environment is to proactively look for system breakdowns and identify ways to improve systems.

HEALTH CARE DELIVERY SYSTEMS

- The health care system is complex and fragmented; complexity science provides a framework to understand, design, and structure change.
- Focus is on the interaction of the parts and relationships
- Nonlinear process

ACCESS TO CARE

Access to care is a client-centered care model based on the principle that health care services should be coordinated and directed by a single physician or other provider. In this model, clients can access services from multiple entry points. Services can be located in the same facility or in an integrated care network of providers in different locations that can be accessed when needed.

QUALITY OF CARE

The National Committee for Quality Assurance (NCQA) has developed the Health Effectiveness Data and Information Set (HEDIS) to measure health outcomes. Race and ethnicity stratifications have been added to measurements related to substance use. Currently, 13 HEDIS measures exist for behavioral health:

1. Follow-Up Care for Children Prescribed ADHD Medication
2. Antidepressant Medication Management
3. Metabolic Monitoring for Children and Adolescents on Antipsychotics
4. Use of First-Line Psychosocial Care for Children and Adolescents on Antipsychotics
5. Follow-Up After Emergency Department Visit for Substance Use Disorder
6. Follow-Up After Hospitalization for Mental Illness
7. Follow-Up After High-Intensity Care for Substance Use Disorder
8. Follow-Up After Emergency Department Visit for Mental Illness
9. Initiation and Engagement of Substance Use Disorder Treatment
10. Adherence to Antipsychotic Medications for Individuals with Schizophrenia
11. Diabetes Screening for People with Schizophrenia or Bipolar Disorder Who Are Using Antipsychotic Medications

12. Cardiovascular Monitoring for People with Cardiovascular Disease and Schizophrenia
13. Diabetes Monitoring for People with Diabetes and Schizophrenia

ORGANIZATION OF PRACTICES

The Patient Protection and Affordable Care Act (ACA, 2010) emphasized care integration to address co-occurring disorders. Practices are encouraged to reorganize and redesign to provide integrated care, including medical and psychiatric care. The client-centered medical (health) home has the support of the Health Resources and Services Administration (HRSA) and initiatives to provide client-centered, evidence-based, coordinated, and quality care are moving forward.

Patient-Centered Care Model (PCC)

- Welcoming environment: Provide a physical space and an initial personal interaction that is welcoming and familiar, not intimidating.
- Respect for clients' values and expressed needs: Obtain information about the client's care preferences and priorities; inform and involve the client and family or caregivers in decision-making; tailor care to the person; and promote a mutually respectful, consistent client–provider relationship.
- Client empowerment or activation: Educate and encourage the client to expand their role in decision-making, health-related behaviors, and self-management.
- Sociocultural competence: Understand and consider culture, economic and educational status, health literacy level, family patterns and situation, and traditions (including alternative and folk remedies); communicate in language and at a level that the client understands.
- Coordination and integration of care: Assess the client's need for formal and informal services that may affect health or treatment; provide team-based care, care management, and referrals as needed; advocate for the client and family; and ensure smooth transitions between different providers and phases of care.
- Comfort and support: Emphasize physical comfort, privacy, emotional support, and involvement of family and friends.
- Access and navigation skills: Provide what the client can consider a medical home; keep waiting times to a minimum; provide convenient service hours; promote access and client flow; and help client attain skills to better navigate the health care system.
- Community outreach: Make demonstrable, proactive efforts to understand and reach out to the local community (Silow-Carroll et al., 2006).

Health Care Home (Substance Abuse and Mental Health Services Administration [SAMHSA], 2015)

- Defined in the ACA as an approach to primary care that provides coordinated care to persons with multiple chronic health conditions, including mental health and substance use
- Offers team-based care
- Builds on community supports

CONFLICT OF INTEREST

A conflict of interest (COI) is a situation in which a person's financial, professional, or personal situation may affect or appear to affect the person's judgment in their professional responsibilities, including health care decisions, research, and other matters, with the potential for personal or professional gain or advantage—or, conversely, loss or disadvantage—of any kind and the possibility of potential harm to clients.

- Disclosure of potential COIs should be done at least annually and whenever new significant financial interests arise.
- Disclosure must be reported to employers, boards, professional agencies, and wherever there is potential for a COI.
- Action should be carried out to resolve potential or actual COIs and reduce bias.
- Health care agencies and educational and research institutions have policies to require the disclosure of any potential COI and to define the limits allowed in any relationship with external organizations and companies.
- A COI form indicating any financial or other relationship with the products being discussed must be completed prior to any professional presentation. In addition, if any off-label uses of medications or medical devices will be discussed, this information must also be disclosed.
- Types of COIs
  - Relationships with pharmaceutical, medical supply, or insurance companies
  - Money, gifts in kind
  - Referrals
  - Fee splitting

RIGHTS OF CLIENTS

- Confidentiality
- Least-restrictive treatment
- Give consent for treatment and withdraw consent at any time

HEALTH POLICY DEVELOPMENT

Health policy consists of decisions, actions, and plans to achieve specific health care goals (Moutselos & Maglogiannis, 2020).

- Four components of health policy
    1. Process: Formulation, implementation, and evaluation
    2. Policy reform: Changes in programs and practices
    3. Policy environment: Arena in which the process takes place (government, media, public)
    4. Policy makers: Key players and stakeholders
- Health policies are developed through law and regulations.
    - Branches of law: Executive (implement law), legislative (initial formulation), and judicial (interpret law)

The Role of the NP in Health Policy Development

Advanced practice nurses are key stakeholders in health policy and have a professional responsibility to be involved in influencing policy as they are able. The NP has information on the effects of current policy from the clients and their experiences, their personal health care experiences, and their professional dealing with the health care system. This includes

- Access to care and insurance coverage for care;
- Cost of care to the client and to the system;
- Ability of the NP to prescribe the most appropriate treatment for client's condition and have that still be affordable; and
- Availability of health care resources, especially in rural or underserved areas.

The psychiatric-mental health nurse practitioner (PMHNP) has three specific issues related to client care: the cost of psychotropic medications, the availability of providers (both psychiatric and therapists), and the local and state statutes related to mental health care.

How to be involved in influencing health care policy:

- Know your local and federal statutes and policy related to the following:
    - Mental health care—especially involuntary care and client rights
    - Medicaid coverage—state level—for individuals and services
    - Medicare coverage—federal level—for individuals and services; this information is available online
- Know your state and federal representatives and senators:
    - Their stance on issues and their legislative committee responsibilities
    - Upcoming legislation that affects health care policy
- Keep in contact with your representatives and let them know your stance and reasons for such. As a constituent, you have access to them through phone or email. Information is online. Take advantage of any ability to meet them and talk face to face—town meetings and constituent events. In some local areas, it is possible to go to the legislative offices and make appointments to meet with them.
- Vote at every opportunity; understand the issues.

CASE STUDY

A PMHNP who is working at a federally qualified health center (FQHC) is asked to implement routine depression screening for all clients who present to the clinic. The PMHNP is excited about the project but has never implemented a system change and is not sure how to proceed. The PMHNP does have access to the quality improvement department and the clinical manager to get guidance.

1. What depression screening measures are in the public domain and have been found to be sensitive to and specific for depression screening?
2. What is the first step the PMHNP should complete to begin their system change process?
3. Who are key players that should be part of the PMHNP's quality improvement team?
4. What model or framework can the PMHNP use to guide their quality improvement project?
5. When conducting a literature review on depression screening in an FQHC, the PMHNP finds two reports of randomized controlled trials (RCTs) and two expert opinion articles. Which type has the highest level of evidence?

ANSWERS TO CASE STUDY DISCUSSION QUESTIONS

1. The screening measures in the public domain that are sensitive to and specific for depression screening are Patient Health Questionnaire–2 (PHQ-2) and Patient Health Questionnaire–9 (PHQ-9).
2. The first step in beginning a systems-change project is to conduct a systemic needs assessment of the organization.
3. The key players that need to be part of the team include all members of the clinic who will be affected by implementation of the depression screening project.
4. Frameworks for quality improvement include evidence-based practice (EBP), quality improvement (QI), and the Model for Improvement using the Plan-Do-Study-Act (PDSA) process.
5. The highest level of evidence in the literature when evaluating quantitative research studies is an RCT.

REFERENCES AND RESOURCES

American Nurses Association. (2010).Position statement: Just culture. https://www.nursingworld.org/~4afe07/globalassets/practiceandpolicy/health-and-safety/just_culture.pdf

Burke, S. (2016). Influence through policy: Nurses have a unique role. Nursing Centered. https://nursingcentered.sigmanursing.org/commentary/more-commentary/Vol42_2_nurses-have-a-unique-role

Croft, B., & Parish, S. L. (2012). Care integration in the Patient Protection and Affordable Care Act: Implications for behavioral health. Administration and Policy in Mental Health Services Research, 40, 258–263. http://doi: 10.1007/s10488-012-0405-0

Fineout-Overholt, E., Melnyk, B. M., & Schultz, A. (2005). Transforming health care from the inside out: Advancing evidence-based practice in the 21st century. Journal of Professional Nursing, 21(6), 335–344.

Institute for Healthcare Improvement (n.d.). How to improve. Resources. https://www.ihi.org/library/model-for-improvement

Institute of Medicine. (2001). Crossing the quality chasm: A new health system for the 21st century. National Academies Press.

Institute of Medicine Committee on the Robert Wood Johnson Foundation Initiative on the Future of Nursing. (2011). The future of nursing: Leading change, advancing health. National Academies Press. https://doi.org/10.17226/12956

Melnyk, B. M., & Fineout-Overholt, E. (2023). Making the case for evidence-based practice and cultivating a spirit of inquiry. In B. M. Melnyk & E. Fineout-Overholt (Eds.), Evidence-based practice in nursing and healthcare: A guide to best practice (5th ed.). Wolters Kluwer.

Moutselos, K., & Maglogiannis, I. (2020). Evidence-based public health policy models development and evaluation using big data analytics and web technologies. Medical Archives (Sarajevo, Bosnia and Herzegovina), 74(1), 47–53. https://doi.org/10.5455/medarh.2020.74.47-53

Northouse, P. G. (2007). Leadership theory and practice (4th ed.). Sage Publications.

Patient Protection and Affordable Care Act, Pub. L. No. 111–148 (2010). https://www.congress.gov/111/plaws/publ148/PLAW-111publ148.pdf

Perese, E. F. (2012). Psychiatric advanced practice nursing: A biopsychosocial foundation for practice. F. A. Davis.

Sherwood, G. D., & Horton-Deutsch, S. (2012). Reflective practice transforming education and improving outcomes. Sigma Theta Tau International.

Silow-Carroll, S., Alteras, T., & Stepnick, L. (2006). Patient-centered care for underserved populations: Definitions and best practices. https://www.issuelab.org/resources/10547/10547.pdf

Substance Abuse and Mental Health Services Administration. (2014). Advancing behavioral health integration with NCQA recognized patient-centered medical homes. U.S. Department of Health and Human Services. https://www.integration.samhsa.gov/integrated-care-models/Behavioral_Health_Integration_ and_the_Patient_Centered_Medical_Home_FINAL.pdf

Substance Abuse and Mental Health Services Administration. (2015). What is a health home? U.S. Department of Health and Human Services. https://www.integration.samhsa.gov/integrated-care-models/Health_Homes_ Fact_Sheet_FINAL.pdf

World Health Organization. (2016). Health policy. https://www.who.int/topics/health_policy/en/

CHAPTER 5

NEUROANATOMY, NEUROPHYSIOLOGY, AND BEHAVIOR

A tremendous expansion of knowledge about the brain has occurred in the past two decades. As more has been learned about the brain and its complex functioning, assessment and treatment for psychiatric disorders have been altered dramatically. Increasingly, the links among genetics, altered brain anatomy and physiology, and the symptoms of psychiatric disorders have been identified (Sadock et al., 2017).

This growing knowledge base will continue to alter the treatment of psychiatric disorders. As new knowledge is disseminated, it is helping diminish the stigma long associated with psychiatric illness.

This chapter reviews the basics of neuroanatomy and physiology that provide the scientific rationale for many of the psychiatric-mental health nurse practitioner (PMHNP) care practices, including psychopharmacological interventions described elsewhere in this review manual. PMHNPs need a solid foundation in neurobiology. Increasingly, the roles of the PMHNP require the application of this knowledge to clinical practice.

THE NERVOUS SYSTEM

- All human thoughts, feelings, and actions are seated in and start with actions of the nervous system.
- Necessary for the PMHNP's role functioning is an understanding of the following basic neuroanatomy and physiology principles:
  - ◊ Neurodeficits that underlie psychiatric disorders
  - ◊ Actions of and client responses to psychopharmacological treatment agents
  - ◊ The nervous system's primary function is to transfer and exchange information.

THE NEURON ("NERVE CELL")

- The basic cellular unit of the nervous system
- The microprocessor of the brain responsible for conducting impulses from one part of the body to another

- Components of the neuron
  - Cell body: Also known as soma; made up of the nucleus and cytoplasm within the cell membrane
  - Axon: Transmits signals away from the neuron's cell body to connect with other neurons and cells
  - Dendrites: Collect incoming signals from other neurons and send the signal toward the neuron's cell body

NERVOUS SYSTEM

- Composed of two separate, interconnected divisions
  - Central nervous system (CNS)
    - Composed of the spinal cord and the brain
  - Peripheral nervous system (PNS)
    - Composed of the peripheral nerves that connect the CNS to receptors, muscles, and glands
    - Includes the cranial nerves just outside the brainstem
    - Comprises the somatic nervous system and the autonomic nervous system:
      - Somatic nervous system: Conveys information from the CNS to skeletal muscles; responsible for voluntary movement
      - Autonomic nervous system: Regulates internal body functions to maintain homeostasis; conveys information from the CNS to smooth muscle, cardiac muscle, and glands; responsible for involuntary movement; divided into the sympathetic nervous system and the parasympathetic nervous system
        - Sympathetic nervous system: The excitatory division; prepares the body for stress (fight, flight, or freeze); stimulates or increases activity of organs
        - Parasympathetic nervous system: Maintains or restores energy; inhibits or decreases activity of organs

NEUROANATOMY AND THE BRAIN

- Brain tissue is categorized as either white matter or gray matter.
  - White matter is the myelinated axons of neurons.
  - Gray matter is composed of nerve cell bodies and dendrites; it is the working area of the brain and contains the synapses, the area of neuronal connection.

- The outermost surface of the brain is structured to contain grooves and dips of corrugated wrinkles within the brain tissue that provide anatomic landmarks or reference points.
  - Functions to increase brain's surface area
  - Increases working area and cell communication area
  - Grooves and dips named by size and depth
    - Sulci: Small shallow grooves
    - Fissures: Deeper groves extending into the brain
    - Gyri are the raised tissue areas.
- Distinct anatomic areas of brain
  - The brain is subdivided into the cerebrum and the brainstem.

CEREBRUM

- Largest part of the brain, which is divided into two halves, the right and left cerebral hemispheres
  - Left hemisphere: Dominant in most people; controls most right-sided body functions
  - Right hemisphere: Controls most left-sided body functions
  - Normal functioning requires effective coordination of two hemispheres.
  - Both hemispheres connected by a large bundle of white matter, the corpus callosum, an area of sensorimotor information exchange between the two hemispheres
  - Each hemisphere is divided into four major lobes, which work in an interactive and integrated manner, and each with a distinct function
- Frontal lobe: Largest and most developed lobe. Functions include:
  - Motor function: Responsible for controlling voluntary motor activity of specific muscles
  - Premotor area: Coordinates movement of multiple muscles
  - Association cortex: Allows for multimodal sensory input to trigger memory and lead to decision-making
  - Seat of executive function: Working memory, reasoning, planning, prioritizing, sequencing behavior, insight, flexibility, judgment, impulse control, behavioral cueing, intelligence, abstraction
  - Language (Broca's area): Expressive speech
  - Personality variables: The most focal area for personality development

  - ◊ Problems in the frontal lobe can lead to personality changes and emotional and intellectual changes.
- ♦ Temporal lobe: Second largest lobe. Functions include:
  - ◊ Language (Wernicke's area): Receptive speech or language comprehension
  - ◊ Primary auditory area
  - ◊ Memory
  - ◊ Emotion
  - ◊ Integration of vision with sensory information
  - ◊ Problems in the temporal lobe can lead to visual or auditory hallucinations, aphasia, and amnesia.
- ♦ Occipital lobe: Smallest and most rear of the lobes. Functions include:
  - ◊ Primary visual cortex
  - ◊ Integration area: Integrates vision with other sensory information
  - ◊ Problems in the occipital lobe can lead to visual field defects, blindness, and visual hallucinations.
- ♦ Parietal lobe: Sensory processing center. Functions include:
  - ◊ Taste
  - ◊ Reading and writing
  - ◊ Problems in the parietal lobe can lead to sensory–perceptual disturbances and agnosia.
- ♦ Cerebrum includes the cerebral cortex, limbic system, thalamus, hypothalamus, and basal ganglia.
  - ◊ Cerebral cortex
    - Controls a wide array of behaviors
    - Controls the contralateral (opposite) side of the body: The right hemisphere controls the left side of the body, and the left hemisphere controls the right side of the body.
    - Sensory information is relayed from the thalamus and then processed and integrated in the cortex.
    - Responsible for much of the behavior that makes us human: Speech, cognition, judgment, perception, and motor function
  - ◊ Limbic system
    - Essential system for the regulation and modulation of emotions and memory
    - Composed of the hypothalamus, thalamus, hippocampus, and amygdala

- ◊ Hypothalamus: Plays key roles in various regulatory functions such as appetite, sensations of hunger and thirst, water balance, circadian rhythm, body temperature, libido, and hormonal regulation
- ◊ Thalamus: Sensory relay station except for smell; modulates flow of sensory information to prevent overwhelming the cortex; regulates emotions, memory, and related affective behaviors
- ◊ Hippocampus: Regulates memory and converts short-term memory into long-term memory
- ◊ Amygdala: Responsible for mediating mood, fear, emotion, and aggression; also responsible for connecting sensory smell information with emotions
- ◊ Basal ganglia: Also known as the corpus striatum
    - Serves as a complex feedback system to modulate and stabilize somatic motor activity (information conveyed from the CNS to skeletal muscles)
    - Plays a role in movement initiation; complex motor functions with associated connections
    - Functions in learning and automatic actions such as walking or driving a car
    - Contains extrapyramidal motor system or nerve tracts
    - Functions in involuntary motor activities (e.g., muscle tone, posture, coordination of muscle movement, common reflexes)
    - Many psychotropic medications can affect the extrapyramidal motor nerve track, causing involuntary movement side effects.
    - Contains both the caudate and the putamen
    - Problems in the basal ganglia can lead to bradykinesia, hyperkinesia, and dystonia.

BRAINSTEM

- ♦ Made up of cells that produce neurotransmitters
- ♦ Includes the midbrain, pons, medulla, cerebellum, and reticular formation
    - ◊ Midbrain: Houses the ventral tegmental area and the substantia nigra (areas of dopamine synthesis)
    - ◊ Pons: Houses the locus ceruleus (area of norepinephrine synthesis)
    - ◊ Medulla: Together with the pons, contains autonomic control centers that regulate internal body functions
    - ◊ Cerebellum: Responsible for maintaining equilibrium; acts as a gross movement control center (e.g., control movement, balance, posture)
        - Each hemisphere of cerebellum has ipsilateral control (same side of body).

- Problems with the cerebellum can lead to ataxia (uncoordinated and inaccurate movements).
- The Romberg test is important for detecting deficiencies in cerebellar functioning.

◊ Reticular formation system: The primitive brain

- Receives input from cortex, an integration area for input from post-sensory pathways
- Innervates the thalamus, hypothalamus, and cortex
- Regulation functions include:
  - Involuntary movement
  - Reflex
  - Muscle tone
  - Vital sign control
  - Blood pressure
  - Respiratory rate
  - Critical to consciousness and ability to mentally focus, to be alert, and to pay attention to environmental stimuli

NEUROPHYSIOLOGY AND THE BRAIN

♦ Two classes of cells are in the nervous system: glia and neurons.

◊ Glia: Structures that form the myelin sheath around axons and provide protection and support

◊ Neurons: Nerve cells responsible for conducting impulses from one part of the body to another

♦ Components of a neuron include:

◊ Cell body: Also known as soma; made up of the nucleus and cytoplasm within the cell membrane

◊ Dendrites: Receive information to conduct impulse toward the cell body

◊ Axon: Sends or conducts information away from the cell body

◊ Synapse or synaptic cleft: The connection site and area of communication between neurons where neurotransmitters are released

- The synapse converts an electrical signal (action potential) from the presynaptic neuron into a chemical signal (neuron transmitter) that is transferred to the postsynaptic neuron.
- Neurotransmitters are released at the synaptic cleft as the result of electrical activity (action potential).

- The two phases of an action potential are
  - Depolarization: The initial phase of the action potential (an excitatory response), when sodium and calcium ions flow into the cell; and
  - Repolarization: The restoration phase (an inhibitory response), when potassium leaves the cell or chloride enters the cell.
- Problems in either the structure or chemistry of the synapse interrupt normal flow of impulses and stimuli, which then contribute to symptoms commonly seen in psychiatric disorders.

♦ Neurotransmitters: Chemicals synthesized from dietary substrates that communicate information from one cell to another.

◇ The neurotransmitter will be released from the presynaptic neuron, cross the synapse, and then bind to a specific receptor on the postsynaptic neuron.

◇ Specific criteria must be met for a molecule to be classified as a neurotransmitter (see Table 5–1).

◇ Categories of neurotransmitters: Monoamines, amino acids, cholinergics, neuropeptides

- Monoamines: "Biogenic amines"—dopamine, norepinephrine, epinephrine, serotonin
  - Dopamine: Known as a catecholamine; produced in the substantia nigra and the ventral tegmental area; precursor is tyrosine; removed from the synaptic cleft by monoamine oxidase (MAO) enzymatic action
    - ■ Four dopaminergic pathways: Mesocortical, mesolimbic, nigrostriatal, tuberoinfundibular (see Chapter 10)

TABLE 5–1.
CLASSIFICATION REQUIREMENTS FOR NEUROTRANSMITTERS

CRITERIA
1. Neurotransmitter must be present at the nerve terminal.
2. Stimulation of neuron must cause release of neurotransmitter in sufficient quantities to cause an action to occur at the postsynaptic membrane.
3. Effects of exogenous transmitter on postsynaptic membrane must be similar to those caused by stimulation of the presynaptic neuron.
4. A mechanism for inactivation or metabolism of the neurotransmitter must exist in the area of the synapse.
5. Exogenous drugs should alter the dose–response curve of the neurotransmitter in a manner similar to that of the naturally occurring synaptic potential.

Note. Adapted from Sadock, B. J., Sadock, V. A., & Ruiz, P. (2017). Kaplan and Sadock's comprehensive textbook of psychiatry (10th ed.). Wolters Kluwer.

  - Norepinephrine: Also known as a catecholamine; produced in the locus ceruleus of the pons; precursor is tyrosine; removed from the synaptic cleft and returned to storage via an active reuptake process; major neurotransmitter implicated in mood, anxiety, and concentration disorders
  - Epinephrine: Also known as a catecholamine; produced by the adrenal glands; the epinephrine system also referred to as the adrenergic system
  - Serotonin: Known as an indole; produced in the raphe nuclei of the brainstem; precursor is tryptophan; removed from the synaptic cleft and returned to storage via an active reuptake process; major neurotransmitter implicated in mood and anxiety disorders
- Amino acids: Glutamate, aspartate, γ-aminobutyric acid (GABA), glycine
  - Glutamate: Universal excitatory neurotransmitter; major neurotransmitter involved in process of kindling, which is implicated in seizure disorders and possibly bipolar disorder; imbalance implicated in mood disorders and schizophrenia
  - Aspartate: Another excitatory neurotransmitter; works with glutamate
  - GABA: Universal inhibitory neurotransmitter; site of action of benzodiazepines, alcohol, barbiturates, and other CNS depressants
  - Glycine: Another inhibitory neurotransmitter; works with GABA
- Cholinergics: Acetylcholine
  - Acetylcholine: Synthesized by the basal nucleus of Meynert; precursors are acetyl coenzyme A and choline
- Neuropeptides: Nonopioid type (substance P, somatostatin); opioid type (endorphins, enkephalins, dynorphins)
  - Modulate pain; decreased amount of neuropeptides is thought to cause substance use

◊ See Table 5–2 for identification of neurotransmitters' role in symptom expression in common psychiatric disorders.

◊ Recovery and degradation of neurotransmitters

- After the neurotransmitter reaches the postsynaptic neuron, it may then diffuse from its receptor to be destroyed by enzymes or to be transported back to the presynaptic neuron for reuse.
- Enzymatic destruction occurs either in the cytosol or in the synapse. The neurotransmitter can be destroyed by the enzymes monoamine oxidase (MAO) in the cytosol or catechol-O-methyl transferase (COMT) intracellularly or in the synapse.
- Reuptake pumps can remove the neurotransmitter from acting in the synapse. The neurotransmitter will be reloaded into the presynaptic neuron and will be recycled.

◊ See table 5–3 for the function of neurotransmitters.

TABLE 5–2.
COMMON PSYCHIATRIC DISORDERS AND NEUROTRANSMITTERS IMPLICATED IN THE COMPLEX PATHOPHYSIOLOGY OF COMMON PSYCHIATRIC DISORDERS

NEUROTRANSMITTER	SUSPECTED IMBALANCE	PSYCHIATRIC PRESENTATION
Acetylcholine	Decrease	Alzheimer's disease
	Increase	Impaired memory
		Parkinsonian symptoms
Dopamine	Increase	Schizophrenia
	Decrease	Psychosis
		Substance use
		Anhedonia
		Parkinson's disease
Norepinephrine	Decrease	Depression
	Increase	Anxiety
Serotonin	Decrease	Depression
		Obsessive–compulsive disorder
		Anxiety disorders
		Schizophrenia
γ-Aminobutyric acid (GABA)	Decrease	Anxiety disorders
Glutamate	Increase	Bipolar affective disorder
	Decrease	Psychosis from ischemic neurotoxicity or excessive pruning
		Memory and learning difficulty
		Negative symptoms of schizophrenia
Opioid neuropeptides	Decrease	Substance use

Note. Adapted from Sadock, B. J., Sadock, V. A., & Ruiz, P. (2017). Kaplan and Sadock's comprehensive textbook of psychiatry (10th ed.). Wolters Kluwer.

NEUROIMAGING ASSESSMENT AND DIAGNOSTIC PROCEDURES

- Techniques that permit observation of the brain can be divided into three categories:
  - Structural imaging
  - Functional imaging
  - Combined structural and functional imaging

TABLE 5–3.
COMPARISON OF COMMON CNS NEUROTRANSMITTERS

NEUROTRANSMITTER	RECEPTORS	GENERAL FUNCTION	SYMPTOMS OF DEFICIT	SYMPTOMS OF EXCESS
Dopamine	D1-like D2-like	Thinking Decision-making Reward-seeking behavior Fine muscle action Integrated cognition	Mild: Poor impulse control Poor spatiality Lack of abstractive thought Severe: Parkinson's disease Endocrine alterations Movement disorders	Mild: Improved creativity Improved ability for abstract thinking Improved executive functioning Improved spatiality Severe: Disorganized thinking Loose association Tics Stereotypic behavior
Norepinephrine	$\alpha 1$ $\alpha 2$	Alertness Focused attention Orientation Primes fight, flight, or freeze Learning Memory	Dullness Low energy Depressive affect	Anxiety Hyperalertness Increased startle Paranoia Decreased appetite
Serotonin	5-HT1A 5-HT1D 5-HT2 5-HT2A 5-HT3 5-HT4	Regulation of sleep Pain perception Mood states Temperature Regulation of aggression Libido Precursor for melatonin	Irritability Hostility Depression Sleep dysregulation Loss of appetite Loss of libido	Sedation Increased aggression Hallucinations (rare)

(Continued)

TABLE 5-3. (CONTINUED)

NEUROTRANSMITTER	RECEPTORS	GENERAL FUNCTION	SYMPTOMS OF DEFICIT	SYMPTOMS OF EXCESS
Acetylcholine	Nicotinic Muscarinic	Attention Memory Thirst Mood regulation REM sleep Sexual behavior Muscle tone	Lack of inhibition Decreased memory Euphoria Antisocial action Speech decrease Dry mouth, blurred vision, constipation	Over-inhibition Anxiety Depression Somatic complaints Self-consciousness Drooling Extrapyramidal movements
GABA	GABAA GABAB	Reduces arousal Reduces aggression Reduces anxiety Reduces excitation	Irritability; Hostility Tension and worry Anxiety Seizure activity	Reduced cellular excitability Sedation, impaired memory
Glutamate	AMPA NNDA	Memory Sustained automatic functions	Poor memory Low energy Distractible	Kindling Seizures Anxiety or panic
Peptides: Opioid type	μ (mu) K (kappa) ε (epsilon) δ (delta) σ (sigma)	Modulate emotions Reward-center function Consolidation of memory Modulate reactions to stress	Hypersensitivity to pain and stress Decreased pleasure sensation Dysphoria	Insensitivity to pain Catatonic-like movement disturbance Auditory hallucinations Decreased memory

Note. Adapted from Sadock, B. J., Sadock, V. A., & Ruiz, P. (2017). Kaplan and Sadock's comprehensive textbook of psychiatry (10th ed.). Wolters Kluwer.

- Structural imaging: Provides evidence of the size and shape of anatomic structures
  - Common structural imaging tests
    - Computed tomography (CT): Provides a three-dimensional view of the brain structures; differentiates structures based on density; provides suggestive evidence of brain-based problems but no specific testing for psychiatric disorders
      - Advantages: Widely available, relatively inexpensive
      - Disadvantages: Lack of sensitivity, cannot differentiate white matter from gray matter; cannot view structures close to the bone tissue; underestimation of brain atrophy; inability to image sagittal and coronal views
    - Magnetic resonance imaging (MRI): Provides a series of two-dimensional images that represent the brain
      - Advantages: Can view brain structures close to the skull and can separate white matter from gray matter; readily available; resolution of brain tissue is superior to CT scanning
      - Disadvantages: Expensive; many contraindications to its use (e.g., clients with pacemakers or any metallic implants such as orthopedic screws or plates, clients on ventilators); clients with claustrophobia often are unable to complete study because of design of machinery (an enclosed tubelike structure with a confining environment)
- Functional imaging: Technique that measures functional of areas of the brain and bases the resulting assessment on blood flow; may use radioactive pharmaceuticals to cross the blood–brain barrier; used mainly for research
  - Common functional imaging tests
    - Electroencephalography (EEG) and evoked potential testing: Least expensive tests that convey information on electrical functioning of the CNS
    - Magnetoencephalography (MEG): Similar to EEG but detects different electrical activities; often used in a complementary fashion with EEG testing
    - Single-photon emission computed tomography (SPECT): Provides information on the cerebral blood flow; limited availability; expensive but less expensive than positron emission tomography
    - Positron emission tomography (PET): Provides images of the brain when positron-emitting radionuclei interact with electrons; expensive procedure that requires extensive resources and support team
- Combined structural and functional imaging: The newest imaging; attempts to examine structure in conjunction with function; currently mainly used for research

- ◇ Available tests include:
    - Functional MRI (fMRI)
    - Three-dimensional, event-related functional MRI (3fEMRI)
    - Fluorine magnetic spectroscopy
    - Dopamine D2 receptor binding

GENOMICS

FAMILY HISTORY, FAMILY TREE, OR PEDIGREE

- Tool in determining the likelihood of genetic disorder in family, inheritance patterns, and risk of recurrence in family members
- The Surgeon General recommended that families know their family history (U.S. Department of Health and Human Services [HHS], n.d.)
- Pedigree symbols in drawing a family tree indicate male, female, marriage, divorce, adoption, twins, pregnancy, consanguinity (relatives having children), conditions
- Family history starts with current family and moves back to grandparents.
- Autosomal-dominant conditions may be present in more than one generation and in up to 50% of offspring when one parent is affected (e.g., Marfan syndrome).
- Recessive conditions appear only in one generation, affecting people who have two copies of a gene mutation, one from each (unaffected) parent (e.g., hemochromatosis, cystic fibrosis).
- X-linked disorders are caused by a gene mutation on a specific X chromosome (e.g., fragile X syndrome, color blindness).
- Risk assessment is based on inheritance patterns and may be by percentage of risk.

GENETIC COUNSELING

- Genetic counseling is a communication process used when a client has a genetic risk and often involves offering a test that could provide information about the genetic status of the person and possible implications for the family.
- A genetic counselor is someone whose primary role is to offer information and support to people concerned about an illness that may have a genetic basis.
- A referral to a genetic counselor may be needed when a client is anticipating a pregnancy and is concerned for the health of the fetus.

GENETIC TERMS

- Chromosomes are structures of DNA (deoxyribonucleic acid) in the nucleus of cells; there are normally 46 total (23 pairs) in humans.
- DNA is made up of two twisted, paired strands composed of sugars linked by four nucleotide bases—adenine (A), thymine (T), cytosine (C), and guanine (G)—specifying the amino acids that make proteins. A is always paired with T and G is always paired with C.
- Genes are a sequence of DNA that cause human characteristics to be passed to the next generation; genes direct the production of proteins.
- Messenger RNA (mRNA) is a molecule in cells that transports DNA code in the nucleus to the site of protein synthesis.
- The Human Genome Project mapped the entire nucleotide sequence of the human genome in 2003. The genome is a complete set of genetic instructions.
- A phenotype is the observable characteristic of a specific trait and is connected to the genetic contributions to that trait (e.g., fast metabolizer of cytochrome P450 2D6 [CYP2D6] medications).
- Gene therapy involves replacing a faulty copy of a gene with a healthy copy of the same gene.
- Personalized medicine is health care based on genetic variability.

STUDIES OF POPULATION GENETICS

- Family studies investigate the occurrence of disorders in first-degree relatives (parents, siblings, and offspring) and second-degree relatives (grandparents, cousins, aunts, and uncles).
- Twin studies survey the concordance rate (presence) of a disorder in monozygotic (identical) and dizygotic (fraternal) twins.
- Adoption studies investigate the risk of a disorder developing in children raised in an environment different from the biological parent with a specific disorder.
- Strong genetic contributions have been found for most psychiatric disorders, with a range of 40% to 90% heritability for some disorders (e.g., attention-deficit/hyperactivity disorder, bipolar disorder).
- Genes are risk factors that make a person vulnerable to developing the illness when combined with certain environmental risk factors that increase susceptibility to developing the disorder.

- Environmental risk factors include prenatal insults, stress, infection, poor nutrition, exposure to toxins, catastrophic loss, and physical and sexual abuse.
- Most diseases are multifactorial, caused by both environmental and genetic factors; single-gene disorders are rare.

GENE EXPRESSION AND DISEASE

- Single nucleotide polymorphisms (SNPs) detect single base changes in a DNA sequence.
- Reduced penetrance of a gene decreases the chance of disease in a person at genetic risk.
- Variable expression of a gene for a disorder occurs at the cellular level.

PHARMACOGENOMICS

- Genes account for differences in the way enzymes metabolize drugs.
- Medications may act differently based on how genes affect metabolism.
- Genetic testing or profiling helps identify the presence of gene variants that may help determine dosing of medication (e.g., CYP test of CYP2D6, CYP2C19, and methylene tetrahydrofolate reductase [MTHFR] genes; see Chapter 7 for further information on pharmacokinetics).
- Testing for presence of HLA-B*1502 allele, an inherited variant of the HLA-B gene, is required by the U.S Food and Drug Administration (FDA) in people of Asian descent prior to prescribing the anticonvulsant carbamazepine due to risk of Stevens-Johnson syndrome and toxic epidermal necrolysis (TEN).

CASE STUDY 1

H.F. is a 24-year-old salesclerk who has a strong family history of mental illness and is worried that they may experience some problems in life because of their family history. H.F. presents to their local primary care provider complaining of the following symptoms:

- Hyperalertness
- Increased startle response
- Concern that people are staring and watching what they eat
- Decreased appetite
- Difficulty falling asleep

H.F. is trying to determine if these experiences are the beginning of a mental illness and wants to have a brain scan done to determine the answer. H.F. is getting married soon and wants to know what the risk is for future children, since it is believed mental illness runs in the family. In working with this client, the PMHNP must consider many issues.

1. Are the symptoms described consistent with a psychiatric disorder?
2. Do psychiatric disorders run in families, as the client believes?
3. Do the symptoms as described by H.F. link with any known neuroanatomic or neurophysiologic deficit?
4. Is a brain scan warranted?
5. Can the risk of the client's future children developing psychiatric disorders be determined?

CASE STUDY 2

J.A. is an 18-year-old, first-year college student who developed symptoms of hearing voices, being distressed, fearful, and thinking others are out to hurt him, which necessitated a brief hospitalization. He was given haloperidol 5 mg IM with lorazepam 1 mg IM and diphenhydramine 50 mg IM upon admission and started on risperidone. One day after admission, the client presents to the nurses' station complaining of a painful "stiff neck" and "thick tongue."

1. What is the best description of the presentation?
2. What is the best explanation for the presentation?
3. Which neurotransmitters are involved in the presentation?
4. How should the PMHNP address this scenario?
5. In formulating diagnostic conclusions about J.A., what should the PMHNP consider?

ANSWERS TO CASE STUDY DISCUSSION QUESTIONS

CASE STUDY 1

1. More assessment would be needed to determine whether symptoms are consistent with a psychiatric disorder or a side effect of medication.
2. Most psychiatric illnesses have been shown to have, in part, a genetic link and, therefore, do tend to run in families.
3. The symptoms are consistent with excessive levels of norepinephrine.
4. No. There are insufficient data to warrant the cost of a brain scan at this time.
5. Yes. The risk of future children developing psychiatric disorders can be determined but only if the client meets criteria for an actual psychiatric illness. Once this is determined, the genetic risk to future children can be identified through the use of such things as concordant rate tables.

CASE STUDY 2

1. The presentation is consistent with acute dystonia.
2. Both haloperidol and risperidone are high-potency D_2 antagonists. Although the client received prophylactic diphenhydramine, adding risperidone, particularly with aggressive dosing, increases the risk of extrapyramidal side effects.
3. CNS dopamine and acetylcholine have a reciprocal relationship. Because dopamine receptors are antagonized by antipsychotic medication, acetylcholine levels increase, giving rise to extrapyramidal side effects. This is particularly true of first-generation antipsychotics, but also of high-potency, second-generation agents.
4. Administer diphenhydramine or benztropine (Cogentin) IM immediately and hold subsequent doses of risperidone until dystonia resolves completely. Resume risperidone at a lower dose along with an oral anticholinergic medication. Adjust the dose of the antipsychotic as indicated. If J.A. continues to experience extrapyramidal side effects, switching to a lower-potency antipsychotic may be necessary.
5. The client may have experienced a sentinel episode of schizophrenia. The symptoms may also have been substance induced.

REFERENCES AND RESOURCES

Alexander, E., Chen, K., Pietrini, P., Rapoport, S. I., & Reiman, E. M. (2002). Longitudinal PET evaluation of cerebral metabolic decline in dementia: A potential outcome measure in Alzheimer's disease treatment studies. American Journal of Psychiatry, 159, 238–245.

Amen, D. G. (1998). Brain SPECT imaging in psychiatry. Primary Psychiatry, 5, 83–87.

Amen, D. G. (2010). Brain SPECT imaging in clinical practice. American Journal of Psychiatry, 167(9), 1125–1126.

American Nurses Association, American Psychiatric Nurses Association, & International Society of Psychiatric-Mental Health Nurses. (2022). Psychiatric-mental health nursing: Scope and standards of practice (3rd ed.). American Nurses Association.

Bartolomeis, A. (2014). Glutamatergic postsynaptic density protein dysfunctions in synaptic plasticity and dendritic spines morphology: Relevance to schizophrenia and other behavioral disorders pathophysiology, and implications for novel therapeutic approaches. Molecular Neurobiology, 49(1), 484–511.

Boyd, M. A. (2022). Psychiatric nursing: Contemporary practice (7th ed.). Lippincott, Williams & Wilkins.

Burhan, A. M., Bartha, R., Bocti, C., Borrie, M., Laforce, R., Rosa-Neto, P., & Soucy, J. P. (2013). Role of emerging neuroimaging modalities in patients with cognitive impairment: a review from the Canadian Consensus Conference on the Diagnosis and Treatment of Dementia 2012. Alzheimer's Research & Therapy, 5(Suppl 1), S4. https://doi.org/10.1186/alzrt200

Carlson, N. R. (2012). Physiology of behavior (11th ed.). Allyn & Bacon.

Goff, D., & Coyle, J. (2001). The emerging role of glutamate in the pathophysiology and treatment of schizophrenia. American Journal of Psychiatry, 158, 1367–1377.

Gong, Q., Dazzan, P., Scarpazza, C., Kasai, K., Hu, X., Marques, T. R., . . . Mechelli, A. (2015). A neuroanatomical signature for schizophrenia across different ethnic groups. Schizophrenia Bulletin, 41(6), 1266–1275.

Lee, Y., & Song, G. (2014). Genome-wide pathway analysis in attention-deficit/hyperactivity disorder. Neurological Science, 35(8), 1189–1196.

Matrisciano, F., Panaccione, I., Grayson, D. R., Nicoletti, F., & Guidotti, A. (2016). Metabotropic glutamate 2/3 receptors and epigenetic modifications in psychotic disorders: A review. Current Neuropharmacology, 14(1), 41–47.

McLeod, T. M., Lopez-Figueroa, A., & Lopez-Figueroa, M. O. (2001). Nitric oxide, stress, and depression. Psychopharmacology Bulletin, 35, 24–41.

Mujica-Parodi, L. R., Corcoran, C., Greenberg, T., Saceim, H. A., & Malaspina, D. (2002). Are cognitive symptoms of schizophrenia mediated by abnormalities in emotional arousal? CNS Spectrums, 7(1), 58–69.

Power, B. D., Nguyen, T., Hayhow, B., & Looi, J. (2015). Neuroimaging in psychiatry: An update on neuroimaging in the clinical setting. Australasian Psychiatry, 24(2), 157–163. https://doi.org/10.1177/1039856215618525

Sadock, B. J., Sadock, V. A., & Ruiz, P. (2017). Kaplan and Sadock's comprehensive textbook of psychiatry (10th ed.). Wolters Kluwer.

Stahl, S. M. (2021). Essential psychopharmacology: Neuroscientific basis and practical applications (5th ed.). Cambridge University Press.

Stuart, G. W. (2013). Principles and practice of psychiatric nursing (10th ed.). Mosby.

U.S. Department of Health and Human Services. (n.d.). Surgeon General's family health history initiative. http://www.hhs.gov/familyhistory

Yuta, A., Inokuchi, R., Nakao, T., & Yamasue, H. (2013). Neural bases of antisocial behavior: A voxel-based meta-analysis. Social Cognitive and Affective Neuroscience, 9(8), 1223–1231.

CHAPTER 6

ADVANCED HEALTH AND PHYSICAL HEALTH ASSESSMENT

This chapter reviews the role of psychiatric-mental health nurse practitioners (PMHNPs) in physical health and advanced health assessment. In this chapter you will review information on the process of completing a physical exam and differential diagnosis and the appropriate use of diagnostic and laboratory testing in providing competent nursing care for clients and families experiencing psychiatric disorders. The chapter specifically highlights the PMHNP role in the identification of physical health problems.

PHYSICAL EXAM

- Reasons to be familiar with the physical exam in psychiatry
  - To be able to detect underlying medical problems
  - To be familiar with a screening neurological exam and to be able to rule out neurological problems that may manifest as symptoms of a psychiatric problem
  - To be able to differentiate normal and abnormal signs and symptoms
  - To know when to refer
- Completed by the PMHNP in the context of their primary psychiatric care role
- Goals are identifying the presence of psychiatric disorders, assessing general health status, and screening for other nonpsychiatric disorders
- Focuses on a physical assessment required to accomplish differential diagnoses to determine client health needs
- Specifically focuses on assessing for disorders or conditions that explain client presentation
  - Psychiatric disorders
  - Nonpsychiatric disorders
- Not intended to replace the role of the primary health care provider for the client
  - The PMHNP should assist clients to establish a primary care provider if they do not already have one.

- Avoids highly personal or intrusive procedures (e.g., Pap exam, male genital exam, rectal exam, breast exam) that may make the formation of a therapeutic alliance more difficult, but it is important to be familiar with these exams and to be able to differentiate normal from abnormal
- Requires the PMHNP to have depth of knowledge regarding the common health disorders that can mimic symptoms of a psychiatric disorder
  - Differential diagnostic considerations
- Requires the PMHNP to have depth of knowledge regarding the common psychiatric disorders that can mimic or produce symptoms of other disorders
  - Differential diagnostic considerations
  - Comorbid conditions and clinical management issues
- Generally, if a client's health issues are determined to be nonpsychiatric, the client is referred to primary care providers other than the PMHNP.
- Because of the brain-based nature of psychiatric disorders, the PMHNP role requires the ability to perform an in-depth neurological exam.
- Neurological exam
  - Reflexes (biceps, triceps, brachioradialis, patellar, Achilles, plantar)
  - Grade reflexes and note asymmetry between the right and left sides.
  - Check primitive reflexes in infants (head lag, flexion, rooting, grasping, Moro, glabellar, Babinski).
  - A positive Babinski sign (fanning of toes and dorsiflexion of the great toe) is normal in infants up to age 2 years.
- Cranial nerves (Mnemonic: On Old Olympus Towering Top A Finn And German Viewed Some Hops. Italicized below in parentheses)
  - Olfactory: I (On)
    - Test sense of smell and ensure patency of the nasal passages.
    - Have the client close their eyes and test each nostril separately while the other is occluded, asking the client to identify familiar odors.
  - Optic: II (Old)
    - Test vision using the Snellen chart or other suitable chart depending on the client's acuity and ability to cooperate.
    - Examine the inner aspect of the eyes with the ophthalmoscope.
    - Test peripheral vision using the confrontation test.
  - Oculomotor: III (Olympus)
    - This is the motor nerve to the five extrinsic eye muscles. Test together with cranial nerve IV (trochlear) and cranial nerve VI (abducens).

- Test the extraocular movements (EOMs).
- Check the equality of pupil size, reaction to light, and ability to accommodate.
- Test the corneal light reflex. (When a light is shined at the bridge of the nose, the light should appear symmetrically in both eyes).

◊ Trochlear: IV (Towering)

- Use the same process as for cranial nerve III (oculomotor) and cranial nerve VI (abducens).

◊ Trigeminal: V (motor division; Top)

- Palpate the masseter muscles with the fingertips while the client clenches their teeth.
    - Look for disparity in tension between the two muscles, which can indicate paralysis on the weak side.
- Look for tremor of the lips, involuntary chewing movements, and spasm of the masticatory muscles.

◊ Trigeminal: V (sensory division; Top)

- Test tactile perception of the facial skin by touching with a wisp of cotton.
- Test corneal reflex with a wisp of cotton.
- Test superficial pain of the skin and mucosa with pinpricks.
- Test the sense of touch in the oral mucosa.

◊ Abducens: VI (A)

- Use the same process as for cranial nerves III (oculomotor) and IV (trochlear).

◊ Facial: VII (motor division; Finn)

- Inspect the face in repose for evidence of flaccid paralysis.
- Test by asking the client to elevate eyebrows, wrinkle forehead, close eyes, frown, smile, and puff cheeks.

◊ Facial: VII (sensory division)

- Test taste for sugar, vinegar, and salt.

◊ Acoustic: VIII (And)

- Check hearing with the audiometer or by the whisper test.
- Check for hearing loss using the Weber and the Rinne tests.

◊ Glossopharyngeal: IX (German)

- Test together with cranial nerve X.

◊ Vagus: X (Viewed)

- Test for elevation of the uvula by having the client open their mouth and say "ah."

        - Test the gag reflex by tickling the back of the throat with a soft cotton tip applicator.
    - ◊ Accessory spinal: XI (Some)
        - Test the strength of the sternocleidomastoid and trapezius muscles against resistance of your hands.
    - ◊ Hypoglossal: XII (Hops)
        - Look for tremors and other involuntary movement when the client protrudes their tongue.
- ♦ Coordination and fine-motor skills include:
    - ◊ Equilibrium: Check by administering the Romberg test: have the client stand up straight with feet together, arms by their sides, and eyes closed. Only slight swaying would be normal, and the client will be able to sustain this pose for approximately 5 seconds. More than slight swaying suggests cerebellar ataxia or vestibular dysfunction.
    - ◊ Diadochokinesia: Ability to perform rapid alternating movements (such as patting knees alternating palm and back of hands, touching thumb to each finger); the client should be able to smoothly execute these movements and maintain the rhythm.
    - ◊ Dyssynergia: Finger-to-nose test, heel-to-knee test
    - ◊ Handwriting: Grasp, finger, hand, and wrist mobility, spacing, line use, letter formation
    - ◊ Gait: Observe client walking
- ♦ Sensory functions include:
    - ◊ Pain: Check sensation to pain with pinprick and compare on each side of body
    - ◊ Temperature: Check temperature if sensation to pain is abnormal.
    - ◊ Superficial touch: Test with a wisp of cotton.
    - ◊ Two-point discrimination: Apply pins to skin simultaneously; ask the client if they feel one or two pinpricks.
    - ◊ Stereognosis: Tests the ability to distinguish forms by placing objects in the client's hands while their eyes are closed
    - ◊ Graphesthesia: Tests the ability to identify figures, letters, or words by tracing the figure on the skin of the palm of the hand
- ♦ Motor functions include:
    - ◊ Muscle mass: Measure muscle mass to check for atrophy or hypertrophy.
    - ◊ Muscle tone: Tension is present when the muscle is resting.
    - ◊ Muscle strength: Check muscular strength against resistance. Be aware of abnormal muscle movements.

- Neurological soft signs include:
  - Dysdiadochokinesia: Inability to perform rapid alternating movements; result of a lesion to the posterior lobe of the cerebellum
  - Astereognosis: Inability to discriminate between objects based on touch alone; result of a lesion in the parietal lobe
  - Choreiform movements: Irregular, brief, repetitive, rapid involuntary movements starting in one part of the body and moving to another
  - Tics: Irregular, repetitive vocalizations or motor movements
  - Agraphesthesia: Inability to recognize letters or numbers "drawn" on the client's hand with a pointed object
  - Facial grimacing: Uncontrollable facial expressions of disgust, disapproval, or pain
  - Impaired fine-motor skills: Limitations in preforming coordinated movements of the fingers and hands
  - Abnormal blinking: Excessive or infrequent blinking of the eyes
  - Abnormal motor tone: Reduced or increased muscle tone
- Be alert for extrapyramidal symptoms (as in Parkinsonism, dystonia, akathisia) in the client taking antipsychotics.
  - Vital signs
  - Measure height, weight, blood pressure (in children age 2 or older), pulse, respirations, temperature, and head circumference (during the first 2 years).
  - Use growth charts for infants and children.
    - Greater than 85th percentile for body mass index (BMI) places a child at increased risk for being overweight.
  - Use BMI charts
    - Normal: 18.5 to 24.9
    - Overweight: 25.0 to 29.9
    - Obese: ≥30
  - High BMI is a risk factor for diabetes, heart disease, stroke, hypertension, osteoarthritis, and some forms of cancer.
- Be alert for high BMI if the client also is being prescribed psychotropic medications with a propensity for weight gain, especially atypical antipsychotics.
  - If a client is presenting with elevated temperature and also is taking psychotropic medications such as carbamazepine (Tegretol) or clozapine (Clozaril), be alert for agranulocytosis.
- Head, skin, nails
  - Note the color and integrity of the skin and whether lesions are present.
  - Note if the skin is well hydrated, dry, or scaly.

  - ◊ Assess skin turgor.
  - ◊ Palpate the skin's temperature.
  - ◊ Note any unusual moles or other lesions.
  - ◊ Look at hair texture and distribution.
  - ◊ Determine the quality of the nails, noting splitting, clubbing, or onychomycosis.
  - ◊ Check capillary refill.
  - ◊ Examine head, scalp, sutures, and fontanelles (if infant).
  - ◊ Check cranial nerve VII (facial nerve) for symmetry (have client smile, frown, wrinkle forehead, puff cheeks).
  - ◊ Be alert for Stevens-Johnson syndrome (life-threatening rash), especially if the client is taking carbamazepine or lamotrigine (Lamictal).
  - ◊ Cancerous moles can be detected by using the acronym ABCDE—asymmetry, border irregularity, color variation, diameter greater than 6 mm, and elevation.

- ♦ Eyes
  - ◊ Check visual acuity using the Snellen chart (tests cranial nerve II: optic nerve).
  - ◊ Test peripheral vision using the confrontation test (tests cranial nerve II: optic nerve).
  - ◊ Note the symmetry of eyes and the appearance of orbits, eyelids, and brows.
  - ◊ Inspect the sclera.
  - ◊ Assess corneal sensation with wisp of cotton (tests cranial nerves V and VII).
  - ◊ Assess papillary reaction to light and accommodation (tests cranial nerves III, IV, and VI).
  - ◊ Assess the six cardinal fields of gaze (extraocular movements; tests cranial nerves III, IV, and VI).
  - ◊ Assess corneal light reflex. Light reflections should appear symmetrically in both pupils (tests cranial nerves III, IV, and VI).
  - ◊ Examine the inner aspect of the eyes with the ophthalmoscope (tests cranial nerve II).
  - ◊ Be aware that many psychotropics can cause blurry vision (an anticholinergic side effect).
  - ◊ Quetiapine may cause cataracts.

- ♦ Ears
  - ◊ Check for configuration, position, and alignment of auricles.
  - ◊ Test auditory acuity (cranial nerve VIII) with the whisper test or audiometer.
  - ◊ Inspect external auditory canals with an otoscope for redness, swelling, or excess cerumen.

- ◊ Tympanic membrane should be translucent pearly gray without retractions or bulges.

- ♦ Nose and sinuses
  - ◊ Note the appearance of the external nose and whether it is smooth, intact, symmetric, midline, has discharge, or is flaring.
  - ◊ Assess nasal patency.
  - ◊ Assess sense of smell.
  - ◊ Inspect internal nasal cavity for patency and septal deviation.
  - ◊ Palpate maxillary and frontal sinuses.
- ♦ Neck
  - ◊ Palpate the lymph nodes (preauricular, postauricular, tonsillar, submandibular, submental, and anterior cervical) for swelling or masses.
  - ◊ Palpate thyroid (usually not palpable except in very thin people).
  - ◊ Palpate and auscultate carotid pulse and note any bruits.
- ♦ Back
  - ◊ Inspect skin and respiratory pattern on posterior chest.
  - ◊ Palpate cervical, thoracic, lumbar, and sacral spine.
  - ◊ Palpate thoracic expansion.
  - ◊ Percuss posterior chest for tympany.
  - ◊ Auscultate posterior chest for vesicular or bronchovesicular sounds and note any adventitious breath sounds.
- ♦ Thorax and lungs
  - ◊ Assess respiratory rate and depth, regularity, and ease of respiration.
  - ◊ Note anterior–posterior (AP) diameter, which should be less than the transverse diameter.
  - ◊ Percuss anterior chest for resonance and note the quality and symmetry of percussion notes.
  - ◊ Auscultate anterior chest for lung sounds; normal breath sounds include vesicular over peripheral lung, bronchovesicular over first and second intercostal spaces at the sternal border, and bronchial over the trachea.
- ♦ Breasts
  - ◊ Inspect breasts in different positions: with client arms relaxed and by side, with arms elevated above head, and with hands on hips. Look for dimpling, retractions, and orange-peel appearance.
  - ◊ Palpate breasts for lumps, including tail of Spence.

- Palpate axillary and epitrochlear lymph nodes.
- Palpate supraclavicular lymph nodes (also known as sentinel or Virchow nodes).
- Be aware that typical antipsychotics as well as atypical antipsychotics may cause galactorrhea.

- Heart
  - Inspect, palpate, and auscultate the carotid pulse.
  - Palpate peripheral pulses and check for symmetry (carotid, brachial, radial, femoral, popliteal, pedal, and posterior tibial).
  - Assess heart rate, rhythm, amplitude, and contour.
  - Assess anatomic location of the apical pulse.
  - Palpate precordium for pulsations, thrills, heaves, and lifts.
  - Auscultate heart sounds with bell and diaphragm and note characteristics of the first and second heart sounds.
  - Assess for jugular venous distention (JVD).
  - Be alert for possible electrocardiogram (ECG) changes if the client is taking tricyclic antidepressants or antipsychotics.
  - Be aware that lithium and anorexia nervosa can cause peripheral edema.
- Abdomen
  - Inspect the contour of the abdomen and check for scars, abdominal aortic pulsations, and the umbilical cord in the newborn.
  - Auscultate for bowel sounds and the abdominal aorta for bruits.
  - Percuss the abdomen and note areas of tympany and dullness. It is normal to hear tympany over the small and large intestines and dullness over organs and a distended bladder.
  - Percuss the size of the liver and spleen.
  - Palpate the abdomen for masses and tenderness. Also palpate the liver and spleen, which are not normally palpable (sometimes the liver can be palpable in thin clients).
- Musculoskeletal
  - Assess client's posture for alignment of extremities and spine and for symmetry of body parts.
  - Test muscle strength of upper and lower extremities.
  - Note symmetry of muscle mass, tone, and strength.
  - Assess active range of motion in the neck and upper and lower extremities, and note any presence of pain with movement.

- ◊ Palpate muscles and joints to elicit pain, deformities, crepitus, and passive range of motion.
- ◊ Check for hip dysplasia in infants.
- ◊ Check for scoliosis in children and adolescents.

- Common indicators of physical child abuse include:
    - ◊ History of unexplained multiple fractures
    - ◊ Burns, hand marks, or bite marks
    - ◊ Injuries at various stages of healing
    - ◊ Evidence of neglect
    - ◊ Bruising on padded parts of body

DIAGNOSTIC AND LABORATORY TESTING

- Assessment of diagnostic and laboratory testing is an essential element of the PMHNP role. It is important for the PMHNP to know when to order such tests, how to interpret the findings, and how to appropriately alter care based on the findings.
- Reasons to assess diagnostic and laboratory testing in psychiatry include:
    - ◊ To assist in the establishment of a diagnosis; as knowledge of underlying pathophysiology grows, diagnostic and laboratory testing use will grow as well
    - ◊ Used to rule out other disorders such as medical causes of psychiatric symptoms; helpful in differential diagnostic assessment
    - ◊ Used to determine whether a client's symptoms are better explained by a nonpsychiatric disorder or by factors such as substance use or misuse
    - ◊ For routine ongoing monitoring such as general health screening, monitoring drug levels of certain psychotropic medications, and assessment and monitoring for complications of psychiatric disorders or adverse effects of drugs

Thyroid Function Tests

- The function of the thyroid gland is to take iodine from the circulating blood, combine it with the amino acid tyrosine, and convert it to the thyroid hormones triiodothyronine (T3) and thyroxine (T4).
- The thyroid gland also stores T3 and T4 until they are released into the bloodstream under the influence of thyroid-stimulating hormone (TSH), which is released from the pituitary gland.

- Only a small amount of T3 and T4 are bound to protein.
- The free portion of the thyroid hormones is the true determinant of thyroid status.
- Free T4 (FT4; normal values 0.8 to 1.8 ng/dL; may vary by lab)
  - FT4 makes up a small portion of the total thyroxine, is available to the tissues, and is the metabolically active form of this hormone.
  - The FT4 test is commonly done to determine thyroid status, to rule out hypo- and hyperthyroidism, and to evaluate thyroid therapy.
  - Elevated FT4 indicates a decreased thyroid function (hypothyroidism), while low FT4 indicates increased thyroid function (hyperthyroidism).
    - Diseases that have increased FT4 levels include:
      - Graves' disease
      - Thyrotoxicosis due to T4
      - Acute thyroiditis
    - Diseases that have decreased FT4 levels include:
      - Hashimoto's thyroiditis
      - Primary hypothyroidism
      - Secondary hypothyroidism (pituitary insufficiency)
      - Tertiary hypothyroidism (hypothalamic failure)
      - Thyrotoxicosis due to high circulating levels of T3 and/or T4
      - Renal failure
      - Cushing's syndrome (normal to low FT4 levels)
      - Cirrhosis (slightly lower or normal FT4 levels)
    - Interfering factors
      - Values can be increased during treatment with heparin, aspirin, and propranolol.
      - Values can be decreased during treatment with furosemide (Lasix) or methadone.
- TSH (normal values 0.4 to 4.0 mIU/L; may vary by lab)
  - Stimulation of the thyroid gland by TSH causes release and distribution of stored thyroid hormones.
    - When T4 and T3 are high, TSH secretion decreases.
    - When T4 and T3 are low, TSH secretion increases.

        - In primary hypothyroidism, TSH levels rise because of low levels of thyroid hormone.
        - If the pituitary gland fails, TSH is not secreted and blood levels of TSH fall.
    - ◇ TSH testing is commonly performed to establish the diagnosis of primary hypothyroidism.
- ♦ Diseases that have increased TSH levels include:
    - ◇ Primary hypothyroidism
    - ◇ Thyroiditis
- ♦ Diseases that have decreased TSH levels include:
    - ◇ Hyperthyroidism
    - ◇ Secondary and tertiary hypothyroidism (low to normal TSH levels)
- ♦ Interfering factors
    - ◇ Values can be decreased during treatment with T3, acetylsalicylic acid, corticosteroids, and heparin.
    - ◇ Values can be increased during drug therapy with lithium.
- ♦ Systemic effects of hypothyroidism (decreased T4, increased TSH)
    - ◇ Mimics symptoms of unipolar mood disorders
        - Confusion
        - Decreased libido
        - Impotence
        - Decreased appetite
        - Memory loss
        - Lethargy
        - Constipation
        - Headaches
        - Slow or clumsy movements
        - Syncope
        - Weight gain
        - Fluid retention
        - Muscle aching and stiffness
        - Slowed reflexes
        - Somatic discomfort including joint aching and stiffness
        - Slowed speech and thinking
        - Sensory disturbances, including hearing

- Cerebellar ataxia
- Loss of amplitude on ECG

- Systemic effects of hyperthyroidism (increased T4, decreased TSH)
  - May mimic symptoms of bipolar affective disorders
    - Motor restlessness
    - Emotional lability
    - Short attention span
    - Compulsive movement
    - Fatigue
    - Tremor
    - Insomnia
    - Impotence
    - Weight loss
    - Increase in appetite
    - Abdominal pain
    - Excessive sweating
    - Flushing
    - Elevated upper eyelid leading to decreased blinking, staring, fine tremor of eyelid
    - Tachycardia
    - Dysrhythmias

Electrolytes

- Carried out as a part of routine screening in acute and critical illness or where there is a known or suspected disorder associated with fluid, electrolyte, or acid–base balance.
- Calcium (Ca; normal values 8.8–10.5 mg/dL)
  - Abnormal values
    - <7.0 mg/dL associated with tetany
    - >11.0 mg/dL associated with hyperparathyroidism
    - >13.5 mg/dL associated with hypercalcemic coma and metastatic cancer.
  - Most calcium (99%) is located in bone and the remainder is in the plasma and body cells.
  - Of the calcium in the plasma, 50% is bound to plasma proteins and 40% is in the free or ionized form. The remaining fraction circulates in the blood.
  - Calcium is the major cation for the structure of bones and teeth.

- ◊ Functions
  - Enzymatic cofactor for blood clotting
  - Required for hormone secretion
  - Required for function of cell receptors
  - Required for plasma membrane stability and permeability
  - Required for transmission of nerve impulses and the contraction of muscles
- ◊ Calcium balance is mediated by interactions among three hormones: parathyroid hormone, vitamin D, and calcitonin.
- ◊ Acting together, these substances determine the amount of dietary calcium absorbed and the renal reabsorption and excretion of calcium by the kidney.
- ◊ Increased levels of calcium can be associated with the following:
  - Acidosis
  - Hyperparathyroidism
  - Cancers (e.g., of bone, leukemia, myeloma)
  - Drugs (such as thiazide diuretics, hormones, vitamin D, Ca)
  - Vitamin D intoxication
  - Addison's disease
  - Hyperthyroidism
- ◊ Decreased levels of calcium can cause the following:
  - Alkalosis
  - Hypoparathyroidism
  - Renal failure
  - Pancreatitis
  - Inadequate dietary intake of calcium, vitamin D
  - Drugs, including barbiturates, anticonvulsants, acetazolamide, adrenocorticosteroids
- ◊ Interfering factors
  - Values are higher in children because of growth and active bone formation.
  - Values can be increased by excessive ingestion of milk or during treatment with lithium, thiazide diuretics, alkaline antacids, or vitamin D.
  - Values can be decreased during treatment with anticonvulsants, aspirin, calcitonin, corticosteroids, heparin, laxatives, diuretics, albuterol, or oral contraceptives.
- ◊ Systemic effects of hypocalcemia (Ca <8.5 mg/dL)
  - Increase in neuromuscular excitability
  - Confusion

        - Paresthesias around the mouth and in the digits
        - Muscle spasms in the hands and feet
        - Hyperreflexia
        - Convulsions
        - Tetany
        - Continuous severe muscle spasm
        - ECG changes: Prolonged QT interval
        - Intestinal cramping
        - Hyperactive bowel sounds
    - ◊ Systemic effects of hypercalcemia (Ca >12.0 mg/dL)
        - Fatigue
        - Weakness
        - Lethargy
        - Anorexia
        - Nausea
        - Constipation
- ♦ Sodium (Na; normal values 135–148 mEq/L)
    - ◊ Changes in sodium levels may result in the following:
        - Behavioral changes
        - Impaired renal function
        - ECG changes: shortened QT interval, depressed T waves
        - Bradycardia
        - Heart block
    - ◊ Sodium accounts for 90% of the extracellular fluid cations and is the most powerful cation in the extracellular fluid.
    - ◊ Sodium regulates osmolality (interstitial and intravascular fluid volume).
    - ◊ Sodium works with potassium and calcium to maintain neuromuscular irritability for conduction of nerve impulses.
    - ◊ Sodium regulates acid–base balance.
    - ◊ Sodium participates in cellular chemical reactions and membrane transport.
    - ◊ Sodium regulates renal retention and excretion of water.
    - ◊ Sodium maintains systemic blood pressure.
    - ◊ Increased levels of sodium are associated with the following:
        - Dehydration
        - Diabetes insipidus

        - Excessive salt ingestion
        - Gastroenteritis
    - Decreased levels of sodium are associated with the following:
        - Addison's disease
        - Renal disorder
        - Gastrointestinal (GI) fluid loss from vomiting, diarrhea, nasogastric suction, ileus
        - Diuresis
    - Systemic effects of hyponatremia (Na <135 mEq/L)
        - Lethargy
        - Headache
        - Confusion
        - Apprehension
        - Seizures
        - Coma
        - Hypotension
        - Tachycardia
        - Decreased urine output
        - Weight gain
        - Edema
        - Ascites
        - Jugular vein distention
    - Systemic effects of hypernatremia (Na >147 mEq/L)
        - Convulsions
        - Pulmonary edema
        - Thirst
        - Fever
        - Dry mucous membranes
- Magnesium (Mg; normal values 1.3–2.1 mEq/L)
    - Changes in magnesium levels may result in the following:
        - Hypotension
        - Tachycardia
        - Low jugular venous pressure
        - Restlessness

- ◊ Magnesium is a major intracellular cation; 40% to 60% is stored in bone and muscle, with 30% in cells.
- ◊ A small amount is in the serum, where one-third is bound to plasma proteins and the rest is in ionized form.
- ◊ Regulation of Mg metabolism is primarily by the kidney.
- ◊ Low serum levels cause renal conservation of Mg.
- ◊ Magnesium is a cofactor in intracellular enzymatic reactions.
- ◊ Magnesium is a cause of neuromuscular excitability.
- ◊ Increased levels of magnesium are associated with the following:
    - Addison's disease
    - Dehydration
    - Adrenalectomy
    - Hypothyroidism
    - Renal failure
    - Hyperthyroidism
    - Diabetic ketoacidosis
- ◊ Decreased levels of magnesium are associated with the following:
    - Hyperaldosteronism
    - GI loss from vomiting
    - Hypokalemia
    - Diabetic ketoacidosis
    - Malnutrition
    - Excessive alcohol use
    - Acute pancreatitis
- ◊ Interfering factors
    - Diarrhea, nasogastric suction, and fistula
    - Malabsorption syndrome
    - Pregnancy-induced hypertension
    - Hemolysis of a sample leads to falsely elevated levels.
    - Numerous drugs can alter levels.
    - Values can be increased by drugs such as antacids and laxatives containing Mg, salicylates, and lithium.
    - Values can be decreased by drugs such as thiazide diuretics, calcium gluconate, insulin, amphotericin B, neomycin, aldosterone, and ethanol.

- Systemic effects of hypomagnesemia (Mg <1.5 mEq/L)
    - Depression
    - Confusion
    - Irritability
    - Increased reflexes
    - Muscle weakness
    - Ataxia
    - Nystagmus
    - Tetany
    - Convulsions
- Systemic effects of hypermagnesemia (Mg >2.5 mEq/L)
    - Nausea and vomiting
    - Muscle weakness
    - Hypotension
    - Bradycardia

- Chloride (normal values 98–106 mEq/L)
    - Changes in chloride levels may result in the following:
        - Respiratory depression
        - Depressed skeletal muscle contraction and nerve function
    - Chloride is the major anion in the extracellular fluid.
    - It provides electroneutrality in relation to sodium.
        - Transport of chloride is passive and follows the active transport of sodium so that increases or decreases in chloride are proportional to changes in sodium.
    - Increased levels of chloride are associated with the following:
        - Acidosis
        - Hyperkalemia, hypernatremia
        - Dehydration
    - Decreased levels of chloride are associated with the following:
        - Alkalosis
        - Hypokalemia
        - Hyponatremia
        - GI loss from vomiting, diarrhea, nasogastric suction, and fistula

- Interfering factors
  - Renal failure
  - Cushing's syndrome
  - Hyperventilation
  - Anemia
  - Diuresis
  - Overhydration
  - Addison's disease
  - Burns
  - Elevated serum triglyceride levels and myeloma proteins may lead to falsely decreased levels.
  - Values can be increased by potassium chloride, acetazolamide, methyldopa, diazoxide, and guanethidine.
  - Values can be decreased by ethacrynic acid, furosemide, thiazide diuretics, and bicarbonate.
  - No specific symptoms are associated with chloride increase or decrease.

- Potassium (K+; normal values 3.5–5.1 mEq/L)
  - Potassium is the major intracellular electrolyte.
  - Total body potassium is about 4,000 mEq, with most of it located in the cells.
  - Intracellular concentration of potassium is 150 to 160 mEq/L; extracellular concentration is 3.5 to 4.5 mEq/L.
  - As the predominant intracellular ion, potassium regulates intracellular fluid osmolality and provides the balance for intracellular electrical neutrality.
  - Potassium is required for glycogen deposition in liver and skeletal muscle cells.
  - Potassium maintains resting membrane potential and assists in transmission and conduction of nerve impulses for the contraction of cardiac, skeletal, and smooth muscle contraction.
  - Potassium balance is regulated by the kidney, aldosterone levels, insulin secretion, and changes in pH.
  - Increased levels of potassium are associated with the following:
    - Acidosis
    - Insulin deficiency
    - Addison's disease
    - Acute renal failure
    - Hypoaldosteronism

- Infection
- Dehydration

◊ Decreased levels of potassium are associated with the following:

- Alkalosis
- Excessive insulin
- GI loss
- Laxative abuse
- Burns
- Trauma

◊ Interfering factors

- Surgery
- Cushing's syndrome
- Hyperaldosteronism
- Thyrotoxicosis
- Anorexia nervosa
- Diet deficient in meat and vegetables
- False elevations can occur with vigorous pumping of the hand during venipuncture, hemolysis of the sample, or high platelet counts during clotting.
- False decreases are seen in anticoagulated samples left at room temperature.
- Values can be decreased by drugs such as furosemide, ethacrynic acid, thiazide diuretics, insulin, aspirin, prednisone, cortisone, gentamycin, lithium, and laxatives.
- Values can be increased by drugs such as amphotericin B, tetracycline, heparin, epinephrine, potassium-sparing diuretics, and isoniazid.
- Chronic marijuana use can elevate potassium level.

◊ Systemic effects of hyperkalemia (potassium >5.5 mEq/L)

- Muscle weakness
- Paralysis
- Tingling of lips and fingers
- Restlessness
- Intestinal cramping
- Diarrhea
- ECG changes: Narrow and taller T waves
- Mild hyperkalemia: Shortened QT interval

        - Severe hyperkalemia: Depressed ST segment, prolonged PR interval, and widened QRS complex leading to cardiac arrest
    - ◊ Systemic effects of hypokalemia (potassium <3.5 mEq/L)
        - Impaired carbohydrate metabolism
        - Impaired renal function
        - Polyuria
        - Polydipsia
        - Skeletal muscle weakness
        - Smooth muscle atony
        - Cardiac dysrhythmias
        - Paralysis and respiratory arrest
        - Liver function tests
    - ◊ Used to monitor liver disease or damage caused by hepatotoxic drugs, as confirmed by elevated levels
- ♦ Alanine aminotransferase (ALT; normal values 5–35 U/L)
    - ◊ Formerly known as serum glutamic-pyruvic transaminase (SGPT), ALT is an enzyme produced by the liver that acts as a catalyst in the transamination reaction necessary for amino acid production.
    - ◊ ALT is found in liver cells in high concentrations and in moderate amounts in body fluid, heart, kidney, and skeletal muscle.
    - ◊ When liver damage occurs, serum levels of ALT rise to as much as 50 times normal.
    - ◊ Pronounced elevated levels (>300 U/L)
        - Liver disease or damage, such as hepatic cancer, hepatitis, or infectious mononucleosis
    - ◊ Moderately elevated levels (100–300 U/L)
        - Biliary tract obstruction
        - Recent cerebrovascular accident
        - Muscle injury from intramuscular injections, trauma, infection, and seizures
        - Muscular dystrophy
        - Acute pancreatitis
        - Intestinal injury
        - Myocardial infarction
        - Congestive heart failure

- Renal failure
- Severe burns

◇ Interfering factors

- Uremia and hemodialysis can cause falsely decreased levels.
- Values can be increased with acetaminophen, allopurinol, aspirin, ampicillin, carbamazepine, cephalosporins, codeine, digitalis, indomethacin, heparin, isoniazid, methotrexate, methyldopa, oral contraceptives, phenothiazines, propranolol, tetracycline, and verapamil.

◆ Aspartate aminotransferase (AST; normal values 5–40 U/L)

◇ Previously known as serum glutamate oxaloacetate transaminase (SGOT), AST is the enzyme that catalyzes the reversible transfer of an amino group between the amino acid, aspartate, and α-ketoglutaric acid.

◇ AST exists in large amounts in both liver and myocardial cells and in smaller but significant amounts in skeletal muscle, kidney, pancreas, and brain.

◇ Serum AST level increases when there is cellular damage to the tissues in which the enzyme is found.

◇ Pronounced elevation (>5 times normal)

- Acute hepatocellular damage
- Myocardial infarction
- Shock
- Acute pancreatitis
- Infectious mononucleosis

◇ Moderate elevation (3–5 times normal)

- Biliary tract obstruction
- Cardiac arrhythmias
- Congestive heart failure

◇ Slight elevation (2–3 times normal)

- Pericarditis
- Cirrhosis, fatty liver
- Pulmonary infarction
- Delirium tremens
- Cerebrovascular accident
- Hemolytic anemia

- ◊ Interfering factors
    - Liver tumors
    - Chronic hepatitis
    - Muscular dystrophy
    - Dermatomyositis
- ◊ Numerous drugs may elevate levels, including antihypertensives, cholinergic agents, anticoagulants, digitalis, erythromycin, isoniazid, methyldopa, oral contraceptives, opiates, salicylates, hepatotoxic medications, and verapamil.
- ◊ Exercise can cause increased levels.

- ♦ Gamma-glutamyl transpeptidase (GGT; normal values 10–38 IU/L)
    - ◊ GGT is an isoenzyme of alkaline phosphatase and assists with the transfer of amino acids and peptides across cellular membranes.
    - ◊ Hepatobiliary tissues and renal tubular and pancreatic epithelium contain large amounts of GGT.
    - ◊ Other sources of GGT include the prostate gland, brain, and heart.
    - ◊ GGT is used to evaluate and monitor a client with known or suspected excessive alcohol use because levels increase even after ingestion of small amounts of alcohol.
        - Also used to evaluate elevated alkaline phosphatase of uncertain etiology.
        - Pronounced, early increases in GGT are found in in hepatic disease.
        - Modest elevation in GGT occurs in cirrhosis and in pancreatic or renal disease.
    - ◊ Elevated GGT
        - Hepatobiliary tract disorders
        - Hepatocellular carcinoma
        - Hepatocellular degeneration such as cirrhosis
        - Hepatitis
        - Pancreatic or renal cell damage or neoplasm
        - Congestive heart failure
        - Acute myocardial infarction (after 4–10 days)
        - Hyperlipoproteinemia
        - Diabetes mellitus with hypertension
        - Seizure disorder
        - Significant alcohol ingestion
    - ◊ Interfering factors
        - Alcohol, barbiturates, and phenytoin can elevate GGT levels.
        - Late pregnancy, oral contraceptives, and clofibrate can lower GGT levels.

DISEASE PREVENTION ACTIVITIES

IMMUNIZATION

Immunizations are critical to preventing disease according to the Centers for Disease Control and Prevention (CDC). Immunizations protect individual children and adults from developing potentially serious diseases while also protecting the community by reducing the spread of infectious diseases.

- Schedules for children and adults are available on the CDC website at www.cdc.gov/vaccines/
- Seasonal influenza vaccination (as live attenuated influenza vaccine [LAIV] or as inactivated type)
- All persons 6 months of age or older should receive annual influenza vaccination.
  - Children 6 months to 8 years of age require two doses of influenza vaccine (4 weeks apart) during their first season of vaccinations.
  - LAIV should not be used in persons younger than 2 years of age or older than 49 years of age.
  - Persons with egg allergy should always receive the vaccination from a health care provider familiar with the potential reaction and should be observed for at least 30 minutes post injection for signs of reaction.
  - Immunocompromised persons should not receive live vaccination.
  - Use live vaccine or inactivated vaccine for healthy nonpregnant adults younger than 50 years of age with no high-risk medical conditions. All others should receive the inactivated vaccine only (Grohskopf et al., 2022).
- Coronavirus disease 2019 (COVID-19) www.cdc.gov/coronavirus/2019-ncov/vaccines/different-vaccines/overview-COVID-19-vaccines.html
  - Based on age, last dose administered, and level of immunocompromised
  - Safe for individuals 6 months or older
  - Yearly booster recommended after initial series is complete
  - Updated or bivalent vaccines protect against the original virus and variants that have been identified
  - COVID-19 vaccine is contraindicated for individuals who experienced a severe reaction to ingredients in the vaccine or have a known allergy to an ingredient in the vaccine.
- Human papillomavirus (HPV) vaccination for girls is recommended at age 11 or 12 years with catch-up vaccination at ages 13 through 26 years to prevent genital HPV infection, which can cause genital warts and cervical cancer.

- ◊ HPV4 may be administered to male clients from age 9 through 26 years to prevent genital warts.

- ♦ Measles, mumps, rubella (MMR; live vaccine)
  - ◊ Recommended first dose at 12 to 15 months of age, second dose at 4 to 6 years of age
  - ◊ Not for pregnant women; people with cancer, weakened immune systems, or HIV or AIDS with T-cell counts below 200; or people currently being treated with high-dose steroids or who have received a blood transfusion within the previous 2 weeks
- ♦ Diphtheria, tetanus, acellular pertussis
  - ◊ Td (tetanus, diphtheria) vaccine should be given every 10 years beginning at age 11 years, with Tdap (tetanus, diphtheria, acellular pertussis) substituted once for Td but no less than 5 years after the last DTaP dose was given. DTaP should not be given to anyone 7 years of age or older.
- ♦ Shingles (Shingrix; also known as herpes zoster) vaccine www.cdc.gov/vaccines/vpd/shingles/public/shingrix
  - ◊ Recommended two doses for individuals age 50 years or older and adults 19 years or older who have a weakened immune system
  - ◊ Shingrix is contraindicated for individuals who
    - Experienced a severe allergic reaction to any component of the vaccine or after a dose of Shingrix;
    - Currently have shingles; or
    - Are currently pregnant.
  - ◊ Shingles is a viral inflammatory condition (caused by herpes zoster virus) with painful vesicular eruptions along the distribution of the nerves from one or more dorsal root ganglia.
- ♦ Varicella (chickenpox) vaccine www.cdc.gov/vaccines/vpd/varicella/hcp/recommendations.html
  - ◊ This vaccine is contraindicated for individuals who
    - Have a history of anaphylactic/anaphylactoid reaction to gelatin, neomycin, or any component of the vaccine;
    - Have blood dyscrasia, leukemia, lymphomas, malignant neoplasms affecting bone marrow or lymphatic system;
    - Have primary or acquired immunodeficiency;
    - Are receiving prolonged, high-dose, systemic immunosuppressive therapy;
    - Have moderate or severe concurrent illness;

- Have a family history of congenital hereditary immunodeficiency (first-degree relative) unless determined to be immunocompetent; or
- Are or may be pregnant.

ANTICIPATORY GUIDANCE

Anticipatory guidance is a framework for implementation of prevention strategies.

- ♦ Based on the premise that information can be provided to people to help them cope more effectively with events that occur through the life span. Within the framework of anticipatory guidance, the practitioner seeks to determine the specific informational needs of the client in a systematic, standard way.
- ♦ Pediatrics considerations: This includes soliciting information from guardians about their concerns in parenting and providing information specific to their concerns as well as teaching guardians about health hazards and strategies to prevent harm, such as car seat safety, water safety, wearing helmets, and so forth.
- ♦ Bright Futures (www.aap.org/en/practice-management/bright-futures) is a national health promotion initiative (launched by the Health Resources and Services Administration in partnership with other agencies) dedicated to the principle that every child deserves to be healthy and that optimal health involves trusting relationships among the health professional, the child, the family, and the community as partners in health practice. Expansion of the model includes screening, care management, and education about mental health problems and disorders in a developmental context.
- ♦ In specific health care situations, anticipatory guidance can be used to assist people in meeting health care challenges across the life span. Some examples include:
    - ◊ Coping with terminal illness or death and dying (anticipatory grief)
    - ◊ Coping with disease progression, such as with Alzheimer's dementia, in a loved one
    - ◊ Coping with change and limitations resulting from spinal cord injuries
    - ◊ Can be implemented in each "well check" to identify information needs pertinent to the client's current life situation. Some examples:
        - Responsible alcohol use for the adolescent going off to college
        - Domestic violence
        - Life after the loss of a loved one (through divorce or death)
        - Planning for retirement

GENDER-BASED MEDICAL TESTING AND SCREENING RECOMMENDATIONS FOR THE GENERAL PUBLIC

TANNER STAGES ASSESSMENT (BICKLEY, 2021)

Defines physical measurements of development in children, adolescents, and adults. The development of primary and secondary sex characteristics (breasts, genitalia, and pubic hair) is assessed by stages to describe the onset and progression of puberty in both male and female clients. Because of natural variability, individuals pass through the stages at different rates based on puberty.

GIRLS: BREAST DEVELOPMENT

Stage 1: Prepubertal

Stage 2: Breast bud stage with elevation of breast and papilla; enlargement of areola

Stage 3: Further enlargement of breast and areola; no separation of their contour

Stage 4: Areola and papilla form a secondary mound above the level of breast

Stage 5: Projection of papilla only, related to recession of areola

BOYS: DEVELOPMENT OF EXTERNAL GENITALIA

Stage 1: Prepubertal

Stage 2: Enlargement of scrotum and testes; scrotum skin reddens and changes in texture

Stage 3: Enlargement of penis (length at first); further growth of testes

Stage 4: Increase in size of penis with growth in breadth and development of glans; testes and scrotum larger, scrotum skin darker

Stage 5: Adult genitalia

BOYS AND GIRLS: PUBIC HAIR

Stage 1: Prepubertal (can see vellus hair similar to that on the abdomen)

Stage 2: Sparse growth of long, slightly pigmented hair, straight or curled, at base of penis or along labia

Stage 3: Darker, coarser, and curlier hair, spreading sparsely over junctions of pubes

Stage 4: Adult-type hair, but covering smaller area than in adult, no spread to medial surface of thighs

Stage 5: Adult type and quantity, with horizontal distribution

WOMEN

Ages 18–39

- Monthly: Skin and oral self-exams
- Yearly: Blood pressure; blood tests and urinalysis; physical exam; Pap smear (beginning at age 21 or within 3 years of sexual activity, whichever comes first), pelvic exam, sexually transmitted infection (STI) detection
- All persons ages 13 to 64 should be tested at least once for HIV (CDC, 2021)

Ages 40–49

- Monthly: Skin and oral self-exams
- Yearly: Blood pressure; blood tests and urinalysis; physical exam; Pap smear (every 2 or 3 years after three consecutive negative smears), pelvic exam, STI detection; ECG every 4 years

Ages 50+

- Monthly: Skin and oral self-exams
- Yearly: Blood pressure; blood tests (complete blood count, metabolic panel, TSH) and urinalysis; physical exam; Pap smear (65 or older not recommended if person had a recent normal Pap smear and is not at high risk for cervical cancer), pelvic exam, STI detection; mammography every 2 years; routine bone density screening starting at age 65 or older (beginning at 60 if increased risk for osteoporotic fractures)
- Every 4 years: ECG
- Every 5 years through age 75: flexible sigmoidoscopy or double-contrast barium enema or computed tomography (CT) colonography (if any of these tests are positive, a colonoscopy should be done), or colonoscopy every 10 years
- Consult provider: Hearing, vision

Additional Colorectal Cancer Screening for High-Risk Women

The American Cancer Society recommends that some people be screened using a different schedule because of their personal or family history.

MEN

Ages 18–39

- Monthly: Self-exams (testicles, skin, and oral)
- Yearly: Blood pressure; blood tests (complete blood count, metabolic panel, thyroid stimulating hormone) and urinalysis; physical exam
- Screening at least once a year for syphilis, chlamydia, and gonorrhea for all sexually active gay, bisexual, and men who have sex with men. Those with multiple or anonymous partners should be tested more frequently (CDC, 2021)
- All persons ages 13 to 64 should be tested at least once for HIV (CDC, 2021)

Ages 40–49

- Monthly: Testicles, skin, and oral self-exams
- Yearly: Blood pressure; blood tests (complete blood count, metabolic panel, TSH) and urinalysis; physical exam; ECG every 4 years

Ages 50+

- Monthly: Testicles, skin, and oral self-exams
- Yearly: Blood pressure; blood tests (complete blood count, metabolic panel, thyroid stimulating hormone) and urinalysis; physical exam; ECG every 3 years
- Every 5 years through age 75: Flexible sigmoidoscopy or double-contrast barium enema or CT colonography (if any of these tests are positive, a colonoscopy should be done), or colonoscopy every 10 years
- Consult provider: Testosterone blood test; hearing and vision screening

HEALTH BEHAVIOR GUIDELINES

EXERCISE

Exercise benefits both physical and mental health. Inactivity has a direct link to obesity, a major health problem in this country. In results of recent studies, exercise has demonstrated effects comparable to antidepressant therapy in the treatment of depression.

- Key factor in staying healthy: Strengthens bones, heart, and lungs; tones muscles; improves vitality; relieves depression; and helps to improve sleep. It is particularly beneficial to persons with comorbid medical conditions such as diabetes, obesity, and hypertension.
- Mind–body connection: Improves cognition and enhances mood
- Neurobiological explanation: Promotes increased concentrations of serotonin, norepinephrine, and endorphins
- Integrative psychiatry includes strategies to improve lifestyle practices (diet, exercise, smoking cessation, decrease or cease substance use, and reduce stress to prevent illness.
- Client teaching regarding exercise
    - Check with a provider before starting an exercise program.
    - Begin exercising gradually. Do not expect results overnight. If you are consistent, you will see improvement within 3 months.
    - Work hard enough to sweat, but not so hard that you cannot carry on a conversation.
    - Plan an exercise routine that lasts at least 30 minutes and perform the workout at least 3 to 5 days a week. Warming up before exercise helps avoid injury.
    - Include both aerobic and strengthening activities in the exercise program.
    - Exercise programs need to be modified for children, pregnant women, the elderly, clients who are obese or disabled, and heart attack survivors as well as modified for high altitudes and extreme hot or cold conditions.
    - Monitor the intensity of exercise by measuring heart rate. The target heart rate during physical activity should be 60% to 90% of the maximum heart rate. Use the following formula to calculate target heart rate:
        - 220 (beats per minute) minus age = maximum heart rate
        - Maximum heart rate multiplied by the intensity level = target heart rate
        - Physical activity at 60% to 70% of the maximum heart rate is considered moderate-intensity exercise.

  - ◊ CDC recommends 60 minutes (1 hour) or more of physical activity each day for children and adolescents.
  - ◊ CDC recommends 150 minutes of moderate-intensity aerobic activity (such as brisk walking) every week and muscle-strengthening activities 2 or more days a week for adults, including for healthy older adults (CDC, 2022).

SELF-AWARENESS

- Requires reflection on one's personal beliefs, thoughts, emotions, motives, biases, and limitations and being aware of how they influence behavior toward others
- A trusted person who can give open, honest feedback to self-examination is helpful.
- Personal experiences influence communication patterns and responses to clients.
- Social biases, feelings, and beliefs projected onto the client may affect the nurse–client relationship.
- Being nonjudgmental and objective cultivates trust in the relationship.
- Clinical supervision by colleague provides ongoing feedback for therapeutic development of the helper, including supporting change as needed.
- If personal values and beliefs make it difficult to be therapeutic with a particular client, refer the client to another provider.

SELF-DISCLOSURE

- Revealing personal information to the client changes the focus away from the client.
- When personal questions are asked, self-disclosure can be limited by redirecting, giving a vague answer, or reminding the client that you will not share your personal information.
- Self-disclosure may be therapeutic only when it is purposeful and has an identified therapeutic outcome, such as role modeling.

HEALTH PROMOTION AND DISEASE PREVENTION EDUCATION

- Preventative care and screening practices are essential aspects of the PMHNP role.
- Screening for physical health problems in the psychiatric client

- Guided by Healthy People 2030 (U.S. Department of Health and Human Services [HHS], 2023), which identifies national health objectives, including behavioral health. Overarching goals are to "eliminate health disparities, achieve health equity, and attain health literacy to improve the health and well-being of all."
- Objectives include:
  - Increase the proportion of mental health treatment to children, people with substance use, and unhoused adults with mental health disorders
  - Increase preventative mental health care in school
  - Reduce adolescent attempts to end their own life
  - Reduce the proportion of adolescents who use marijuana

PUBLIC HEALTH PRINCIPLES

- Primary prevention: Aimed at decreasing the incidence (number of new cases) of mental disorders
  - Helping people avoid stressors or cope with them more adaptively
  - Example: Stress management classes for graduate students, smoking prevention classes, Drug Abuse Resistance Education (DARE) Keepin' It REAL elementary and middle school curriculum (DARE, 2023)
- Secondary prevention: Aimed at decreasing the prevalence (number of existing cases) of mental disorders
  - Early case finding
  - Screening
  - Prompt and effective treatment
  - Example: Telephone hotlines, crisis intervention, disaster responses
- Tertiary prevention: Aimed at decreasing the disability and severity of a mental disorder
  - Rehabilitative services
  - Avoidance or postponement of complications
  - Example: Day treatment programs; case management for physical, housing, or vocational needs; social skills training

RISK FACTORS

- Predisposing characteristics that make it more likely that a person will develop a disorder
- Biological risk factors: History of mental illness in family, poor nutritional status, poor general health
- Psychological risk factors: Poor self-concept, external locus of control, poor ego defenses
- Social risk factors: Stressful occupation, low socioeconomic status, poor level of social integration

PREVENTATIVE FACTORS

- Factors that prevent or protect the person from the disorder
- Coping mechanisms or resources that facilitate a healthy response to stress
- Biological preventative factors: No history of mental illness in the family, healthy nutritional status, good general health
- Psychological preventative factors: Good self-esteem or self-concept, internal locus of control, healthy ego defenses
- Social preventative factors: Low-stress occupation, higher socioeconomic status, higher level of education

CASE STUDY 1

M.J. is 79 years old, married, and being treated by the PMHNP for symptoms of major depression. M.J. was started on citalopram, 10 mg, 4 weeks ago and has been taking 20 mg, p.o. q.a.m., for the past 3 weeks.

Pertinent medical history includes hypertension, which is well controlled by benazepril and hydrochlorothiazide. M.J. also takes finasteride for benign prostatic hyperplasia.

1. How should the PMHNP think about what may be going on with M.J.?
2. How should the PMHNP intervene?

M.J. and spouse arrive at the follow-up appointment and M.J. reports that the primary care provider checked his sodium level, which was low, and that he was instructed to stop the citalopram. M.J. is not on any antidepressant treatment and reports that he has been feeling progressively more tired, stomach has been upset, and he feels "a little foggy." These symptoms began "about a week ago."

3. How would this presentation change the PMHNP's treatment plan?
4. What is the appropriate intervention for this client?

CASE STUDY 2

S.J., a 27-year-old retail store employee, has been referred by the primary care provider (PCP) to the PMHNP for evaluation and treatment of a chief complaint of "mood swings." The client tells the PMHNP, "I have been feeling pretty good" for the past week after coming through a 3-week period of feeling down, having no motivation, sad, and crying most days. The PCP discontinued fluoxetine, 20 mg, several days ago.

The client is endorsing symptoms of mild euphoria and irritability; speech is pressured, is hyperverbal, but is easily redirected. S.J. reports sleeping "about 4 to 5 hours a night," and describes the energy as "pretty good!" There is no evidence of psychosis. Insight and judgment are intact, and S.J. states, "I think I'm a little high. I'm worried it's going to get me in trouble at work."

Past psychiatric history is significant for depressive episodes beginning in early teens, during which suicidal ideation was experienced. The client has been treated with several selective serotonin reuptake inhibitors (SSRIs) over the years, all prescribed by her primary care provider and in each case, noticed rapid improvement of mood and then discontinued the drug after several months. She denies a history of hypomania until the past year.

Medical history is noncontributory.

Family history is significant for bipolar I disorder in dad and possibly paternal grandmother. Mother has a long history of untreated "depression and anxiety."

The PMHNP and S.J. discuss treatment options and decide to start lithium carbonate.

1. What client teaching should be included in preparation for beginning lithium?
2. What tests should be ordered before beginning this drug?
3. What additional test should be ordered before treating S.J. with lithium?

Three months after beginning lithium, S.J. presents with lethargy, constipation, and bradycardia.

4. What should the PMHNP consider as etiology?
5. What labs tests should be ordered?
6. What adjustment should be made to the client's medication?

ANSWERS TO CASE STUDY DISCUSSION QUESTIONS

CASE STUDY 1

1. All SSRIs and some other antidepressants have been implicated in hyponatremia. Owing to diminished renal functioning and frequent polypharmacy, hyponatremia is more common in the elderly. In addition to citalopram, the client is taking hydrochlorothiazide, which may also cause hyponatremia.
2. The signs and symptoms of hyponatremia vary, depending on how quickly sodium levels drop. Slow decrease in sodium may lead to a subtle presentation such as feeling tired, and slightly "foggy." Clients experiencing a more precipitous drop will present with dramatic changes in level of consciousness and severe headache owing to cerebral edema. The PMHNP should assess for signs and symptoms of hyponatremia and order a sodium level.
3. An assessment should be made if the client has had trials on another SSRI. Assessment of depression symptoms needs to be completed and use of a depression scale, such as the Patient Health Questionnaire-9 (PHQ-9) or Geriatric Depression Scale (GDS) are indicated.
4. If the client has not had another trial on a SSRI, an additional SSRI would be indicated and the PMHNP would follow up on the client's response to the medication.

CASE STUDY 2

1. The client should be taught about the potential risks and benefits of taking lithium. Women of childbearing age should be educated about the risk of birth defects, including Ebstein's anomaly. Consideration of lithium dose and maintenance of blood levels should be included in discussing the relative risk. The signs and symptoms of lithium toxicity must be part of client education.
2. Baseline labs consisting of a metabolic panel, TSH, and complete blood count (CBC) should be done. Women of childbearing age should have a pregnancy test prior to starting lithium.
3. Clients age 65 years of age or older or who have a history of heart disease should have a baseline ECG.
4. Lethargy and constipation may be due to hypothyroidism or hypercalcemia, both of which may be caused by lithium.
5. The client should have TSH, free T4, and electrolytes tested.
6. The lithium should be tapered off and an alternative medication used for mood stabilization.

REFERENCES AND RESOURCES

American Nurses Association, American Psychiatric Nurses Association, & International Society of Psychiatric-Mental Health Nurses. (2022). Psychiatric-mental health nursing: Scope and standards of practice (3rd ed.). American Nurses Association.

American Psychiatric Association. (2010). Practice guidelines for the treatment of patients with major depressive disorder. https://psychiatryonline.org/pb/assets/raw/sitewide/practice_guidelines/guidelines/mdd.pdf

American Psychiatric Association. (2016). Practice guideline for psychiatric evaluation of adults (3rd ed.) https://doi.org/10.1176/appi.books.9780890426760

American Psychiatric Association. (2022). Diagnostic and statistical manual of mental disorders (5th ed., Text rev.).

American Psychiatric Association. (2023). Practice guideline for the treatment of patients with eating disorders (4th ed.). https://doi.org/10.1176/appi.books.9780890424865

Anandarajah, G., & Hight, E. (2001). Spirituality and medical practice: Using the hope questions as a practical tool for spiritual assessment. American Family Physician, 63(1), 81–88.

Bakerman, S. (2002). ABCs of interpretive laboratory data (4th ed.). Interpretive Laboratory Data.

Bickley, L. S. (2023). Bates' guide to physical examination and history taking (13th ed.). LWW.

Centers for Disease Control and Prevention. (2021). STD & HIV screening recommendations. http://www.cdc.gov/std/prevention/screeningreccs.htm

Centers for Disease Control and Prevention. (2022). Physical activity. https://www.cdc.gov/physicalactivity/basics/adults/

Centers for Disease Control and Prevention. (2023). Shingles vaccination. https://www.cdc.gov/vaccines/vpd/shingles/public/shingrix/

Clinical Evidence Organization. (2000). Clinical evidence international sourcebook. BMJ Publishing Group.

DARE. (2023). D.A.R.E.'s Keepin' it REAL elementary and middle school curriculums adhere to lessons from prevention research principles. https://dare.org/

Davidson, J. R. (2000). Trauma: The impact of post-traumatic stress disorder. Journal of Psychopharmacology, 14(Suppl. 1), S5–S12.

Faulkner, G. (2000). Behavioral outcomes and guidelines sourcebook. Faulkner & Gray.

Grohskopf, L. A., Blanton, L. H., Ferdinands, J. M., Chung, J. R., Broder, K. R., Talbot, H. K., Morgan, R. L., Fry, A. M. (2022). Prevention and control of influenza with vaccines: Recommendations of the advisory committee on immunization practices, United States,

2022–23 influenza season. MMWR Recommendations and Reports, 71(No. RR-1), 1–28. http://dx.doi.org/10.15585/mmwr.rr7101a1

Jarvis, C. (2011). Physical health examination and health assessment (6th ed.). Elsevier.

Margolin, G., & Gordis, E. B. (2000). The effects of family and community violence on children. Annual Review of Psychology, 51, 445–479.

National Institutes of Health. (2021). Cultural respect. https://www.nih.gov/institutes-nih/nih-office-director/office-communications-public-liaison/clear-communication/cultural-respect

O'Reilly, D. J. (2000). Thyroid function tests: Time for reassessment. British Medical Journal, 320, 1332–1334.

Sadock, B., Sadock, V., & Ruiz, P. (2017). Kaplan and Sadock's comprehensive textbook of psychiatry (10th ed.). Wolters Kluwer.

Schatsburg, A., Cole, J., & DeBattista, C. (2007). Manual of clinical psychopharmacology (6th ed.). American Psychiatric Association.

Strub, R. (2000). The mental status examination in neurology. Oxford University Press.

Stuart, G. W., & Laraia, M. T. (2004). Principles and practice of psychiatric nursing (8th ed.). Mosby.

U.S. Department of Health and Human Services. (2023). Healthy people 2030. https://www.healthypeople.gov/

CHAPTER 7

PHARMACOLOGICAL PRINCIPLES

Psychopharmacology, one of the most active and developing areas of psychiatric research, is the use of psychotropic medication to treat psychiatric disorders. Psychiatric-mental health nurse practitioners (PMHNPs) must have a thorough understanding of the science and art of prescribing, of the pharmacokinetic and pharmacodynamic actions of a given drug, as well as the client's motivation to take the drug. The basic pharmacological principles are discussed in this chapter.

CONCEPTS IN PHARMACOLOGICAL MANAGEMENT

- Pharmacology: Study of what drugs do and how they do it
- Pharmacokinetics: Study of what the body does to drugs; includes absorption, distribution, metabolism, and excretion
- Pharmacodynamics: Study of what drugs do to the body; target sites for drug actions include receptors, ion channels, enzymes, and carrier proteins

PHARMACOKINETICS

- Absorption: Method and rate at which drugs leave the site of administration
  - With oral medications, absorption normally occurs in the small intestine.
- Distribution: Occurs after the drug leaves the systemic circulation and enters the interstitium and cells
  - Drugs are redistributed in organs according to the fat and protein content of the organs.
  - Most psychotropic medications are lipophilic and highly protein-bound. Only the unbound (free) portion of the drug is active. Therefore, people with low protein (albumin) levels—such as in malnutrition, wasting, or aging—can potentially experience toxicity (see below) from an increased amount of free drug. People with high fat-to-lean body mass ratio (as in older adults) will have erratic amounts of active drug in their system.
- Metabolism: Process by which the drug becomes chemically altered in the body
- First-pass metabolism: Process by which the drug is metabolized by cytochrome P450 (CYP) enzymes in the intestines and liver prior to going to the systemic circulation

- Elimination: Process by which the drug is removed from the body
- Half-life (T½): Time needed to clear 50% of the drug from the plasma
    - The half-life also determines the dosing interval and the length of time to reach steady state.
- Steady state: Point at which the amount of drug eliminated between doses is approximately equal to the dose administered
    - Drugs usually are administered once every half-life to achieve a steady state.
    - It takes approximately five half-lives to achieve a steady state and five half-lives to completely eliminate a drug.
- Alterations in pharmacokinetics
    - Hepatic CYP enzyme interactions can induce or inhibit the metabolism of certain drugs, thus changing their desired concentration levels (see Table 7-1).
    - Approximately 10% of Caucasians are poor metabolizers of the CYP2D6 enzyme.
    - Approximately 20% of Asians may have reduced activity of the CYP2C19 enzyme.

TABLE 7-1.
CYTOCHROME P450 (CYP) INHIBITORS AND INDUCERS

INHIBITORS	INDUCERS
Amiodarone	Broccoli
Cimetidine	Brussels sprouts
Ciprofloxacin	Carbamazepine
Clarithromycin	Chamomile tea
Erythromycin	Charred meat
Corticosteroids	Dexamethasone
Cyclosporine	Modafinil
Diltiazem	Nicotine (as part of tobacco smoke)
Verapamil	Phenobarbital
Fluconazole	Phenytoin
Protease inhibitors	Prednisone
Grapefruit	Primidone
Omeprazole	Rifampin
	St. John's wort
	Topiramate

Note. Adapted from Goldberg, J. F., & Stahl, S. (2021). Practical psychopharmacology. Cambridge University Press.

   - ◊ First-pass metabolism activity of CYP enzymes 2C9, 2C19, 2D6, and 3A4 in young children may exceed the rates in adolescents and adults and give rise to underexposure to certain medications Conversely, the ontogeny of the 1A2 pathway is delayed, possibly leading to toxic effects from drugs that are substrates of this pathway (e.g., some antipsychotics).
   - ◊ Enzyme inducers can decrease the serum level of other drugs that are substrates of that enzyme, thus possibly causing subtherapeutic drug levels.
   - ◊ Enzyme inhibitors can increase the serum level of other drugs that are substrates of that enzyme, thus possibly causing toxic levels.
   - ◊ Liver disease will affect liver enzyme activity and first-pass metabolism, possibly resulting in toxic plasma drug levels.
   - ◊ Kidney disease or drugs that reduce renal clearance, such as nonsteroidal anti-inflammatory drugs (NSAIDs), may increase serum concentration of drugs that are excreted by the kidneys (such as lithium). Older adults are more sensitive to psychotropics because of their decreased intracellular water, protein binding, low muscle mass, decreased metabolism, and increased body fat concentration.
- ♦ Most psychotropics are lipophilic and highly protein-bound. Thus, because older adults have more body fat and less protein, they are more likely to develop toxicity due to accumulation and erratic blood levels of drug.

PHARMACODYNAMICS

- ♦ Target sites for drug actions include receptors. Several types of pharmacodynamics involve receptors:
   - ◊ Agonist effect: Drug binds to receptors and activates a biological response
   - ◊ Inverse agonist effect: Drug causes the opposite effect of agonist; binds to same receptor
   - ◊ Partial agonist effect: Drug does not fully activate the receptors
   - ◊ Antagonist effect: Drug binds to the receptor but does not activate a biological response
- ♦ Another site for drug actions is ion channels, which exist for many ions such as sodium, potassium, chloride, and calcium and can be open at some times and closed at other times. Neurotransmitters or drugs may be excitatory or inhibitory depending on the type of ion channel they gate.
   - ◊ Excitatory response: Depolarization; involves the opening of sodium and calcium channels so these ions go into the cell
   - ◊ Inhibitory response: Repolarization; involves the opening of chloride channels so chloride goes into the cell, potassium leaves, or both

- Another site for drug actions are enzymes, which are important for drug metabolism and play an important role in the chemical alteration of the drug. Some drugs (e.g., monoamine oxidase inhibitors [MAOIs]) inhibit the action of a particular enzyme, thus increasing the availability of the neurotransmitter.
- Another site for drug actions is carrier proteins or reuptake pumps, which transport neurotransmitters out of the synapse and back into the presynaptic neuron to be recycled or reused. Some drugs, such as selective serotonin reuptake inhibitors (SSRIs), will inhibit reuptake pumps, thus increasing the synaptic availability of the neurotransmitter.

OTHER TERMINOLOGY

- Potency: Relative dose required to achieve certain effects
- Therapeutic index: Relative measure of the toxicity or safety of a drug; ratio of the median toxic dose to the median effective dose
    - Drugs with a high therapeutic index (e.g., divalproex, 50–125 mcg/mL) have a high margin of safety; that is, the therapeutic dose and the toxic dose are far apart.
    - Drugs with a low therapeutic index (e.g., lithium, 0.5–1.2 mEq/L) have a low margin of safety; that is, the therapeutic dose and the toxic dose are close together.
- Tolerance: The process of becoming less responsive to a particular drug over time
- Tachyphylaxis: An acute decrease in the therapeutic response

PMHNP PHARMACOLOGICAL MANAGEMENT ROLE

- Pharmacological management process
    - Make a diagnosis and identify the target symptoms.
    - Consider the phase of illness (such as acute, relapse, recurrence).
    - Assess prior personal and family history of response to certain medications.
    - Assess the client's motivation for and any misgivings about treatment.
    - Identify potential interactions between the currently prescribed medications.
    - Identify cultural implications of certain drugs.
    - Discuss the risks, benefits, and alternatives to the treatment.
    - Document informed consent and the client's understanding of target symptoms, benefits, risks, and alternatives to treatment.
    - Monitor response and side effects.

- Follow-up and role of the PMHNP
  - Use of standards of care
    - Assist in determining length of treatment.
    - Do relapse planning.
  - It is helpful and advised to use standardized clinical rating scales to establish the client's baseline and to monitor progress or decompensation over time.
  - Screening tests also will aid in making a diagnosis and ruling out other disorders. (See corresponding chapters for a list of relevant screening tools.)
  - It is important to recognize the large body of evidence-based data supporting the combined use of pharmacological and nonpharmacological treatments, as offering clients the best possibility for significant clinical improvement
  - Inconsistency in commitment and adherance to treatment plan is a common problem with all chronic illnesses, including psychiatric disorders, and should be a continuous focus of concern for the PMHNP.
- Common medications used in the clinical management of psychiatric disorders and usually prescribed by the PMHNP are identified in Table 7–2. See corresponding chapters for specific information on each medication.
- A Drug Enforcement Administration (DEA) number is required for prescription of controlled substances.
  - Schedule of controlled substances
    - Schedule I
      - Nonmedicinal substances
      - High potential for misuse
      - Used for research purposes only
      - Not legally available by prescription
      - Examples include heroin, lysergic acid diethylamide, marijuana, 3,4-methylenedioxymethamphetamine, methaqualone, peyote
      - The U.S. Department of Health and Human Services (HHS) recommended to both the DEA and the U.S. Food and Drug Administration (FDA) that marijuana be rescheduled from Schedule I to Schedule III under the Controlled Substances Act (CSA).
    - Schedule II
      - Medicinal drugs in current use
      - High potential for misuse and dependency
      - Written or electronic prescription only
      - No telephone orders allowed

- No refills allowed on prescription
- Examples include combination products with less than 15 mg of hydrocodone per dosage unit, cocaine, methamphetamine, methadone, hydromorphone, meperidine, oxycodone, fentanyl, morphine, dextroamphetamine amphetamine, methylphenidate

- Schedule III
  - Medicinal drugs with less misuse potential than Schedule II drugs
  - Still greater potential for misuse than Schedule IV drugs
  - Telephone orders if followed by written prescription
  - Prescription must be renewed every 6 months.
  - Refills limited to five
  - Examples include products containing less than 90 mg of codeine per dosage unit, ketamine, anabolic steroids, testosterone, buprenorphine
- Schedule IV
  - Medicinal drugs with less misuse potential than Schedule III drugs
  - Examples include benzodiazepines, carisoprodol, zolpidem, tramadol, propoxyphene, chlordiazepoxide, clorazepate, modafinil, phenobarbital, eszopiclone, temazepam, armodafinil
- Schedule V
  - Medicinal drugs with the lowest misuse potential
  - Handled in a manner similar to that for noncontrolled drugs
  - Examples include cough preparations with less than 200 mg of codeine or per 100 mL, diphenoxylate/atropine, difenoxin/atropine, pregabalin, parepectolin

TABLE 7–2.
MEDICATIONS COMMONLY USED IN THE CLINICAL MANAGEMENT OF PSYCHIATRIC DISORDERS*

MEDICATIONS USED TO TREAT SCHIZOPHRENIA AND OTHER PSYCHOTIC DISORDERS	
Typical antipsychotics	chlorpromazine
	fluphenazine
	haloperidol
	loxapine
	perphenazine
	thioridazine
	thiothixene
	trifluoperazine

(Continued)

TABLE 7–2. (CONTINUED)

MEDICATIONS USED TO TREAT SCHIZOPHRENIA AND OTHER PSYCHOTIC DISORDERS	
Second-generation antipsychotics	aripiprazole
	asenapine
	brexpiprazole
	cariprazine
	clozapine
	iloperidone
	lumateperone
	lurasidone
	olanzapine
	paliperidone
	pimavanserin
	risperidone
	quetiapine
	ziprasidone
MEDICATIONS USED TO TREAT MOOD DISORDERS AND BIPOLAR AFFECTIVE DISORDERS	
Mood stabilizers	carbamazepine
	divalproex
	gabapentin (off label)
	lamotrigine
	lithium carbonate
	oxcarbazepine (off label)
	topiramate (off label)
	valproic acid
MEDICATIONS USED TO TREAT MOOD DISORDERS, UNIPOLAR AFFECTIVE DISORDERS, AND DEPRESSIVE DISORDERS	
Tricyclic antidepressants (TCAs)	amitriptyline
	amoxapine
	clomipramine
	desipramine
	doxepin
	imipramine
	nortriptyline
	protriptyline
	trimipramine

(Continued)

TABLE 7–2. (CONTINUED)

MEDICATIONS USED TO TREAT MOOD DISORDERS, UNIPOLAR AFFECTIVE DISORDERS, AND DEPRESSIVE DISORDERS	
Selective serotonin reuptake inhibitors (SSRIs)	citalopram escitalopram fluoxetine fluvoxamine paroxetine paroxetine mesylate sertraline
Serotonin norepinephrine reuptake inhibitors (SNRIs)	desvenlafaxine duloxetine levomilnacipran milnacipran (indicated for the treatment of fibromyalgia) venlafaxine
Monoamine oxidase inhibitors (MAOIs)	isocarboxazid phenelzine selegiline tranylcypromine
Other agents	brexanolone bupropion bupropion/dextromethorphan esketamine mirtazapine nefazodone trazodone vilazodone vortioxetine zuranolone
MEDICATIONS USED TO TREAT ANXIETY DISORDERS	
Benzodiazepines	alprazolam chlordiazepoxide clonazepam clorazepate diazepam lorazepam oxazepam

(Continued)

TABLE 7–2. (CONTINUED)

MEDICATIONS USED TO TREAT ANXIETY DISORDERS	
Anxiolytics	buspirone
Other agents	atenolol
	gabapentin (off label)
	hydroxyzine
	propranolol
MEDICATIONS USED TO TREAT ATTENTION DEFICIT/ HYPERACTIVITY DISORDER	
Stimulants	amphetamine
	dexmethylphenidate
	dextroamphetamine
	lisdexamfetamine
	methylphenidate
	mixed salt amphetamine
	Serdexmethylphenidate/dexmethylphenidate
Non-stimulants	atomoxetine
	bupropion
	clonidine
	desipramine
	imipramine
	nortriptyline
	guanfacine
	venlafaxine
	viloxazine

*Medications listed in this table are FDA approved for the indicated use unless otherwise indicated as "off label"

OTHER PHARMACOLOGICAL CONSIDERATIONS

- Some common medications can induce depression or mania (see Table 7–3).
- Remember that some medications can possibly cause a false urinary drug screen result (see Table 7–4).
- It is vital to be aware of the teratogenic nature of many psychotropic agents. It is important to discuss the risks versus the benefits of medications during pregnancy.
    - Possible risks of psychotropic medications during pregnancy include:
        - Problems with appetite
        - Transient agitation or sedation

TABLE 7–3.
MEDICATIONS THAT INDUCE DEPRESSION OR MANIA

MEDICATIONS THAT INDUCE DEPRESSION	MEDICATIONS THAT INDUCE MANIA
• Beta blockers • Steroids • Interferon • Isotretinoin • Some retroviral drugs • Antineoplastic drugs • Benzodiazepines • Progesterone	• Steroids • Disulfiram • Isoniazid • Antidepressants in persons with bipolar disorder

        - Premature labor
        - Drug discontinuation symptoms
        - Teratogenic effects of certain psychotropics
    - ◊ Possible risks of not taking psychotropic medications during pregnancy include:
        - Recurrence of symptoms
        - Adverse effects on mother–infant bonding
        - Poor maternal self-care
- ♦ FDA pregnancy ratings for medications
    - ◊ A: Controlled studies show no risk
    - ◊ B: No evidence of risk in humans
    - ◊ C: Risk cannot be ruled out
    - ◊ D: Positive evidence of risk
    - ◊ X: Absolutely contraindicated in pregnancy
- ♦ Teratogenic risks of common psychiatric medications
    - ◊ Benzodiazepines: Floppy baby syndrome, cleft palate
    - ◊ Carbamazepine: Neural tube defects
    - ◊ Lithium: Ebstein's anomaly
    - ◊ Divalproex sodium: Neural tube defects, specifically spina bifida; atrial septal defect; cleft palate; and possible long-term developmental deficits

TABLE 7–4.
MEDICATIONS THAT CAN CAUSE DRUG SCREEN, FALSE-POSITIVE RESULTS

FALSE POSITIVE FOR	DRUG RESPONSIBLE
Amphetamines	• Stimulants (i.e., amphetamine/dextroamphetamine methylphenidate) • Bupropion • Fluoxetine • Trazodone • Ranitidine • Nefazodone • Nasal decongestants • Pseudoephedrine
Alcohol	• Diazepam
Benzodiazepines	• Sertraline
Cocaine	• Amoxicillin • Most antibiotics • Nonsteroidal anti-inflammatory drugs (NSAIDs)
Heroin or morphine	• Quinolones • Rifampin • Codeine • Poppy seeds
Methadone or PCP	• Over-the-counter cough medicine dextromethorphan

CASE STUDY 1

A.S, a 74-year-old client who has been seen by the PHMNP for symptoms of depression presented at the appointment with complaints of tremors, diaphoresis, headache, and nausea over the past week. The client is currently being prescribed amitriptyline (50 mg q.h.s.), which was increased at the last visit, and sertraline (100 mg q.d.). The client denies depression but admits to increased confusion and memory problems.

1. What is the biggest pharmacological concern with the combination of medication the client is being prescribed?
2. What would be the PHMNP's plan of action?
3. What pharmacokinetics should the PHMNP consider when treating older adults?

CASE STUDY 2

S.L., a 30-year-old client, is having first time symptoms of being sad, tearful, hopeless, irritabile, having no energy, trouble concentrating, and problems going to sleep and staying asleep. The client is employed as a grade school teacher but is currently on summer break. Despite participaton in 6 months of cognitive behavioral therapy with an experienced therapist, symptoms have not improved. S.L. continues to describe feeling sad, being tearful, and feeling anxious with trouble shutting thoughts off, particularly when trying to fall asleep at night. The client feels tired upon awakening, despite getting 7 to 8 hours of sleep, and has trouble getting out of bed. Energy remains low throughout the day and S.L. notes a decrease in motivation as well. Weight and appetite are unchanged. The client denies suicidal ideation. After careful evaluation, the PMHNP suggests a trial of fluoxetine and prescribes 20 mg, p.o. q.a.m., with food.

The client calls the PMHNP before the scheduled follow-up appointment, requesting to come in sooner due to "feeling worse." S.L. describes more difficulty falling asleep, feels "revved up" much of the time, and is having mild nausea and headaches.

1. What are possible reasons for the client feeling "worse"?
2. What should the PMHNP suggest as the next intervention?

CASE STUDY 3

B.D. is a 22-year-old who presents to the PMHNP with signs and symptoms of sadness, not being able to fall asleep at night, being tired in the mornings, feeling worthless, and having lack of energy. The client has a strong family history of major depression and both their mother and older sister have been treated with an antidepressant. B.D. has never been treated for depression before, and states, "I am nervous about taking medication because I seem to get side effects from everything."

1. How should the PMHNP respond to B.D.'s concerns about taking medication?
2. How should the PMHNP begin to think about medication management?
3. The client is started on sertraline, 50 mg, and calls within a few days of starting the drug and states, "I am experiencing an upset stomach, headache, difficulty sleeping, and an overall feeling of being edgy."
4. What is the most likely reason for B.D.'s reported side effects?
5. What is the most reasonable intervention by the PMHNP?
6. Other than potential side effects, what information should the PMHNP include in client teaching when starting a person on a new medication?

ANSWERS TO CASE STUDY DISCUSSION QUESTIONS

CASE STUDY 1

1. The SSRI is potentially increasing the concentration of the tricyclic antidepressant (TCA) to toxic levels.
2. Check the blood level of amitriptyline and decrease the dose; consider tapering the client off the TCA.
3. Higher body fat content, decreased gastric acid secretion, and decreased hepatic and renal functioning all predispose an older adult to the potential toxic effects of medications. Anticholinergic effects and orthostasis are particularly common and problematic.

CASE STUDY 2

1. Fluoxetine may cause uncomfortable activation in some clients. In addition, the client appears to be having multiple side effects. Fluoxetine is metabolized primarily by cytochrome P450 (CYP) 2D6. People who have a variant of CYP2D6 are considered "slow metabolizers," and may need significantly lower doses of medications that are substrates of CYP2D6. Finally, all clients started on antidepressants must be monitored closely for a switch from depression to hypomania or mixed mania. Although the client's increase in insomnia and feeling "revved up" and "worse" are likely side effects from fluoxetine, this could signal beginning symptoms of a shift into a bipolar spectrum mood state.
2. Unless agitation is prominent, the first prudent intervention would be to lower the dose of fluoxetine. If this is not helpful in diminishing side effects, prescribing a low dose of lorazepam or other benzodiazepine used as a "bridge" medication until the SSRI is effective may be prudent. If neither of these interventions proves helpful, the medication should be changed.

CASE STUDY 3

1. The PMHNP should ask the client to provide more information about being "nervous" about taking medicine and ask about the medications their immediate family members are taking, whether or not the family members have had problems with side effects, and finally, whether any medication has been particularly helpful to their family members.

2. A genetic polymorphism screening test to determine gene variants may be reasonable. Because mood and anxiety disorders have a genetic component, beginning with a medication that has been beneficial in the treatment of similar symptoms in a first-degree relative is a reasonable starting point of treatment.
3. The sertraline was started at too high a dose.
4. The dose was too high for this person.
5. Lower the dose to 25 mg. Make sure the medication is being taken with food. If the client is not already doing so, switch the time of dosing to after breakfast.
6. During client teaching, the PMHNP should cover the usual course of treatment: typical time until benefit, typical therapeutic dosing, and expected length of treatment. The PMHNP should also emphasize that most side effects are transient and can usually be managed, such as by adjusting the dose.

REFERENCES AND RESOURCES

American Psychiatric Association. (2010). Practice guidelines for the treatment of patients with major depressive disorder. https://psychiatryonline.org/pb/assets/raw/sitewide/practice_guidelines/guidelines/mdd.pdf

Antai-Otong, D. (Ed.). (2008). Psychiatric nursing: Biological and behavioral concepts (2nd ed.). Delmar Cengage Learning.

Boyd, M. A. (2002). Psychiatric nursing: Contemporary practice (2nd ed.). Lippincott.

De Wildt, S. N., Tibboel, D., & Leeder, J. S. (2014). Drug metabolism for the paediatrician. Archives of Disease in Childhood, 99(12), 1137–1142.

Dipiro, J. T., Talbert, R. L., & Yee, G. C. (Eds.). (2002). Pharmacotherapy: A pathophysiological approach (5th ed.). McGraw-Hill.

Goldberg, J. F., & Stahl, S. (2021). Practical psychopharmacology. Cambridge University Press.

Hirschfeld, R., & Holzer, C. (2003). Validity of the mood disorder questionnaire: A general population study. American Journal of Psychiatry, 160, 178–180.

Jones, B. L. (2022). Overview of drug treatment in children. www.merckmanuals.com/professional/pediatrics/principles-of-drug-treatment-in-children/overview-of-drug-treatment-in-children

Kroenke, K., Spitzer, R. L., & Williams, J. B. (2001). The PHQ-9: Validity of a brief depression severity measure. Journal of General Internal Medicine, 16(9), 606–613.

Sacco, L. N., & Sheikh, H. Z. (2023). Department of Health and Human Services recommendation to reschedule marijuana: Implications for federal policy. Congressional Research Service. https://crsreports.congress.gov/product/pdf/IN/IN12240

Sadock, B., Sadock, V., & Ruiz, P. (2017). Kaplan and Sadock's comprehensive textbook of psychiatry (10th ed.). Wolters Kluwer.

Schatsburg, A., Cole, J., & DeBattista, C. (2019). Manual of clinical psychopharmacology (9th ed.). American Psychiatric Association Press.

Stahl, S. M. (2020). Stahl's essential psychopharmacology: Prescriber's guide. (7th ed.). Cambridge University Press.

CHAPTER 8

NONPHARMACOLOGICAL TREATMENT

This chapter discusses nonpharmacological interventions such as individual psychotherapies, group therapy, family therapies, and complementary and alternative therapies. Because medications alone do not treat a person's environment or response to stress, an integrated approach is the most beneficial in treating mental illnesses. Although some people seek counseling for self-discovery, the most common issues for individual therapy are as follows:

- Losses
- Interpersonal conflicts
- Symptomatic presentations such as panic, phobias, and negativity
- Unfulfilled expectations at life transitions
- Characterological issues such as narcissism or aggressiveness

Confidentiality may be broken when there is increased potential for self-harm or harm to others; abuse of a child, older adult, or person with disabilities; when the therapist determines that the person needs hospitalization; and when clients request that their information be released to a third party.

INDIVIDUAL THERAPY (COREY, 2017)

- Psychoanalytic therapy
  - Originated by Sigmund Freud (1856–1939), who believed that behavior is determined by unconscious motivations and instinctual drives (see also Chapter 3)
  - Promotes change by the development of greater insight and awareness of maladaptive defenses
  - Attends to past developmental and psychodynamic factors, which shape present behaviors
- Cognitive therapy
  - Originated by Aaron Beck (1921–2021)
  - Purports that external events do not cause anxiety or maladaptive responses
  - States that a person's expectations, perceptions, and interpretations of events cause anxiety

    - ◊ Allows clients to view reality more clearly through an examination of their central distorted cognitions
    - ◊ Goal is to change clients' irrational beliefs, faulty conceptions, and negative cognitive distortions
- ♦ Behavioral therapy
    - ◊ Originated by Arnold Lazarus (1932–2013)
    - ◊ Focuses on changing maladaptive behaviors by participation in active behavioral techniques such as exposure, relaxation, problem-solving, and role-playing
- ♦ Dialectical behavioral therapy
    - ◊ Originated by Marsha Linehan (born 1943)
    - ◊ Commonly used with people with borderline personality disorder
    - ◊ Focuses on emotional regulation, tolerance for distress, self-management skills, interpersonal effectiveness, and mindfulness, with an emphasis on treating therapy-interfering behaviors
    - ◊ Goals
        - Decrease suicidal behaviors
        - Decrease therapy-interfering behaviors
        - Decrease emotional reactivity
        - Decrease self-invalidation
        - Decrease crisis-generating behaviors
        - Decrease passivity
        - Increase realistic decision-making
        - Increase accurate communication of emotions and competencies
- ♦ Existential therapy
    - ◊ Originated by Viktor Frankl (1905–1997)
    - ◊ A philosophical approach in which reflection on life and self-confrontation are encouraged
    - ◊ Emphasizes accepting freedom and making responsible choices
    - ◊ States that a basic dimension of humans includes finding meaning and purpose in life—"Why am I here? What is my purpose?"
    - ◊ Goals are to live authentically and to focus on the present and on personal responsibility
- ♦ Humanistic therapy
    - ◊ Originated by Carl Rogers (1902–1987)
    - ◊ Also known as person-centered therapy

- ◇ Concepts include self-directed growth and self-actualization; people are born with the capacity to direct themselves toward self-actualization
- ◇ Each person has the potential to actualize and find meaning.

- ♦ Interpersonal therapy
  - ◇ Originated by Gerald L. Klerman (1928–1992) and Myrna M. Weissman (born 1940)
  - ◇ Evidence-based therapy with focus on interpersonal issues that are creating distress
  - ◇ Time-limited, active, focused on the present and on interpersonal distress
  - ◇ Developed to treat aspects of depression and is effective for adults and adolescents
  - ◇ Has been applied to treat interpersonal distress related to other disorders, including bipolar, substance use, and eating disorders
- ♦ Eye movement desensitization and reprocessing (EMDR)
  - ◇ Originated by Francine Shapiro (1948–2019)
  - ◇ A form of behavioral and exposure therapy
  - ◇ Involves the use of bilateral stimulation—moving the eyes back and forth, alternating tapping on hand or knee, or sounds in ears
  - ◇ Used most commonly in posttraumatic stress disorder
  - ◇ Goal is to achieve adaptive resolution
  - ◇ Desensitization phase: The client visualizes the trauma, verbalizes the negative thoughts or maladaptive beliefs, and remains attentive to physical sensations. This process occurs for a limited time while the client maintains rhythmic eye movements. They are then instructed to block out negative thoughts; to breathe deeply; and then to verbalize what they are thinking, feeling, or imagining.
  - ◇ Installation phase: The client installs and increases the strength of the positive thought that they have declared as a replacement of the original negative thought.
  - ◇ Body scan: The client visualizes the trauma along with the positive thought and then scans their body mentally to identify any tension within.
- ♦ Somatic therapy
  - ◇ Originated by Wilheim Reich (1897–1957)
  - ◇ Purports that trauma goes beyond the mind and can result in physical symptoms
  - ◇ Untreated/unprocessed trauma can lead to reactivation and emotional distress
  - ◇ Physical sensations precede emotions; through facilitation of awareness, emotional regulation can be achieved.

GROUP THERAPY (YALOM, 2020)

- Benefits
  - Increases insight about oneself
  - Increases social skills
  - Is cost-effective
  - Develops sense of community
- Irvin Yalom (born 1931) was the first person to put a theoretical perspective on group work and identified 10 therapeutic factors that differentiate group therapy from individual therapy.
  1. Instillation of hope: Participants develop hope for creating a different life. Members are at different levels of growth; thus, they gain hope from others that change is possible.
  2. Universality: Participants discover that others have similar problems, thoughts, or feelings and that they are not alone.
  3. Altruism: This results from sharing oneself with another and helping another.
  4. Increased development of socialization skills: New social skills are learned and maladaptive social behaviors are corrected. The group can provide a "natural laboratory."
  5. Imitative behaviors: Participants can increase their skills by imitating the behaviors of others.
  6. Interpersonal learning: Interacting with others increases adaptive interpersonal relationships.
  7. Group cohesiveness: Participants develop an attraction to the group and other members as well as a sense of belonging.
  8. Catharsis: Participants experience catharsis as they openly express their feelings, which were previously suppressed.
  9. Existential factors: Groups enable participants to deal with the meaning of their own existence.
  10. Corrective refocusing: Participants reexperience family conflicts in the group, which allows them to recognize and change behaviors that may be problematic.
- Group phases (Tuckman, 1965)
  - Pre-group phase: The leader considers the direction and framework of the group.
    - Purpose
    - Goals

    - Membership criteria
    - Membership size
    - Pre-group interview
    - Informed consent
  - ◊ Forming phase: Members are concerned about self-disclosure and being rejected. Goals and expectations are identified, and boundaries are established. The development of trust and rapport is very important.
  - ◊ Storming phase: Members are resistant and may begin to use testing behaviors. Issues related to inclusion, control, and affection begin to surface. Leaders' tasks are to allow expression of both positive and negative feelings, assist the group in understanding the underlying conflict, and examine nonproductive behaviors.
  - ◊ Norming phase: Resistance to the group is overcome by members. A strong attraction to the group and others emerges. Open and spontaneous communication occurs and the group norms are established.
  - ◊ Performing phase: The group's work becomes more focused. Creative problem solving and solutions begin to emerge. Experiential learning takes place. Group energy is directed toward completion of goals.
  - ◊ Adjourning phase: Preparation is made to end the group. (Remember that the work of termination begins during the first stage of the group.) Both members and leaders express their feelings about each other and termination. A discussion and overview of what has been learned, as well as what issues still need to be worked on, takes place.
- ♦ Reminiscence therapy
  - ◊ Characterized by a progressive return of memories of past experiences
  - ◊ Used with older adults
  - ◊ Enables participants to search for meaning in their lives and strive for some resolution of past interpersonal and intrapsychic conflicts

FAMILY THERAPIES (GOLDENBERG & GOLDENBERG, 2016)

- ♦ Family systems concepts
  - ◊ A system is any unit structured on feedback—such as the family.
  - ◊ The process by which all family members operate together is referred to as the family system.
  - ◊ Family systems theory is based on the idea that one could not understand any family member (part) without understanding how all family members operate together (system).
  - ◊ The family system operates based on a set of rules that may be overt or covert.

- ◊ Boundaries: Barriers that protect and enhance the functional integrity of families, individuals, and subsystems. System boundaries can be physical or psychological.
    - Types of boundaries:
        - Clearly defined boundaries: Maintain person's separateness while emphasizing belongingness
        - Rigid or inflexible boundaries: May lead to distant relationships and to disengagement
        - Diffuse boundaries: Blurred and indistinct boundaries; lead to enmeshment
- ◊ Circular causality: An ongoing feedback loop; a series of actions and reactions that maintain a problem. Individuals and emotional problems are best understood within the context of relationships and through assessing interactions within an entire family.
- ◊ Family homeostasis: Tendency of families to resist change and to maintain a steady state
- ◊ Morphogenesis: A family's tendency to adapt to change when changes are necessary
- ◊ Morphostasis: A family's tendency to remain stable in the midst of change

- ♦ Family systems therapy
    - ◊ Originated by Murray Bowen (1913–1990), who believed that a person's problematic behavior may serve a function or purpose for the family or be a symptom of dysfunctional patterns
    - ◊ Focus is on chronic anxiety within families
    - ◊ Treatment goals are to increase the family's awareness of each member's function within the family and to increase levels of self-differentiation (the level at which one's sense of self-worth is not dependent on external relationships, circumstances, or occurrences)
    - ◊ Triangles: Dyads that form triads to decrease stress; the lower the level of family adaptation, the more likely a triangle will develop
    - ◊ Nuclear family emotional system: Level of differentiation of the parents is usually equal to the level of differentiation for the entire family
    - ◊ Multigenerational transmission process: Dysfunction present over several generations
    - ◊ Family projection process: Parents transmitting their own level of differentiation on the most susceptible child
    - ◊ Emotional cutoffs: Attempting to break contact with the family of origin
    - ◊ Sibling position: Influences interactions and personality characteristics

- Structural family therapy
  - Originated by Salvador Minuchin (1913–1990), who placed emphasis on how, when, and to whom family members relate in order to understand and then change the family's structure
  - A person's symptoms are rooted in the context of family transaction patterns. The symptom is a function of the health of the whole family and is maintained by structural problems in the system.
  - The main treatment goal is to produce a structural change in the family organization to more effectively manage problems—changing transactional patterns and family structure.
  - Family structure: An invisible set of functional demands that organize the way members interact with each other, made up of subsystems (e.g., marital, parental, sibling), coalitions (e.g., two members joining forces against a third member), and boundaries
  - Structural mapping (genogram): Mapping relationships using symbols to represent overinvolvement, conflict, coalitions, and so forth
  - Hierarchies: Distribution of power
- Experiential therapy
  - Originated by Virginia Satir (1916–1988)
  - Behavior is determined by personal experience and not by external reality.
  - Focus is on being authentic, on freedom of choice, on human validation, and on experiencing the moment.
  - Treatment goals are to develop authentic, nurturing communication and increased self-worth of each family member; overall goal is growth rather than symptom reduction alone
  - It does not focus on particular techniques.
- Strategic therapy
  - Originated by Jay Haley (1923–2007)
  - Symptoms are viewed as metaphors and reflect problems in the hierarchal structure. Symptoms are a way to communicate metaphorically within a family.
  - Treatment goal is to help family members behave in ways that will not perpetuate the problem behavior
  - Interventions are problem-focused. Strategic therapy is more symptom-focused than structural therapy.
  - Strategic family therapists are concerned mainly with those techniques that change the sequence of interactions that is maintaining the problem.
  - Techniques are straightforward directives, paradoxical directives, and reframing belief systems

- Straightforward directives: Tasks that are designed in expectation of the family member's compliance
- Paradoxical directives: A negative task that is assigned when family members are resistant to change and the member is expected to be noncompliant (use this technique with caution)
- Reframing belief systems: Problematic behaviors are relabeled to have more positive meaning (e.g., jealousy reframed to caring)

- Solution-focused therapy
  - Originated by Steve deShazer (1940–2005), Bill O'Hanlon (born 1952), and Insoo Berg (1934–2007)
  - Focus is to rework for the present situation solutions that have worked previously
  - Treatment goal is effective resolution of problems through cognitive problem solving and use of personal resources and strengths
  - Techniques include the use of miracle questions, exception-finding questions, and scaling questions.
    - Miracle questions: "If a miracle were to happen tonight while you were asleep, and tomorrow morning you awoke to find that the problem no longer existed, what would be different?"; "How would you know the miracle took place?"; "How would others know?"
    - Exception-finding questions: Directing clients to a time in their lives when the problem did not exist, which helps them move toward solutions by assisting them in searching for any exceptions to the pattern. "Was there a time when the problem did not occur?"
    - Scaling questions: "On a scale of 1–10, with 10 being very anxious and depressed, how would you rate how you are feeling now?" This is useful for highlighting small increments of change.

COMPLEMENTARY AND ALTERNATIVE THERAPIES

- Complementary and alternative therapies (CATs) deal with the connection between the mind and the body and are viewed as holistic health care (dealing with the biopsychosocial and spiritual components of the person).
  - Complementary therapies: Used in addition to traditional medical practices
  - Alternative therapies: Used in place of traditional medical practices
  - Integrative therapies: Therapy that is not restricted to one methodology; interventions are tailored to the individual with a goal of improving the efficacy and effectiveness of the treatment.

- Why people use CATs
  - Desire for more control over decision-making
  - Decreased insurance coverage for traditional medical therapies, thereby making the use of CATs cheaper
  - Preference for natural rather than synthetic medications
  - Increased costs of prescriptions and services
  - Failure of conventional medications
- Mind–body interventions
  - Guided imagery
  - Meditation
  - Yoga
  - Biofeedback
- Biologically based therapies
  - Herbal products
  - Vitamins
  - Supplements
  - Aromatherapy
- Manipulative and body-based therapies
  - Acupressure and acupuncture
  - Massage
  - Reflexology
- Acupressure and Acupuncture
  - Based on the basic tenet of Chinese medicine that vital energy (chi) flows along specific pathways that have many points of access and that manipulating these points, by either hands or needles, corrects imbalances by stimulating or removing blockages to energy flow
  - Thought to produce effects by regulating the nervous system and aiding the activity of endorphins and immune system cells at different sites in the body
  - Also thought to alter brain chemistry by changing the release of neurohormones and neurotransmitters
- Biofeedback
  - A process providing a person with visual or auditory information about the autonomic physiologic functions of their body, such as blood pressure, muscle tension, and brain wave activity
  - The person learns to consciously control these processes, which were regarded previously as involuntary.

- ◊ Uses
  - Stress-related symptoms (e.g., anxiety)
  - Pain
  - Insomnia
  - Neuromuscular problems (e.g., migraines, muscular tension, tension headaches, Raynaud's disease, urinary incontinence)
  - Neurobehavioral disorders
  - Enhancement of healing
  - Athletic and work performance
- ◊ Desired outcome
  - Positive change in baseline measures
  - Demonstrated skill at self-regulation
  - Improvement in symptoms
  - Improved use of skills in daily life
  - Reduction of muscle bracing
  - Increased sense of self-efficacy

- ♦ Aromatherapy
  - ◊ Therapeutic use of plants or oils to obtain many therapeutic effects, such as analgesic, psychological, and antimicrobial benefits
  - ◊ In psychiatry, olfactory stimulation used to elicit feelings or memories during psychotherapy
- ♦ Herbal products and supplements
  - ◊ Practice of herbal medicine originated in China and is the oldest system of medicine
  - ◊ Relies on plants to cure illnesses and maintain health
  - ◊ Similar to prescription medications, many plants contain active compounds that produce physiological effects
  - ◊ U.S. Food and Drug Administration (FDA) approval is not required; thus, no uniform standards ensure quality control or potency.
  - ◊ Common supplements and interactions include:
    - Omega-3 fatty acids
      - Used for attention-deficit/hyperactivity disorder, dyslexia, cognitive impairment, dementia, cardiovascular disease, asthma, lupus, and rheumatoid arthritis
      - Interacts with warfarin, increasing anticoagulant effect (people cautioned to stop using before surgery)

- S-adenosyl-L-methionine (SAM-e)
  - Used for depression, osteoarthritis, and liver disease
  - May cause hypomania, hyperactive muscle movements, and possible serotonin syndrome
- Tryptophan
  - Used for depression, obesity, insomnia, headaches, and fibromyalgia
  - Found in high concentrations in turkey
  - Increased risk of serotonin syndrome with use of selective serotonin reuptake inhibitors (SSRIs), monoamine oxidase inhibitors (MAOIs), and St. John's wort
- Vitamin E
  - Used for enhancing the immune system and protecting cells against effects of free radicals
  - Used for neurological disorders, diabetes, and premenstrual syndrome
  - Interacts with warfarin, increasing anticoagulant effect; antiplatelet drugs; and statins, increasing additive effect and risk of rhabdomyolysis
- Melatonin
  - Used for insomnia, jet lag, shift work, and cancer
  - Sets timing of circadian rhythms and regulates seasonal responses
  - Interacts with aspirin, nonsteroidal anti-inflammatory drugs (NSAIDs), beta blockers, corticosteroids, valerian, kava kava, and alcohol
  - Can inhibit ovulation in large doses
- Fish oil
  - Used for bipolar disorder, hypertension, lowering triglycerides, and decreasing blood clotting
    - Interacts with warfarin, aspirin, NSAIDs, garlic, and ginkgo
    - May alter glucose regulation
    - Most supplements are contraindicated during pregnancy because they are secreted in breast milk during lactation.

◊ Common herbals with psychoactive effects include:

- Ayahuasca: Fear, paranoia, disequilibrium, coma, death
- Black cohosh: Menopausal symptoms, premenstrual syndrome, dysmenorrhea
- Belladonna: Anxiety

- Catnip: Sedation
- Chamomile: Sedation, anxiety
- Ginkgo: Delirium, dementia, sexual dysfunction caused by SSRIs
- Ginseng: Depression, fatigue
- Khat: Stimulant
- Kratom: Stimulant at low doses and sedative at higher doses
- Salvia: Hallucinogenic
- Valerian: Sedation

- ♦ Alternative therapy
  - ◊ Massage
    - Believed to increase blood circulation, improve lymph flow, improve musculoskeletal tone, and have a relaxing effect on the mind
  - ◊ Meditation
    - Consciously directing one's attention to alter one's state of consciousness
    - Produces physiological effects such as decreased heart rate, blood pressure, and respiratory rate; decreased anxiety; and increased alpha brain waves
  - ◊ Reflexology
    - Stimulates the body's natural healing power through massaging the feet, hands, and ears
    - Alleviates tension by cleaning crystalline deposits under the skin that may interfere with the natural flow of the body's energy
    - Based on the mapping of body parts on the soles and sides of the feet, hands, and ears
    - Treats disorders related to the represented body parts by application of pressure
    - Used for back pain, migraines, infertility, sleep disorders, digestive disorders, and stress-related conditions
  - ◊ Macrobiotics
    - Foods classified as yin (cold and wet) and yang (hot and dry)
    - Goal is to keep the dietary yin and yang in balance in attempt to live in harmony with nature
  - ◊ Yoga
    - Originated in Indian religious practices
    - Combines mind and body connection
    - Uses breathing, physical movements, and meditation

CASE STUDY

You are a psychiatric-mental health nurse practitioner (PMHNP) working with a client who has a diagnosis of major depressive disorder. In session the client states, "Nothing good ever happens to me. I'm just a failure and should accept that people at work think I'm inadequate to do my job."

1. What therapeutic approach would be most helpful in working with this client?
2. Specifically, what cognitive and behavioral techniques would be helpful?
3. Which scales would be helpful to use in assessing her depression and negative thoughts?
4. If you chose a cognitive behavioral therapy (CBT) approach to work with this client, what is the three question technique?
5. What types of distortions does this client have and, as the therapist, how would you begin to address the distortions?

ANSWERS TO CASE STUDY DISCUSSION QUESTIONS

1. The therapy that would be most helpful is CBT.
2. Having the client complete a thought record to identify situations that lead to automatic thoughts, emotions, and responses would be helpful.
3. Scales that would be useful to track progress in therapy include: Patient Health Questionnaire-9 (PHQ-9), Beck Depression Inventory, and the Schema questionnaire.
4. The three-question technique when using CBT involves Socratic questioning. For example, asking the following: (1) Evidence of negative belief; (2) How else can the client interpret the situation? (3) If it is true, what are the implications?
5. The types of distortions expressed by the client are all-or-nothing thinking and overgeneralization. A technique that would be helpful to address the distortion is using a scale that will help put the distortions on a continuum to help respond differently to low scale items.

REFERENCES AND RESOURCES

Corey, M., Corey, G., & Corey, C. (2017). Groups: Process and practice (10th ed.). Cengage Learning.

Goldenberg, I., & Goldenberg, H. (2016). Family therapy: An overview (9th ed.). Brooks/Cole Cengage Learning.

Lindquist, R., Tracy, M. F., & Snyder, M. (2022). Complementary therapies in nursing promoting integrative care (9th ed.). Springer Publishing.

Miller-Karas, E. (2023). Building resilience to trauma (2nd ed.). Routledge.

Sadock, B., Sadock, V., & Ruiz, P. (2017). Kaplan and Sadock's comprehensive textbook of psychiatry (10th ed.). Wolters Kluwer.

Scharf, R. (2015). Theories of psychotherapy and counseling (5th ed.). Cengage Learning.

Tusaie, K., & Fitzpatrick, J. (2021). Advanced practice psychiatric nursing integrating psychotherapy, psychopharmacology, and complementary and alternative approaches. Springer Publishing.

United Nations Office on Drugs and Crime. (2013). Factsheet "new psychoactive substances." www.unodc.org/documents/scientific/FACTSHEET_NPS.pdf

Weisz, J., & Kazdin, A. (2010). Evidence-based psychotherapies for children and adolescents (2nd ed.). Guilford Press.

Wheeler, K. (2022). Psychotherapy for the advanced practice psychiatric nurse (3rd ed.). Springer Publishing.

Yalom, I. (2020). Theory and practice of group psychotherapy (6th ed.). Basic Books.

CHAPTER 9

DEPRESSIVE DISORDERS AND BIPOLAR DISORDERS

This chapter reviews the mood disorders and evidence-based practice guidelines that psychiatric-mental health nurse practitioners (PMHNPs) use in treating clients who have these disorders. As a childhood disorder, disruptive mood dysregulation disorder will be discussed in Chapter 15.

Mood disorders are the most common of all psychiatric illnesses. It has become increasingly common for mood disorders to be treated in primary care settings, and often clients first present in such settings because of the high degree of somatic symptomatology that accompanies these disorders.

Sadness is a common, normal human emotion. PMHNPs caring for clients who present for evaluation of depression must distinguish between normal levels of sadness and pathological levels that are symptomatic of an underlying brain-based illness called major depression. Major depression requires treatment and generally will not fully abate without therapeutic intervention. Untreated, major depression predisposes people to other serious health problems, so pathological levels of depression should not go untreated.

SADNESS AS A COMMON EMOTIONAL STATE

- Sadness, one of the most common human emotions, exists on a continuum ranging from the absence of depression at one end to pathological levels that produce significant symptoms of a psychiatric disorder called major depression at the other.
- Cultural differences affect behavioral manifestations of depression.
- Mild depression can be a healthy reaction to life stressors that motivates a person to deal with events and emotions.
    - Sadness can be pathological if
        - It is disproportionate to events and sustained over a significant time period;
        - It significantly impairs normal functioning (e.g., occupational, social, school, relational functioning);
        - It significantly impairs normal somatic functioning (e.g., loss of appetite, altered sleep, altered self-care activities, altered sexual functioning); or
        - It is apparently unrelated to any identifiable event or situation in a person's life.

MAJOR DEPRESSIVE DISORDER (MDD)

DESCRIPTION

- One of the most common psychiatric disorders; the primary unipolar affective disorder
- A complex brain-based illness with a primary characteristic of a persistent disturbance in mood
- An excessive or distorted degree of sadness that manifests with behavioral, affective, cognitive, and somatic symptoms
- May have a known precipitating event, situation, or concern but often occurs without any precipitating stressor identified
- Interferes significantly with daily functioning and goal attainment
- Has complex genetic, biochemical, and environmental etiological factors

ETIOLOGY

- The multiple theories of the etiology of depression fall into two categories: psychological and neurobiological.
- Psychodynamic theories
  - Object loss theory (Ronald Fairbairn)
    - This theory assumes that early psychological developmental issues lay the foundation for depressive responses in later life; that the accomplishment of the first stage of development in which the child is able to form relationships is normal; and that, during the second stage of development, the child experiences traumatic separation from significant objects of attachment (usually a maternal object).
    - Loss may be related to maternal death, illness, or emotional lack of availability and is unexpected and overwhelming.
    - Depth of loss produces a constellation of responses dominated by separation anxiety, grief, mourning, and despair.
    - This critical object loss event predisposes the child to respond in similar ways to any future losses or significant separation.
  - Aggression-turned-inward theory (Sigmund Freud)
    - This theory assumes that early psychological developmental issues lay the foundation for depressive responses in later life; that the accomplishment of the first stage of development in which the child is able to form relationships is normal; and that during the second stage of development, the child experiences the loss of the significant mothering person.

- The loss can be real or imagined and is unexpected and overwhelming.
- The loss may be related to maternal death, illness, or emotional lack of availability, or to the birth of a new sibling and the child's perception of losing undivided, individualized attention from the mother. The child's initial reaction is anger; however, the child feels unsafe to express this anger openly and directly. This may relate to the child's fear of further loss if they respond with anger or their subjective perception that anger is unacceptable.
- The child uses defense mechanisms to deal with conflict created by desire for the love object but co-occurring with anger for the love object.
- Instead of anger being expressed outward at the maternal figure, it turns inward because it is more acceptable and safer to be angry at oneself than at one's mother.
- Anger at oneself is rationalized as the child assumes that the loss of the mother was related to something bad that they did rather than to the caregiver's actions.
- Excessive guilt becomes a manifestation of the process of dealing with aggression experienced with the loss of the mother's attention.
- A similar emotional reaction (such as low self-esteem, excessive guilt, inability to cope with anger, self-destructive impulses) occurs as an adult whenever a loss is experienced.

◊ Cognitive theory (Aaron Beck)

- This theory represents a cognitive diathesis–stress model in which developmental experiences sensitize a person to respond to stressful life events in a depressed manner.
- Cognitive theory assumes that people with a tendency to be depressed think about the world differently than nondepressed people and that depressed people are more negative and believe that bad things are going to happen to them because of their own personal shortcomings and inadequacies.
- This thinking promotes low self-esteem and beliefs that the person deserves to have bad things happen to them and promotes pessimistic perceptions about the world at large and about their future, as well as globalizes the negativity to all events, situations, and people in their life.
- When confronted by stressful events, these people tend to appraise them and the potential consequences in a negative, hopeless manner and, therefore, are more depressed than people with different cognitive styles.

◊ Learned helplessness–hopelessness theory (Martin Seligman)

- This theory is a modified version of cognitive theory, which assumes that a person becomes depressed due to perceptions of lack of control over life events and experiences. These perceptions are learned over time, especially as the person perceives others seeing them as inadequate.
- Perceptions of lack of control lead to the person not adapting or coping.

- The person's behavior becomes passive and nonreactive because of self-perceptions of personal characteristics of being helpless, hopeless, and powerless.

♦ Biological theories

◊ Genetic predisposition

- There is a clear genetic predisposition to depressive disorders; one assumption is a polygenic single nucleotide polymorphism (SNP) disorder.
- Having a depressed parent is the single strongest predictor of depression. Children of depressed parents are three times more likely than the general population to experience MDD in their lifetimes and have a 40% chance of having a depressive episode before age 18.
- The earlier the age at onset for MDD and the more severe the symptoms, the more likely it is that a person has a strong genetic predisposition for depression.

◊ Endocrine dysfunction

- MDD has symptoms that suggest endocrine abnormalities as part of the etiologic picture.
- Neurovegetative symptoms commonly seen in MDD (e.g., sleep disturbances, appetite disturbances, libido disturbances, lethargy, anhedonia) are related to functions of the hypothalamus and pituitary and the hormones they secrete.
- A high incidence of postpartum mood disturbances is suggestive of endocrine dysfunction.
- Dysphoria is often triggered by changes in levels of sex steroids that occur during the menstrual cycle.
- Deregulation of the hypothalamic–pituitary–adrenal (HPA) axis—which controls the physiological response to stress and consists of interconnected feedback pathways between the hypothalamus, pituitary gland, and adrenal glands—is another theory of an endocrine basis for MDD. In this theory, MDD is presumed to be, at least in part, a result of an abnormal stress response related to HPA axis dysregulation.
    - In response to stress, the hypothalamus releases corticotropin-releasing hormone (CRH), which then stimulates the pituitary to release adrenocorticotropic hormone (ACTH). This then stimulates the adrenals to release cortisol.
    - Hyperactivity of the HPA axis has been shown to be present in people with MDD, as have possibly elevated cortisol levels.
    - Over time, elevated cortisol levels damage the central nervous system (CNS) by altering neurotransmission and electrical signal conduction.
    - Evidence supports that cortisol over time can cause changes in size and function of brain tissue.

    - Evidence supports that major depression may be associated with proinflammatory cytokine activation.
- HPA axis dysregulation is the rationale and scientific basis for the dexamethasone suppression test (DST), a screening test for depression, which has proved to be too nonspecific and is not commonly used in clinical practice.

◇ Abnormalities of neurotransmitter function

- All of the following are possible neurotransmitter function abnormalities causing depression:
    - Dysregulation of one or more biogenic amine neurotransmitters: dopamine, serotonin, norepinephrine
    - Low levels of endogenous catecholamines in specific areas of the brain
    - Serotonin levels were shown to be low in postmortem studies in people who die by suicide and in people with MDD.
    - Low level of the serotonin precursor tryptophan
    - Low levels of the serotonin metabolite 5-hydroxyindoleacetic acid (5-HIAA)
    - Receptor sensitivity for neurotransmitters set unusually high in specific areas of the brain
- A stronger neurotransmitter receptor cascade is required to induce neuronal activity.
    - Low density of receptor sites in specific areas of the brain
    - Hypometabolism in specific areas of the brain regulating mood, appetite, and cognition
    - The complexity of brain functions implies that the etiology of complex disorders such as MDD involves the relative balance of available neurotransmitters and not just a low level of one neurotransmitter.
    - Structural brain changes
- Neuroimaging has shown consistent abnormalities in certain structures of the brain in people with chronic and severe depression.
    - Hypovolemic hippocampus
    - Hypovolemic prefrontal cortex–limbic striatal regions
- MDD is a common comorbidity in people who have experienced brain damage, including damage from stroke and trauma.
    - Chronobiological theory

- Desynchronization of circadian rhythms produces the symptom constellation collectively called MDD.
- Circadian rhythms control biological processes that are frequent problems in depressed persons:
  - Interrupted sleep–rest cycle
  - Rapid eye movement (REM) sleep abnormalities
  - Frequent waking
  - Intensified dreaming
  - Diurnal variations to circadian-related behaviors
  - Decreased arousal and energy levels
  - Decreased activity patterns
  - Increased cortisol secretion
  - Increased emotional reactivity

INCIDENCE AND DEMOGRAPHICS

- MDD is a common illness, with ~5% of the U.S. population 18 years of age or older in a given year, or 15 million U.S. adults, having the disorder.
- MDD is the leading cause of disability in the United States and is the most common psychiatric illness seen in primary care practices; however, only 50% of people with MDD ever receive treatment.
- MDD can occur at any age; however, the average age at onset is the mid-20s.
- During the reproductive years, the lifetime risk for MDD varies with gender—25% for women and 12% for men; the risk is equal for the genders before puberty and after menopause.
- MDD is a greater source of morbidity for women than any other illness.
- MDD is associated with high mortality; 15% of people with MDD will die by suicide. People with MDD have a four times greater risk of premature death than the control population.
- The disease course is variable and can involve isolated episodes separated by many years, clusters of episodes, or a severe episode with some remission of symptoms but with chronic symptoms persisting over time.
- If left untreated, an episode of MDD usually lasts for 4 months or longer.

- MDD tends to be a chronic, recurrent illness.
- One year after an initial diagnosis of MDD, symptoms often persist.
  - 40% of clients have enough significant symptoms to meet full Diagnostic and Statistical Manual of Mental Disorders, Fifth Edition, Text Revision (DSM-5-TR; American Psychiatric Association [APA], 2022) criteria for MDD.
  - 20% of clients do not meet full DSM-5- TR criteria but still have a significant symptom level that impairs functioning.
  - 40% have no symptoms.
- The number of prior episodes predicts the likelihood of future episodes (Judd et al., 2000).
- People with a first episode of major depression have an ~60% risk of a second episode.
  - People who experience a second episode have an ~70% risk of a third episode.
  - People who experience a third episode have an ~90% risk of a fourth episode.

RISK FACTORS

- Genetic loading
  - Family history, especially a first-degree relative
- Prior episode of MDD
- Female sex
- Postpartum period
- Medical comorbidity
- Single marital status
- Significant environmental stressors, especially multiple losses

PREVENTION AND SCREENING

- Provide at-risk family education.
- Provide community education to help reduce stigma, to convey signs and symptoms of illness, and to emphasize the treatment potential for the control of symptoms.
- Provide significant screening efforts to help recognize, intervene, and initiate treatment early.

- Provide health care provider with education to facilitate early recognition and effective treatment.
- A significant and protracted prodromal symptom period is usually noted before full onset of illness.

ASSESSMENT

Conduct baseline screening with a tool such as the Patient Health Questionnaire 9 (PHQ-9); the Edinburgh Postnatal Depression Scale (EPDS; Siu & U.S. Preventive Task Force, 2016); the Beck Depression Inventory (BDI); or the Hamilton Depression Rating Scale (HAM-D) and repeat throughout the course of treatment to evaluate initial symptoms and response to treatment.

Client History

- Detailed history of present illness, including time frame, progression, and any associated symptoms
- Social history, including present living situation, relationship status, education, occupation, spirituality, and substance use/misuse history to include tobacco, alcohol, prescription drugs, and illicit substances
- Medication use, including prescription, over-the-counter, alternative, supplements, and home remedies
- Recent medical illness or surgery
- Initial and periodic functional history and assessment
- Validation of history with family member
    - Initial presentation often manifests as vague somatic complaints
        - Bodily aches, pains
        - Headaches
        - Muscle pains
        - Lack of energy
        - Gastrointestinal problems
- When mood is the presenting complaint, often client word choice may be vague or indirect.
    - The person may describe mood as depressed, discouraged, sad, "blue," "blah," or "down in the dumps."

  - ◊ Irritable mood is a frequent subjective state validated by a significant person in the client's life.
- ♦ Characteristic low energy is seen, so assess for individual activity intolerance without other apparent cause.
- ♦ Anhedonia is almost always present to some degree.
- ♦ Sleep disturbance is almost always present.
  - ◊ Typically problems occur with middle or terminal insomnia.
  - ◊ Hypersomnia can be present.
  - ◊ Diurnal variations can be present.
- ♦ A prodromal episode consisting of a high level of subjective anxiety and mild depressive symptoms often develops over days to weeks before onset of a full episode.
- ♦ Women often report symptoms occurring in a fixed pattern around several days before onset of menses, so assess for menstrual history.
- ♦ Psychotic features can be present, so always assess for their presence.
- ♦ Assess for client's symptoms according to diagnostic criteria for MDD:
  - ◊ Anhedonia or a depressed mood, or both
  - ◊ Depressed mood most of the day, nearly every day, as indicated by subjective reports or observations of others
    - In children, irritable mood
  - ◊ Marked anhedonia in all or almost all activities of daily living
  - ◊ At least three or more significant symptoms present during the same 2-week period that represent a change in previous functioning
  - ◊ Significant, unintentional weight loss or gain of more than 5% of body weight with increased appetite and usually a concurrent craving for specific foods, such as carbohydrates or sweets
  - ◊ Hypersomnia or insomnia nearly every day
  - ◊ Psychomotor agitation or retardation
  - ◊ Fatigue or loss of energy
  - ◊ Self-deprecating comments or thoughts
  - ◊ Feelings of worthlessness or excessive or inappropriate guilt nearly every day
  - ◊ Decreased concentration and memory
  - ◊ Recurrent morbid thoughts or suicidal ideation
  - ◊ Symptoms that begin within 2 months of significant loss such as death of a loved one and do not persist beyond 2 months are generally considered bereavement and not MDD.

Physical Exam Findings

- There are no specific physical findings.
- People with certain other disorders (such as diabetes, myocardial infarction, carcinomas, stroke) have a statistically significant increased risk for MDD.
    - Prognosis for treatment of other disorders is poor if MDD is not recognized and effectively treated.
- Clients with MDD may have trouble participating in assessments related to the cognitive problems of the disorder.
    - Impaired ability to report chronological timeline of illness
    - Poor decision-making
    - Slowed thought processes
    - Poor concentration
- Clients with MDD often have psychomotor findings.
    - Agitation
    - Retardation

Mental Status Exam Findings

- Appearance
    - Unkempt
    - Tired-looking
    - Clothing showing little attention or care about how the person looks
    - Dark-colored, loose-fitting clothing
    - Significant weight change from baseline
- Mood
    - Sad
    - "Depressed"
    - Anxious
    - Irritable
- Affect
    - Constricted or blunted
    - Sad, tearful

    - ◊ Anxious
    - ◊ Irritable
- ♦ Speech
    - ◊ Underproductive
    - ◊ Slowed response times
    - ◊ Monotonal intonation
- ♦ Thought process
    - ◊ Usually organized but may be disorganized if psychosis present
    - ◊ Slowing
    - ◊ Distractible
    - ◊ Ruminative
- ♦ Thought content
    - ◊ Morbid preoccupation
    - ◊ Suicidal ideation exists on continuum of severity:
        - Guilt for not being able to overcome the depression or for what they are "putting loved ones through"
        - Thoughts that others would be better off if the person was "gone"
        - Transient recurrent thoughts of suicide
        - Nonspecific thoughts of active action to end their own life
        - Specific plan for suicide
        - Specific plan with timeline for completion
        - Specific plan with acquisition of the means to carry out plan
    - ◊ Suicidal motivation differs for different clients:
        - Desire to give up struggle
        - Attempt to end significant emotional pain
        - Lack of any visible options for dealing with stressors, hopeless, helpless
        - Anger and frustration with poor impulse control
    - ◊ Research evidence supports that it is not possible to predict accurately whether or when a person will attempt to end their life by suicide (see Table 9–1 for review of suicide assessment).
    - ◊ Suicide risk is especially high for persons with certain symptoms or history:
        - Presence of psychotic symptoms
        - History of past attempts

            - History of first-degree relative who died by suicide
            - Concurrent substance use or dependency
            - Current serious health problem (see the following sections for clinical management of suicidality)
- ♦ Orientation
    - ◊ Client is usually oriented to person, place, and time unless psychosis is present.
- ♦ Memory
    - ◊ Usually impaired recent and short-term memory
- ♦ Concentration
    - ◊ Usually significantly impaired
- ♦ Abstraction
    - ◊ Abstract ability on proverb testing usually intact
    - ◊ If concrete, assess for other psychotic findings
- ♦ Insight
    - ◊ May be intact or impaired
- ♦ Judgment
    - ◊ May be impaired for self-welfare

TABLE 9–1.
ASSESSING FOR SUICIDAL BEHAVIOR

Past history of client attempts to end their own life or suicide death in family
Negativity and morbidity
Suicidal ideation currently
Plan and intent for suicide action
Means and access to suicide
Perceived social supports
Lethality of intended suicide action:
High lethality: Jumping from significant height, gun, hanging
Moderate lethality: Overdose of toxic agents (such as aspirin, sleeping pills)
Low lethality: Superficial wrist-cutting, breath-holding
Impulsivity
Substance use or dependence
History of psychiatric disorder

Diagnostic and Laboratory Findings

- No laboratory findings specific to MDD exist
- Complete blood count (CBC), chemistry profile, thyroid function tests, B_{12} and folate levels to rule out metabolic causes or unidentified conditions
- Consider referral for sleep study if snoring, apnea, or suspicion of other sleep disorder
- Drug toxicity screening, if indicated by history
- Depression related to a differential diagnosis

DIFFERENTIAL DIAGNOSIS

- Endocrine disorders
    - Hypothyroidism
    - Diabetes
    - Hyperaldosteronism
    - Cushing's or Addison's disease
- Neurological disorders
    - Stroke
    - Epilepsy
    - Dementia
    - Huntington's disease
    - Sleep apnea
    - Wilson's disease
    - Neoplasms
    - Head trauma
    - Multiple sclerosis
    - Parkinson's disease
- Cardiac disorders
    - Myocardial infarction
    - Congestive heart failure
    - Hypertension

- Infectious and inflammatory states
  - Mononucleosis
  - AIDS
  - Pneumonia: viral and bacterial
  - Systemic lupus erythematous
  - Temporal arteritis
  - Tuberculosis
- Nutritional disorders
  - Pernicious anemia
  - Pellagra
- Other disorders
  - Fibromyalgia
  - Chronic fatigue syndrome
  - Bereavement or grief reaction
  - Electrolyte imbalance
  - Uremia and other renal conditions
- Psychiatric disorders
  - Anxiety disorders
  - Eating disorders
  - Bipolar affective disorder
  - Substance dependence–related disorders
- Medications that can cause altered mood states as side effects
  - Steroids
  - Estrogen compounds
  - Antihypertensive agents
  - Anti-Parkinson's agents
  - Antineoplastic agents
  - Antibacterial and antifungal agents
  - Analgesics
  - Isotretinoin (Accutane)
  - Benzodiazepines

CLINICAL MANAGEMENT

- The top goal in the acute phase of MDD is ensuring client safety.
- A general consideration is to rule out or treat any conditions that may contribute to depression and cognitive impairment.
- Assess for the acuity level of client presentation.

Reasons for brief hospitalization during acute episodes of MDD include the following:

- Ensure client safety
- Initiate medication change, when doing so as an outpatient poses undue risk
- Restabilize on medication
- Monitor suicidality
- Ensure client adherence with treatment to reach stabilization

Clinical management during nonacute episodes occurs most often in community settings.

- Obtain baseline labs as indicated before initiation of treatment.
  - Pharmacological management
  - Nonpharmacological management (psychotherapy)

Pharmacological Management

- Inform client that a therapeutic effect may take at least 4 to 6 weeks.
- Once started, continue antidepressants for a minimum of 6 to 12 months.
  - If client has more than two prior episodes of MDD, consider continuing antidepressants indefinitely.
- Not all symptoms of MDD will respond to pharmacological interventions.
  - Identify clear, measurable target symptoms and educate the client about these symptoms (see Table 9–2).
- Research has found that the most effective intervention is a combination of medication and psychotherapy.
- Antidepressant rebound is common when stopping antidepressants abruptly, particularly when drugs with short half-lives are involved.
- Antidepressants may induce mania or mixed mania in susceptible persons.

- All antidepressants have FDA box warnings regarding suicidality for children, adolescents, and young adults.
- Classes of antidepressants
    - Selective serotonin reuptake inhibitors (SSRIs)
        - Act primarily to increase serotonin levels in the CNS by inhibiting their presynaptic reuptake
        - See Table 9–3 for examples.
    - Tricyclic antidepressants (TCAs)
        - Elevate serotonin and norepinephrine levels primarily by inhibiting their presynaptic reuptake
        - See Table 9–4 for examples.
    - Monoamine oxidase inhibitors (MAOIs)
        - Elevate serotonin and norepinephrine levels primarily by inhibiting MAO, the enzyme that breaks down monoamine neurotransmitters
        - See Table 9–5 for examples.
    - Serotonin norepinephrine reuptake inhibitors (SNRIs)
        - Inhibit dual reuptake of norepinephrine and serotonin
        - Action very selective on neurotransmitters
        - Elevate serotonin and norepinephrine levels by inhibiting their presynaptic reuptake
        - See Table 9–6 for examples.

TABLE 9–2.
TARGET SYMPTOMS OF ANTIDEPRESSANT TREATMENT

Target symptoms
Depressed mood
Sleep–rest disturbances
Anxiety
Irritability
Impaired concentration
Impaired memory
Appetite disturbance
Agitation
Anhedonia
Impaired energy and motivation

TABLE 9–3.
DRUGS FOR MOOD DISORDERS: ANTIDEPRESSANTS—SELECTIVE SEROTONIN REUPTAKE INHIBITORS AND SEROTONIN MODULATORS

AGENT SSRIS	DOSAGE	SIDE EFFECTS	COMMENTS
Citalopram	20–40 mg/day	Sedation, sexual dysfunction, agitation, yawning, GI disturbance, weight gain	QTc interval in doses above 40 mg (20 mg in older adults) and in those susceptible to prolonged QTc Pregnancy Category C Lactation Category L2
Escitalopram	10–20 mg/day	Somnolence, headache, sexual dysfunction, GI disturbances	Pregnancy Category C Lactation Category L2
Fluoxetine	20–80 mg/day	Insomnia, headache, GI disturbance, sexual dysfunction	Long half-life Discontinuation syndrome unlikely Pregnancy Category C Lactation Category L2
Fluvoxamine	100–300 mg/day	Sedation, sexual dysfunction, agitation GI disturbances	Doses above 150 mg should generally be given b.i.d. Pregnancy Category C Lactation Category L2
Paroxetine	20–60 mg/day	Headache, GI disturbances, somnolence, sexual dysfunction	Discontinuation syndrome very common Pregnancy Category D Lactation Category L2
Sertraline	50–200 mg/day	Nausea, headache, sleep disturbance, GI disturbance	Pregnancy Category C Lactation Category L2
Serotonin Modulators			
Nefazodone	50–250 mg/day	Headache, nausea, constipation	Pregnancy Category C Lactation Category L4
Trazodone	50–300 mg/day	Somnolence, nausea, diarrhea	Pregnancy Category C Lactation Category L2
Vilazodone	20–40 mg/day	Diarrhea, nausea	Pregnancy Category C Lactation Category L3
Vortioxetine	5–20 mg/day	Diarrhea, nausea, sexual dysfunction	Pregnancy Category C Lactation Category L3

GI, gastrointestinal; QTc, corrected QT (interval); SSRI, selective serotonin reuptake inhibitor

TABLE 9–4.
TRICYCLIC ANTIDEPRESSANTS

AGENT	DOSAGE	COMMENTS
Amitriptyline	50–300 mg/day	Also used for chronic pain (particularly neuropathic), insomnia Pregnancy Category C Lactation Category L2
Amoxapine	200–300 mg/day	Do not use with increased QTc intervals or acute myocardial infarction or history of seizures Pregnancy Category C Lactation Category L2
Clomip-ramine	100–250 mg/day	Approved for obsessive–compulsive disorder; 250 mg/day maximum because of increased seizure risk Pregnancy Category C Lactation Category L2
Desipramine	100–300 mg/day	Also used for ADHD (off-label for pediatric clients and for ADHD) Pregnancy Category C Lactation Category L2
Doxepin	100–300 mg/day	Also used for insomnia Pregnancy Category C Lactation Category L5 Avoid
Imipramine	100–300 mg/day	Also used for enuresis and separation anxiety Pregnancy Category D Lactation Category L2
Nortriptyline	50–150 mg/day	Also used for enuresis and ADHD Pregnancy Category D Lactation Category L2
Protriptyline	15–60 mg/day	Pregnancy Category C Lactation Category: Inadequate data
trimipramine	100–300 mg/day	Pregnancy Category C Lactation Category: Inadequate data

ADHD, attention-deficit/hyperactivity disorder; QTc, corrected QT (interval)

TABLE 9–5.
MONOAMINE OXIDASE INHIBITORS

DRUG	DOSAGE	COMMENTS
Isocarboxazid	20–60 mg/day	Also used for panic disorder, phobic disorders, selective mutism
Phenelzine	45–90 mg/day	Caution: High-tyramine diet; sympathomimetic agents Divided dosing: b.i.d. and q.i.d.
Tranylcypromine	30–60 mg/day	All Pregnancy Category C Lactation Category: Inadequate Information
Selegiline	Transdermal patch 6–12 mg	No dietary restrictions with 6 mg dose; may need higher dose to see antidepressant effect Pregnancy Category C Lactation Category L4 Avoid

TABLE 9–6.
SEROTONIN NOREPINEPHRINE REUPTAKE INHIBITORS

AGENT	DOSAGE	SIDE EFFECTS	COMMENTS
Desvenlafaxine	50 mg/day	Nausea, diaphoresis, dizziness	Can raise blood pressure Pregnancy Category C Lactation Category L3
Duloxetine	30–120 mg/day	Dizziness, headache, GI disturbances	Can elevate blood pressure Can elevate liver function test results Has significant discontinuation syndrome if stopped abruptly Pregnancy Category C Lactation Category L3
Levomilnacipran	40–120 mg/day	Nausea, hypotension, erectile dysfunction, constipation	Pregnancy Category C Lactation Category: No data available
Venlafaxine	112.5–225 mg/day	Diaphoresis, headache, dizziness, GI disturbance	Can increase blood pressure Safer in overdose than TCAs Significant discontinuation syndrome if stopped abruptly Pregnancy Category C Lactation Category L3

GI, gastrointestinal; TCA, tricyclic antidepressant

- ◊ Norepinephrine dopamine reuptake inhibitors (NDRIs)
  - Inhibit dual reuptake of norepinephrine and dopamine
  - Action very selective on neurotransmitters
  - Elevate dopamine and norepinephrine levels by inhibiting their presynaptic reuptake
- ◊ Serotonin agonist and reuptake inhibitors (SARIs)
  - Dual action
  - Agonist of serotonin 5-hydroxytryptamine (5-HT2) receptors
  - Action very selective on neurotransmitters
  - Elevate serotonin levels by inhibiting serotonin reuptake

- ♦ The various antidepressants differ markedly in characteristics such as
  - ◊ Cost
  - ◊ Side-effect profile
  - ◊ Safety in overdose
  - ◊ Safety in clients with other disorders
  - ◊ Drug–drug interactions
  - ◊ Cytochrome P450 (CYP) enzyme liver effects
- ♦ To achieve the best control of symptoms, match the client's symptom profile to the pharmacodynamic and pharmacokinetic properties of specific antidepressant agents.

SSRIs

- ♦ First-line treatment for first episode of major depression with mild to moderate symptoms
- ♦ Serious side effects are rare
- ♦ Much safer in overdose than TCAs
- ♦ Also effective for panic disorder, obsessive–compulsive disorder, bulimia, generalized anxiety disorder, social phobia, posttraumatic stress disorder, and premenstrual dysphoric disorder

TCAs

- ♦ Considered second-line drugs for treating MDD (see Table 9–4)

- Affect many neurotransmitters, leading to more side effects and possibly poor adherence
  - Anticholinergic: Dry mouth, blurred vision, constipation, memory problems (from muscarinic receptor blockade)
  - Antiadrenergic: Orthostatic hypotension (from alpha 1 receptor blockade)
  - Antihistaminergic: Sedation and weight gain (from histamine receptor blockade)
  - Electrocardiogram (ECG) changes and cardiac dysrhythmias possible; avoid in clients known to have susceptibility (personal or family history). Monitor ECG before treatment and annually in older adults.
  - Unsafe in many co-occurring disorders (such as cardiac disease)
  - Known to induce hypomania in susceptible clients
- Well-identified serum blood levels guide dosing (particularly with nortriptyline) and predict toxicity.
- Inexpensive and available in generic forms.
- Anticholinergic properties may be highly problematic but may also be useful in clients with significant bowel irritability.
- Avoid abrupt withdrawal because of significant discontinuation syndrome.
- Avoid prescribing to people who are at high risk for suicide; the lethal dose is 1,000 mg or more (a week's supply of an average dose). Combination of TCAs with MAOIs can cause lethal serotonin syndrome, hypertensive crisis, or both; adhere to 2-week washout period (5 weeks for fluoxetine) before switching between the two classes of medications.
- Use caution if the person is taking both a TCA and an SSRI, because the SSRI can elevate TCA concentrations because of pharmacodynamic or pharmacokinetic interactions. Monitor TCA levels.

MAOIs

- MAOIs are unsafe in many co-occurring disorders.
- Can be fatal in overdose
- Side-effect profile and stringent dietary restrictions often lead to poor client adherence.
- Clinically significant side effects of MAOIs include
  - Insomnia
  - Hypertensive crisis

- ◊ Weight gain
- ◊ Anticholinergic side effects
- ◊ Lightheadedness and dizziness
- ◊ Sexual dysfunction

- ♦ Not first- or second-line agents for MDD because of dangerous food and drug interactions (see Tables 9–5 and 9–7)
  - ◊ Hypertensive crisis occurs when MAOIs are taken in conjunction with foods containing tyramine, a dietary precursor to norepinephrine.
    - When MAO is inhibited, tyramine exerts a strong vasopressor effect, stimulating the release of catecholamines, epinephrine, and norepinephrine, which can increase blood pressure and heart rate.
    - Hypertensive crisis is life-threatening and cannot be reversed unless more MAO is produced by the body.
  - ◊ Hypertensive crisis and death also can occur when MAOIs are taken in conjunction with certain medications:
    - Meperidine
    - Decongestants
    - TCAs
    - Atypical antipsychotics
    - St. John's wort
    - L-tryptophan
    - Stimulants and other sympathomimetics
    - Asthma medications

TABLE 9–7.
TYRAMINE-FREE DIETARY CONSIDERATIONS

CATEGORY OF FOOD	SPECIFIC FOODS TO AVOID
Cheeses	Aged cheeses, such as blue, brie, Camembert, and Roquefort
Meat	Smoked, aged, and cured meats such as sausages, pastrami, and salami
Fish	Smoked, aged, and cured fish such as pickled herring and salted fish
Beverages	Any aged and fermented beverages such as red wine, aged liquors, whiskey (gin and vodka permissible), beer (bottled and pasteurized permissible)
Other	Bean curd (tofu), soy products, sauerkraut, miso, yeast extract, monosodium glutamate (MSG), ripe bananas, avocado

- ◊ Symptoms of hypertensive crisis
  - Sudden, explosive-like headache, usually in occipital region
  - Elevated blood pressure
  - Facial flushing
  - Palpitations
  - Pupillary dilation
  - Diaphoresis
  - Fever
- ◊ Treatment of hypertensive crisis
  - Discontinue the MAOI.
  - Give phentolamine (binds with norepinephrine receptor sites, blocks norepinephrine).
  - Stabilize fever.
  - Reevaluate the person's diet and adherence and reiterate medication guidelines, as necessary.
- ◊ People taking MAOIs must follow a tyramine-free diet and must avoid many medications, including most over-the-counter cold and allergy preparations.
- ◊ Combining an MAOI with a serotonergic agent is contraindicated because this may cause serotonin syndrome.
  - Symptoms of serotonin syndrome
    - Agitation, restlessness
    - Rapid heart rate and elevation in blood pressure
    - Headache
    - Sweating, shivering, and goose bumps
    - Myoclonic jerking and loss of coordination
    - Confusion, fever, seizures, unconsciousness
  - Treatment of serotonin syndrome includes discontinuing the offending agents and supportive treatment of symptoms. Mild symptoms such as restlessness may respond to removal of the offending agent, close monitoring, and judicious use of a benzodiazepine. More severe symptoms constitute a medical emergency necessitating hospitalization and treatment such as cyproheptadine, anticonvulsants, and autonomic support.

♦ Clients who are taking MAOIs must be educated to recognize the signs and symptoms of hypertensive crisis and serotonin syndrome and understand that they must seek immediate medical attention should they suspect either one of occurring.

OTHER ANTIDEPRESSANTS

- Other antidepressants used in the treatment of MDD may be classified as SNRIs, NDRIs, and SARIs (see Tables 9-6 and 9-8).
- Psychotic features can be present with MDD and bipolar I disorder.
  - Routinely assess for the presence of psychotic symptoms during periods of symptom exacerbation.
  - Features are usually mood congruent.
  - Can be managed with short-term use of antipsychotic medications (see Chapter 11)
- Comorbidities are common and include various medical conditions (as noted earlier in the chapter) as well as psychiatric comorbidities such as panic disorder, obsessive–compulsive disorder, and substance use or dependence.
- Altered appetite and sleep–rest patterns predispose clients with MDD to decreased overall health status.
- Increased mortality exists in people with MDD.

TABLE 9–8.
OTHER ANTIDEPRESSANT AGENTS

AGENT	DOSAGE	SIDE EFFECTS	COMMENTS
Brexanolone	30–90 mcg/kg/hour IV	Sedation, dizziness, xerostomia	Restricted distribution, indicated for postpartum depression Pregnancy Category: No available data Lactation Category L2
Bupropion	IR 150–450 mg/day SR 150–400 mg/day ER 150–450 mg/day	Headache, nervousness tremors, tachycardia, insomnia, decreased appetite	Contraindicated if client has seizures, eating disorder Can increase energy level Also used for attention-deficit/hyperactivity disorder (off label) and smoking cessation Pregnancy Category C Lactation Category L3
Esketamine	56–84 mg twice a week for 4 weeks	Dissociative effects, sedation, dizziness, nausea	Pregnancy Category: No data available Lactation Category: No available data

AGENT	DOSAGE	SIDE EFFECTS	COMMENTS
Mirtazapine	15–45 mg/day	Sedation, weight gain, increased cholesterol	Inverse relationship between dose and sedation Pregnancy Category C Lactation Category L3
Nefazodone	300–600 mg/day	Headache, drowsiness, GI disturbances	Must monitor liver function test results Can cause liver failure Safer in overdose than TCAs CYP 3A4 inhibitor Pregnancy Category C Lactation Category L4 Avoid
Trazodone	200–600 mg/day	Sedation, nausea, headache, hypotension	Safer in overdose than TCAs Priapism possible Not well tolerated at antidepressant dose because of sedation Most commonly used for sleep May prolong QTc interval Pregnancy Category B Lactation Category L2
Vilazodone	20–40 mg/day	Diarrhea, nausea, headache, xerostomia	Pregnancy Category C Lactation Category L3
Vortioxetine	20 mg/day	Nausea, diarrhea, dizziness, xerostomia	Pregnancy Category C Lactation Category L3
Zuranolone	50 mg q.p.m. × 14 days	Somnolence, dizziness, nasopharyngitis, diarrhea	Indicated for postpartum depression Pregnancy Category A Lactation Category L2

CYP, Potent cytochrome P450; ER, extended release; GI, gastrointestinal; IR, immediate release; QTc, corrected QT (interval); SR, sustained release; TCA, tricyclic antidepressant

Nonpharmacological Management

- Electroconvulsive therapy (ECT)
    - Generalized tonic-clonic seizure induced in anesthetized person
    - Usual course is 6 to 12 treatments
    - Mechanism of action
        - Neurotransmitter theory: Increases dopamine, serotonin, and norepinephrine
        - Neuroendocrine theory: Releases hormones such as prolactin, thyroid-stimulating hormone, pituitary hormones, endorphins, and adrenocorticotropic hormone
        - Anticonvulsant theory: Exerts an anticonvulsant effect, which then produces an antidepressant effect
    - APNA ECT Treatment Considerations Checklist
    - Situations in which ECT is used
        - Client preference
        - Need for rapid response because of severity of illness
        - MDD with psychotic features
        - Risk of other treatment outweighs risk of ECT
        - Treatment resistance
    - Possible contraindications
        - Cardiac disease
        - Compromised pulmonary status
        - History of brain injury or brain tumor
        - Anesthesia medical complications
    - Adverse effects
        - Possible cardiovascular effects
        - Systemic effects (e.g., headaches, muscle aches, drowsiness)
        - Cognitive effects (e.g., memory disturbance and confusion)
- Transcranial magnetic stimulation (TMS)
    - Option for clients who have not had adequate response to medications and psychotherapy (treatment-resistant depression)
    - Involves placement of small wire coil on scalp to conduct electrical current, creating a magnetic field through the tissues of the head
    - Performed in office setting, without anesthesia
    - Sessions typically last 40 minutes and the typical course is five sessions per week for 6 weeks.

  - Side effects are minimal but may include headache, scalp discomfort, tingling or twitches to facial muscles, lightheadedness, and hearing discomfort from procedure noise.
  - Seizures, although rare, have been reported.
- Vagus nerve stimulation (VNS)
  - Option for clients who have not had an adequate response to medications and psychotherapy (treatment-resistant depression)
  - Pacemaker-like device implanted in left side of chest to stimulate left branch of vagus nerve; transcutaneous devices being tested
  - Generally done as outpatient procedure but anesthesia is required
  - Side effects generally occur as the pulse generator stimulates the vagus nerve and include voice changes, hoarseness, cough, throat or neck pain, chest spasms, dyspnea on exertion, tingling of skin, dysphagia
  - Intended for use along with traditional treatments
- Phototherapy
  - 2,500 to 10,000 lux for 30 minutes up to 2 hours, one to two times per day (Sadock et al., 2017)
- Individual therapy (see Chapter 8, Nonpharmacological Treatment)

Psychodynamic psychotherapy

Cognitive behavioral therapy (CBT)

- Modify perceptions
- Decrease negativity
- Increase sense of internal control
- Enhance coping skills
- Modify environmental factors contributing to illness

Brief therapy (solution-focused therapy)

- Focus on precipitant stressor
- Cope with immediate impact of MDD on personal life
- Modify contributory environmental factors

Group therapy

- Improve decision-making
- Improve socialization skills

- Improve assessment of individual strengths
- Gain new coping skills

Family therapy

- Enhance family coping
- Improve knowledge base
- Plan for relapse
- Gain insight into the effects of MDD on the family unit
- Undertake psychoeducation for family members about the illness state of MDD

Clinical Management of Suicidality

- Pay significant attention to positive assessments for suicidality.
- Always assume client is serious when they vocalize suicidal thoughts.
- Identify current stressors that may be contributing to crisis.
- May manage in community setting for clients with low to moderate risk; generally do not manage in community setting during acute suicidal ideation periods unless client is able to make a collaborative safety plan.
- Consider hospitalization.
- Consider mobilizing available social resources.

Risk factors for suicide

- Age 45 or older if male
- Age 55 or older if female
- Divorced, single, or separated
- White
- Living alone
- Psychiatric disorder
- Physical illness
- Substance use

- Previous attempt(s) to end their own life
- Family history of suicide
- Recent loss
- Male sex

LIFE SPAN CONSIDERATIONS

Children

- Core symptoms of MDD are the same for children. However, some symptoms are more pronounced in children.
    - Irritability
    - Somatic complaints
    - Social withdrawal
- Some core symptoms are less common in children before the onset of puberty:
    - Psychosis
    - Motor retardation
    - Hypersomnia
    - Increased appetite
- MDD often has a strong separation anxiety component in children.
- Children usually do not respond well to TCAs; however, they do respond well to SSRIs.
- All antidepressants indicated for children, adolescents, and young adults carry a FDA box warning about an increase in suicidal thoughts; monitor closely for suicidal thoughts, behavior, agitation, and aggression in children taking antidepressants.

Older Adults

- Persons with MDD admitted to a long-term care facility have significantly shorter life spans than the control population.
- Sixty-five percent are more likely to die within the first year in a long-term care facility.

- Cognition and memory symptoms of MDD in the older adult population often are confused with dementia-related symptoms (pseudodementia).
  - Clients with dementia usually have a premorbid history of slowly declining cognition.
  - In MDD, cognitive changes have a relatively acute onset and are significant when compared to premorbid functioning.
- It is important to complete a functional assessment for older adults.
  - Determines the degree to which the person's abilities and performance match the demands of their life
  - Determines the impact of illness on overall functioning
  - Skill deficit: Inability to perform a functional skill despite the physical ability, as in dementia
  - Performance deficit: Ability to perform a functional skill but lacks the motivation to do so, as in depression
- Reasons for performing functional assessment
  - To correctly diagnose (e.g., to differentiate depression from dementia)
  - To track client improvement or decompensation
  - To help families set realistic expectations
- Components of functional assessment
  - Activities of daily living (ADLs): Basic self-care skills, such as bathing, dressing, eating, and toileting
  - Instrumental activities of daily living (IADLs): Complex activities needed for independent functioning, such as shopping, cooking, driving, and housekeeping
  - Executive functioning: Judgment and planning; ability to maintain calendar, manage money and appointments, and prioritize activities
- The degree of change over time and the speed of change are better observed with objective recording and when the assessment is measured at intervals such as every 6 months.

FOLLOW-UP

- Follow-up care practices for the PMHNP to consider
  - Include teaching client the goals, risks, benefits, and potential side effects of medication treatment
  - Continuously monitor client's response to medication; the treatment goal is complete remission of symptoms.

- ◊ Utilize screening tools such as the PHQ-9 in follow-up appointments.
- ◊ Educate clients about the symptoms of depression and that it is a chronic illness; establish a relapse plan for all clients.
- ◊ Assess for suicidality during every client contact.
- ◊ Assess for the presence of psychotic symptoms during every client contact.
- ◊ Assess and manage client for side effects of treatment, including sexual side effects, in an attempt to increase medication adherence.
- ◊ Observe all clients treated with antidepressants for development of serotonin syndrome (overstimulation of serotonin receptors usually caused by drug–drug interactions).

- ♦ Drug combinations that can cause serotonin syndrome
  - ◊ SSRIs and MAOIs
  - ◊ SSRIs and TCAs
  - ◊ Triptans
  - ◊ Opioids
  - ◊ Drug and herbal interactions
  - ◊ SSRIs and St. John's wort
- ♦ Symptoms of serotonin syndrome
  - ◊ Autonomic instability
  - ◊ Altered sensorium
  - ◊ Restlessness
  - ◊ Agitation
  - ◊ Myoclonus
  - ◊ Hyperreflexia
  - ◊ Hyperthermia
  - ◊ Diaphoresis
  - ◊ Tremor
  - ◊ Chills
  - ◊ Diarrhea and cramps
  - ◊ Ataxia
  - ◊ Headache
  - ◊ Insomnia
- ♦ Monitor for adverse effects over time.

- Some SSRIs are known to increase blood glucose and contribute to hyperlipidemia, and others may elevate liver function test results.
- Discontinue SSRIs slowly to prevent discontinuation syndrome.
- Symptoms of discontinuation syndrome
  - Flu-like symptoms (due to cholinergic rebound; particularly problematic with TCAs)
  - Fatigue and lethargy
  - Myalgia
  - Decreased concentration
  - Nausea and vomiting
  - Impaired memory
  - Paresthesias, including "shock-like" sensations
  - Irritability
  - Anxiety
  - Insomnia
  - Crying without provocation
  - Dizziness and vertigo
- Risk factors for discontinuation syndrome
  - Medications with short half-lives
  - Abrupt discontinuation
  - Inconsistent, irregular use pattern
  - High dose range
  - Long-term treatment
  - Prior history of discontinuation syndrome
- Expected course of MDD
  - Evidence indicates the best treatment outcomes if medications are used in conjunction with appropriate therapy.
  - Evidence indicates that clients should take an antidepressant agent for at least 12 months after remission of symptoms.
  - Clients who have had three or more episodes of MDD usually require lifelong medication.

PERSISTENT DEPRESSIVE DISORDER (DYSTHYMIA)

DESCRIPTION

- A disorder similar to MDD but with less-acute symptoms; with a more protracted, chronic disease course; and without any manifestations of psychotic symptoms
- Less discrete episodes of illness than MDD
- Symptoms often go undetected and, therefore, untreated for years.
- Vegetative symptoms (e.g., sleep, appetite, weight changes) are much less common in dysthymia than in MDD.

ETIOLOGY

- Similar to MDD (see MDD Etiology, page 172)

INCIDENCE AND DEMOGRAPHICS

- Affects 5.4% of the U.S. population ages 18 or older, or 10.9 million Americans
- People with dysthymia have an increased risk for developing MDD; 15% to 25% of people diagnosed with dysthymia will have a lifetime episode of MDD.
- People with onset of symptoms before age 21 have a 75% likelihood of a lifetime episode of MDD.
- Women are two to three times more likely to develop dysthymic disorder than men.

RISK FACTORS

- Genetic predisposition
- A first-degree relative with MDD
- A first-degree relative with dysthymia
- Female sex

PREVENTION AND SCREENING

- At-risk family education
- Community education
- Stigma reduction
- Signs and symptoms of illness
- Treatment potential for control of symptoms
- Early recognition, intervention, and initiation of treatment
- Because of the chronic nature of the disorder, symptoms become a part of a client's day-to-day existence and often go unreported unless solicited by direct questioning.
- Aggressive screening procedure required

ASSESSMENT

Client History

- Assess for the following:
    - Chronically depressed mood that occurs for most of the day, more days than not, for at least 2 years
    - Prominent presence of low self-esteem, self-criticism, and a perception of general incompetence compared to others
    - Other common symptoms
        - Low energy and fatigue
        - Poor concentration
        - Difficulty with decision-making
        - Feelings of hopelessness
        - Feelings of inadequacy
        - Mild anhedonia
        - Social withdrawal
        - Brooding about past issues
        - Subjective irritability or anger
        - Decreased productivity and activity

- ◊ Less common symptoms
    - Alteration in appetite
    - Alteration in sleep–rest patterns

Physical Exam Findings

- Similar to MDD (see MDD Physical Exam Findings, page 180)

Mental Status Exam Findings

- Similar to MDD (see MDD Mental Status Exam Findings, page 180)
- Usually no vegetative findings
- Mood described as sad, "down for all of my life"

Diagnostic and Laboratory Findings

- No specific diagnostic lab findings exist.
- Consider referral for sleep study if snoring, apnea, or suspicion of other sleep disorder

DIFFERENTIAL DIAGNOSIS

- Similar to MDD (see MDD Differential Diagnosis, page 183)

CLINICAL MANAGEMENT

Pharmacological Management

- Because of increased risk for development of MDD, dysthymia is often treated with antidepressant medications in a manner similar to that for MDD (see MDD Pharmacological Management, page 186).

Nonpharmacological Management

- Similar to MDD (see MDD Nonpharmacological Management, page 196)
- Treat any underling sleep disorders as identified by sleep studies.
- Often good clinical outcomes with nonpharmacological management if client is willing

Common Comorbidities

- MDD is often superimposed on dysthymia (double depression)
- The subjective worsening of symptoms or onset of new symptoms such as vegetative ones often brings the person into treatment.
- When dysthymia precedes MDD, clinical management is more complex, and outcomes can be less positive.
- Dysthymic disorder is associated with personality disorders.
  - Borderline
  - Histrionic
  - Narcissistic
  - Avoidant
  - Dependent

LIFE SPAN CONSIDERATIONS

- Similar to MDD (see MDD Life Span Considerations, page 199)
- In children, prevalence rates of dysthymia are equal for boys and girls.
- Associated with several childhood disorders
  - Attention-deficit/hyperactivity disorder
  - Conduct disorder
  - Anxiety disorders
  - Learning disorders
- The period of symptoms required for diagnosis is only 1 year, compared with 2 years for adults.

- In children, the mood is usually described as irritable rather than sad but may report both irritability and sadness
- Low self-esteem, poor social skills, and pessimism

FOLLOW-UP

- Similar to MDD (see MDD Follow-Up, page 201)

GRIEF AND BEREAVEMENT

DESCRIPTION

- Involves a wide range of normal responses that can become abnormal and excessive
- Involves normative emotional, cognitive, and behavioral reactions to death or loss of a significant person or object
- Unlike in major depression, self-esteem is usually preserved in the grieving person.
- Involve nonnormative psychological responses to an identifiable stressor that can result in the development of clinically significant emotional or behavioral symptoms
  - ◊ Stressor encompassing elements of perceived loss
  - ◊ Develops within 3 months of stressor
- Single event
  - ◊ End of relationship
  - ◊ Death of relative or partner
- Recurring event
  - ◊ Living with person with terminal illness
- Developmental event
  - ◊ Leaving home to go away to school
  - ◊ Getting married
  - ◊ Becoming a parent
  - ◊ Retiring from work

- PMHNP assessment is needed to separate normal, healthy grieving from pathological grieving, which may represent an adjustment disorder or major depression. The PMHNP must consider the following factors:
  - Severity of response
  - Duration of response
  - Effects of response on normal daily functioning
  - Person's perception of impact of stressor
- When severity or duration is excessive, grieving may be abnormal.
- In the absence of other significant clinical symptoms, grief usually is classified as an adjustment disorder:
  - Adjustment disorder with depressed mood
  - Adjustment disorder with anxiety
  - Adjustment disorder with mixed anxiety and depression
  - Adjustment disorder with disturbed conduct

ETIOLOGY

- Significant loss
- Limited coping skills
- Limited social supports

INCIDENCE AND DEMOGRAPHICS

- Normal grief is universally experienced.
- Grief is common in older adults as their social sphere begins to decrease.
- Twenty percent of older adults who lose a spouse experience depression within the first year of that loss.
- Lifetime prevalence for adjustment disorder is 2% to 8% in the U.S. population.
- Grief occurs in 12% of general hospital clients.
- Grief occurs in 50% of clients after cardiac surgery.

RISK FACTORS

- Limited social network
- Poor physical health
- Limited coping skills

PREVENTION AND SCREENING

- Ask about losses.
- Identify at-risk persons.
- Do preventative counseling.
- Begin early recognition, intervention, and initiation of treatment.
  - Routine screening in all health care settings

ASSESSMENT

- Often clients will not disclose grieving or bereavement issues unless directly asked.

Client History

- Assess for the following:
  - Recent losses
  - Anniversary dates of past losses
  - Reaction to loss
  - Functional impairment
  - Social and family support systems
  - Insomnia
  - Anorexia
  - Presence of dysfunctional coping
  - Suicidal thoughts
  - Substance use
  - Denial

Physical Exam Findings

- No physical exam findings specific to grief and bereavement

Mental Status Exam Findings

- Depressed mood
- Anxious affect
- Crying uncontrollably

Diagnostic and Laboratory Findings

- CBC, chemistry profile, thyroid function tests, and B_{12} level to rule out metabolic causes or unidentified conditions
- Drug toxicity screening, if indicated by history

DIFFERENTIAL DIAGNOSIS

- Normal grieving
- MDD
- Anxiety disorders (see Chapter 10)
- Substance-related disorders (see Chapter 13)

CLINICAL MANAGEMENT

Pharmacological Management

- If needed
    - Short-term use of anti-anxiety agents
    - Short-term use of sleep-induction agents
- Benzodiazepines
- Nonbenzodiazepine hypnotic such as zolpidem
- Tricyclic or other sedating antidepressants
- Antihistamines

Nonpharmacological Management

- Encourage expression of grief and loss.
- Use support groups.
- Offer community resources.
- Offer psychoeducation on grief reactions and responses.
- With significant functional impairment, consider psychotherapy (e.g., crisis therapy, brief solution-focused therapy, CBT).

LIFE SPAN CONSIDERATIONS

- Can occur at any age
- Older adults are at greater risk because of higher numbers of losses that may become cumulative in their impact.

FOLLOW-UP

- Follow up weekly during acute period.
- Monitor for development of MDD.
- Monitor for impact on general health state.
- Maintain supportive follow-up over time.
- Be sensitive to nontraditional losses that may be significant to the person:
  - Loss of a pet
  - Loss of status in work or school setting

PROLONGED GRIEF DISORDER

DESCRIPTION

- Prolonged grief disorder was added to the DSM-5-TR (APA, 2022) as a new diagnosis. This disorder is distinguished by grief that results in a maladaptive reaction following the death of a person who was close to the individual. Symptoms must be clinically significant and present most days. The symptoms must be present for the following durations:
  - Twelve months or more in adults
  - Six months or more in children and adolescents

- Symptoms include:
    - Intense yearning/longing for and preoccupation with the deceased person
    - Disruption of identity
    - Disbelief
    - Avoidance
    - Emotional pain
    - Unable to engage in previous interests or future planning
    - Emotionally numb
    - Feeling that life is meaningless
    - Intense loneliness
- Clinically significant impairment in social, occupational, or other areas of functioning
- Clearly exceeds the expectation of a grief reaction
- Cannot be better explained by another disorder

INCIDENCE AND DEMOGRAPHICS

- Prevalence is unknown
- Gender difference is not significant

RISK FACTORS

- Level of dependency
- Death of a child
- Violent or unexpected death
- Financial stress

PREVENTION AND SCREENING

- Ask about loss.
- Identify at-risk persons.
- Do preventative counseling.
- Begin early recognition, intervention, and initiation of treatment.

ASSESSMENT

- Often clients will not disclose grieving issues unless directly asked.

Client History

- Assess for the following:
  - Recent losses
  - Anniversary dates of past losses
  - Reaction to loss
  - Functional impairment
  - Social and family support systems
  - Insomnia
  - Anorexia
  - Presence of dysfunctional coping
  - Suicidal thoughts
  - Substance use
  - Denial

Physical Exam Findings

- No physical exam findings specific to prolonged grief disorder

Mental Status Exam Findings

- Depressed mood
- Anxious affect
- Sleep issues
- Crying uncontrollably
- Suicidality

Diagnostic and Laboratory Findings

- CBC, chemistry profile, thyroid function tests, and B_{12} level to rule out metabolic causes or unidentified conditions
- Drug toxicity screening if indicated by history

DIFFERENTIAL DIAGNOSIS

- MDD
- Posttraumatic stress disorder (PTSD)
- Acute grief
- Normative grief

CLINICAL MANAGEMENT

- Rule out or treat any conditions that may contribute to current symptom manifestation.

Pharmacological Management

- Pharmacological management has not been shown to significantly decrease symptoms.
- Depression and anxiety symptoms can be managed with SSRIs.

Nonpharmacological Management

- CBT
- Bereavement support groups
- Targeted grief therapy such as Complicated Grief Therapy (CGT)

LIFE SPAN CONSIDERATIONS

- Can occur at any age

FOLLOW-UP

- Follow-up is determined by severity and level of support.
- Monitor for symptoms of depression, anxiety, and suicidality.
- Monitor impact on general health and sleep.
- Maintain supportive follow-up over time.

PREMENSTRUAL DYSPHORIC DISORDER

DESCRIPTION

- Dysphoric symptoms that occur in response to changing sex steroid hormone levels that occur during the ovulatory menstrual cycle
- Symptoms generally begin during the luteal phase, ~1 week before the onset of menses, and generally lift within a day or two after menses has begun.
- Common symptoms include:
    - Marked lability
    - Irritability
    - Depressed mood
    - Anxiety
    - Low energy
    - Sleep disturbances

ASSESSMENT

Client History

- Symptoms occur repeatedly during each menstrual cycle and there must be a symptom-free period in the follicular phase, after menses has occurred.
- Symptoms cause marked impairment in functioning and sense of well-being.

Differential Diagnosis

- A careful evaluation must be completed to rule out other mood disorder.

CLINICAL MANAGEMENT

Pharmacological Treatment

- Treatment may consist of hormonal contraceptives, SSRIs, or both.

LIFE SPAN CONSIDERATIONS

- Symptoms may worsen as the client becomes perimenopausal.

BIPOLAR DISORDER

DESCRIPTION

- Complex brain-based illness with a primary characteristic of disturbance in mood
- Mood disturbance often of both polarities
  - Depressive
  - Expansive or manic
- Several patterns
  - Single-polarity symptoms only (mania)
  - Distinct symptom patterns of alternating polarity—manic symptoms alternating with depressive symptoms
  - Mixed, co-occurring symptoms
- Presents with excessive or distorted degree of sadness or elation, or both
- Manifests with behavioral, affective, cognitive, and somatic symptoms
- May have precipitating event, situation, or concern but often occurs without any precipitating stressor identified
- Has complex genetic, biochemical, and environmental etiological factors

ETIOLOGY

- Multiple theories ranging from psychological to neurobiological
- Probable multifactorial etiological profile

Biological Theories

- γ-Aminobutyric acid (GABA) deregulation
- Increased noradrenergic activity
- Voltage-gated ion channel abnormalities
- Abnormalities lead to abnormal balances of intracellular and extracellular levels of neurotransmitters, which then cause subsequent disruption of electric signal transmission in brain regions.
- Kindling: Process of neuronal membrane threshold sensitivity dysfunction
    - Long-lasting, epileptogenic changes induced by daily subthreshold brain stimulation
    - Brain becomes overly sensitive to electrical stimuli
    - Neuronal misfiring occurs
    - Process becomes automatic; neuronal firing occurs even without stimuli

INCIDENCE AND DEMOGRAPHICS

- Less common than MDD
- 0.7% of general population at risk
- Affects 2.3 million American adults; 1.2% of the U.S. adult population older than age 18
- Mean age at onset in early 20s
- May present in childhood (rare) or adolescent years
- Prevalence for males and females is the same.

RISK FACTORS

- Genetic loading
- Family history of first-order relative having MDD or bipolar disorder
- A 24% increased risk if relative has bipolar disorder type I (see the following sections)
- A 5% increased risk if relative has bipolar disorder type II (see the following sections)
- A 25% increased risk if relative has MDD
- For bipolar disorder type II, similar to MDD (see MDD Risk Factors, page 204)

PREVENTION AND SCREENING

- At-risk family education
- Community education
  - Stigma reduction
  - Signs and symptoms of illness
  - Treatment potential for control of symptoms
- Early recognition, intervention, and initiation of treatment
  - Significant and protracted prodromal symptom period usually noted before full onset of illness
  - Usually mild manifestations of criteria symptoms before full clinical syndrome is apparent
  - The longer time between onset of symptoms and diagnosis, the more difficult to interrupt the cyclicity of illness.
  - Depressive episodes predominate, making misdiagnosis common.

ASSESSMENT

Client History

- Assess for the following:
  - Detailed history of present illness, including time frame, progression, and any associated symptoms
  - Social history, including present living situation; marital status; occupation; education; and alcohol, tobacco, and illicit drug use
  - Medication use, including prescription, over-the-counter, alternative, supplements, and home remedies
  - Initial and periodic functional history and assessment
  - Corroborative information from family member when possible
- Diagnostic criteria
  - Period of abnormally or persistently elevated, expansive, or irritable mood, lasting for at least 1 week
  - Mood episode has rapid development and escalation of symptoms over a few days
  - Often precipitated by significant environmental stressor
  - Mood disturbance may result in brief psychotic symptoms.

- ◊ Manic episodes last days to several months.
- ◊ Briefer duration and ending more abruptly than major depressive episodes
- ◊ In 60% of people, a major depressive episode immediately precedes or follows the manic episode.
- ◊ Persistence of other suggestive symptoms
    - Decreased need for sleep
    - Feels rested after 3 hours sleep on average
    - Usually a marked difference from normal baseline sleep pattern
    - Inflated self-esteem
    - Grandiosity
    - Increased goal-directed activities
    - Excessive involvement in pleasurable activities with a high potential for painful consequences
    - Unrestrained buying sprees
    - Sexual indiscretions
    - Unsound business ventures
    - Excessive substance use
    - Highly recurrent depressive episodes
- ◊ Recurrent shifts in polarity
    - Major depressive episode shifting to a manic episode
    - Manic episode shifting to a major depressive episode
    - Major depressive episode shifting to a mixed episode
- ◊ Expansive or elated mood symptoms
    - Manic
        - Symptoms as described previously
    - Hypomanic
        - Similar to mania
        - More brief in duration
        - Episode not as severe as mania
        - Does not require hospitalization
        - Does not cause significant functional impairment

- Two common types
    - Type I
        - Clinical history characterized by occurrence of one or more manic or mixed episodes
    - Type II
        - Clinical history characterized by occurrence of one or more major depressive episodes accompanied by at least one manic or hypomanic episode
        - In a small subset of people with bipolar disorder, the recurrent shifts in polarity can occur more frequently and this is called rapid cycling.
            - Occurrence of four or more mood episodes during the previous 12 months
            - Mood episodes are either major depressive or manic.
            - Other than occurring more frequently, mood episodes are the same as non–rapid-cycling episodes.
            - Twenty percent of people with bipolar disorder have rapid cycling.
            - Most rapid cyclers are women (90%).
            - Identifying rapid cycling is important.
            - Antidepressants may accelerate cycling.
            - Persons with rapid cycling have a poorer prognosis.

Physical Exam Findings

- No physical exam findings specific to bipolar disorder
- Clinical findings consistent with thyroid dysfunction

Mental Status Exam Findings in Mania or Hypomania

- Appearance
    - Psychomotor restlessness or agitation
    - Frequent change of dress
    - Prone to bright-colored, often sexualized dress
    - Dramatic or flamboyant dress usually out of character for person when compared to nonsymptomatic periods
- Speech
    - Rapid
    - Loud

    - Pressured
    - Difficult to interrupt
    - Joking, irrelevant, amusing
    - Word clanging in severely ill clients
- Affect
    - Labile
    - Irritable
    - Overly theatrical and dramatic
- Mood
    - Euphoric
    - Cheerful
    - High
    - Expansive
    - Irritable
- Thought process
    - Thoughts racing
    - Flight of ideas
    - Thoughts disorganized and incoherent in severely ill clients
- Thought content
    - Inflated self-esteem
    - Indiscriminate enthusiasm
    - Inflated sense of abilities bordering on delusional
    - Increased sexual content
- Orientation
    - Fully oriented
- Memory
    - Impaired short-term
    - Impaired recall
- Concentration
    - Highly distractible
- Abstraction
    - Generally abstractive
    - Can be concrete on proverb testing during psychotic episodes

- Judgment
  - Poor
  - Prone to imprudent behavioral choices with potential for negative consequences
- Insight
  - The person usually does not recognize that they are ill.
  - Resists treatment options

Diagnostic and Laboratory Findings

- CBC, chemistry profile, thyroid function tests, and B_{12} level to rule out metabolic causes or unidentified conditions
- Drug toxicity screening if indicated by history

DIFFERENTIAL DIAGNOSIS

- If the first onset of manic symptoms occurs after age 40, most likely symptoms are caused by another medical condition.
- Many medical conditions mimic manic symptoms:
  - Endocrine disorders
  - Hyperthyroidism
  - Intoxication or withdrawal from illicit drug use
    - Amphetamines
    - Cocaine
    - Hallucinogens
    - Opiates
- Medications
  - Captopril
  - Cimetidine
  - Corticosteroids
  - Cyclosporine
  - Disulfiram
  - Hydralazine
  - Isoniazid

- Mania can be precipitated by treatment of MDD or other unipolar mood disorders in susceptible persons.
  - Antidepressants
  - ECT
  - Light therapy

CLINICAL MANAGEMENT

- Rule out or treat any conditions that may contribute to current symptom manifestation.
- Assess and identify client's level of acuity.
- Determine severity of illness.
- Determine duration of illness.
- Ascertain history of response to treatment.
- During acute manic episodes or significant depressive episodes, client may require brief hospitalization
  - To ensure client safety,
  - To ensure client adherence with treatment to reach stabilization, or
  - To rapidly stabilize on medication.
- Clinical management during nonacute episodes occurs most often in community settings.

Pharmacological Management

- Pharmacological management should generally not entail the use of an antidepressant agent if a mood-stabilizing agent is not in place.
  - Especially important in clients who are rapid-cycling
  - May precipitate shift from depression to hypomania, mania, or dysphoric hypomania (mixed state)

Mood-stabilizing agents

- Commonly used pharmacological agents

- Lithium
  - Gold standard for treating manic episodes
  - Evidence of anti-suicidal effects
  - Action largely unknown
  - Long history of use; drug profile well established
  - Evidence exists showing some effectiveness on depressive symptoms as well as on manic symptoms
  - Has many clinically significant side effects (see Table 9–9); clients on this drug require careful monitoring (see Table 9–10)
  - Narrow therapeutic window
  - Therapeutic effect and potential for adverse side effects (see Table 9–9); monitored by use of serum lithium level
    - Obtained at trough level
    - Twelve hours post-dose
    - Therapeutic serum range from 0.5 to 1.2 mEq/L
    - Level greater than 1.2 mEq/L increases risk for toxic side effects.
  - Baseline labs before initiation of lithium to ensure safety and efficacy
    - Thyroid panel
    - Serum creatinine
    - Blood urea nitrogen (BUN)
    - Pregnancy test
    - ECG for clients 50 years of age or older
  - Rapid-cycling clients seldom respond to lithium monotherapy
  - Must educate client (and significant others) about side effects and signs and symptoms of lithium toxicity
- Anticonvulsant medication
  - Lamotrigine
    - FDA box warning for lamotrigine: serious rash
  - Carbamazepine
    - FDA box warning for carbamazepine: agranulocytosis and aplastic anemia
  - Valproic acid/divalproex sodium
    - FDA box warning for valproic acid/divalproex sodium: hepatotoxicity and pancreatitis
    - Baseline labs before carbamazepine or valproic acid/divalproex sodium
      - CBC
      - Liver function tests (LFTs)

- Labs drawn 1 week after start of carbamazepine, valproic acid/divalproex sodium
    - Twelve-hour trough serum drug level
    - CBC
    - LFTs

TABLE 9–9.
CLINICALLY SIGNIFICANT SIDE EFFECTS OF LITHIUM

ORGAN SYSTEM AFFECTED	CLINICAL FINDING
Endocrine	Weight gain Impaired thyroid functioning
Central nervous system	Fine hand tremors Fatigue Mental cloudiness Headaches Coarse hand tremors with toxicity Nystagmus
Dermatological	Maculopapular rash Pruritus Acne
Gastrointestinal	Gastrointestinal upset Diarrhea Vomiting Cramps Anorexia
Renal	Polyuria with related polydipsia Diabetes insipidus Edema Microscopic tubular changes
Cardiac	T-wave inversions Dysrhythmias
Hematological	Leukocytosis

TABLE 9–10.
DRUGS FOR MOOD DISORDERS

AGENT	DOSAGE	THERAPEUTIC PLASMA LEVEL	SIDE EFFECTS	COMMENTS
Carbamazepine	10–20 mg/kg/ day	6–12 mcg/mL	Common: Nausea, dizziness, sedation, headache, dry mouth, constipation, skin rash Rare: Agranulocytosis/aplastic anemia, Stevens-Johnson syndrome, particularly in Asians (screen for HLA-B*1502 allele before initiating)	Hepatic enzyme inducer Monitor LFTs Alternative to lithium or valproic acid Pregnancy Category D Lactation Category L2
Divalproex	15–40 mg/kg/ day	50–125 mcg/mL	Common: Nausea, diarrhea, abdominal cramps, sedation, tremor Rare: Increased liver enzymes, Stevens-Johnson syndrome (unlike carbamazepine, divalproex does not carry screening directive for HLA-B*1502 antigen at this time)	Minimizes GI effects More effective than lithium for rapid cycling and mixed bipolar Loading dose: 20 mg/kg Pregnancy Category D Lactation Category L2
Gabapentin	maximum dose 3600 mg/day	2–20 mcg/mL	Common: Dizziness, somnolence, ataxia, fatigue Rare: Suicidal ideation, aggressiveness, hallucinations, mania, panic attacks	Creatinine at baseline Pregnancy Category C Lactation Category L2
Lamotrigine	25–600 mg/ day	Level monitoring not necessary	Common: Dizziness, ataxia, somnolence, diplopia, nausea, headache, hepatotoxicity Rare: Life-threatening rashes, including Stevens-Johnson syndrome (unlike carbamazepine, lamotrigine does not carry directive to screen for HLA-B*1502 antigen at this time), leukopenia	Indication for maintenance only Helps in depressive phase of bipolar affective disorder Titrate slowly: 25 mg p.o. q.d.–x 2 weeks, then 50 mg p.o. q.d. × 2 weeks, etc. Concomitant use with divalproex may double lamotrigine level and should be factored into dosing. Concomitant use with carbamazepine may increase metabolism and should be factored into dosing.

(Continued)

TABLE 9–10. (CONTINUED)

AGENT	DOSAGE	THERAPEUTIC PLASMA LEVEL	SIDE EFFECTS	COMMENTS
Lamotrigine (continued)				Often used in combination with lithium, second-generation antipsychotics, and antidepressants Pregnancy Category: C Lactation Category: L2
Lithium carbonate	1,200–2,400 mg/day (acute) 900–1,200 mg/day (maintenance)	0.8–1.2 mEq/L 0.6–1.2 mEq/L	Common: Nausea, fine-hand tremors, increased urination and thirst Toxicity: Slurred speech, confusion, severe GI effect	Established standard treatment for bipolar disorder Risk of hypothyroidism Avoid in pregnancy, especially first trimester Monitoring kidney functioning is essential Concurrent use of NSAIDs and ACEIs may double lithium level Pregnancy Category D Lactation Category L3
Oxcarbazepine	2400 mg/day	10–35 mcg/mL	Common: Dizziness, headache, nausea, vomiting Serious: Hyponatremia, SIADH, anaphylaxis	Monitor creatinine at baseline, sodium levels throughout treatment Pregnancy Category C Lactation Category L3
Topiramate	400 mg/day	5–20 mcg/mL	Common: Metabolic acidosis, cognitive dysfunction, paresthesia Serious: Nephrolithiasis, osteomalacia, osteoporosis	Monitor creatinine and bicarbonate at baseline and periodically Pregnancy Category C Lactation Category L3
Valproic acid	60 mg/kg/day	50–125 mcg/mL	Common: Headache, nausea, vomiting, asthenia Serious: Hepatotoxicity, pancreatitis, SIADH, hyponatremia	Monitor LFTs at baseline, first 6 months, and throughout treatment. Platelets: coagulation at baseline and periodically. Pregnancy Category D Lactation Category L2

ACEI, angiotensin converting enzyme inhibitors; GI, gastrointestinal; LFT, liver function tests; NSAID, nonsteroidal anti-inflammatory drugs ; SIADH, syndrome of inappropriate antidiuretic hormone secretion

- Response to treatment with lithium or anticonvulsant medications is 1 to 2 weeks.
  - Stevens-Johnson Syndrome (SJS)
    - Rare, potentially life-threatening immune reaction to a foreign antigen that can occur with exposure to any anticonvulsant drug
    - Treatment includes stopping the offending agent with supportive measures, often in a hospital burn unit.
    - Signs and symptoms of SJS include:
      - Facial swelling
      - Tongue swelling
      - Macules, papules, and "burning," confluent erythematic rash
      - Skin sloughing
      - Prodromal headache, malaise, arthralgia, and painful mucous membranes may occur before rash occurs

Nonpharmacological Management

- Somatic treatments
  - Treatment as discussed previously for MDD episodes (see page 185)
- Therapies
  - Treatment as discussed previously for MDD episodes (see page 185)
- During acute phase of manic episode
  - Monitor and help clients meet nutritional needs.
  - Help client meet sleep–rest needs.
  - Monitor for safety.
- During less acute periods
  - CBT
  - Behavioral therapies
  - Interpersonal therapies
  - Supportive groups
  - Milieu therapy
    - Provides for structure and safety needs
    - Provides socialization and interpersonal support
    - Encourages independence

- ◊ Client and family education
  - Explain underlying pathology of illness
  - Discuss signs and symptoms
  - Help identify strategies for living with illness
  - Help understand and make decisions regarding care options
- ◊ Relapse prevention plan
- ◊ Overall health promotion

COMMON COMORBIDITIES

- ♦ Hypothyroidism
- ♦ Substance use

GENERAL HEALTH CONSIDERATIONS

- ♦ High-risk activities from manic behavior
  - ◊ Sexual
    - Client education for sexually transmitted infections (STIs)
    - Assessment and monitoring for STIs
  - ◊ Financial and legal
- ♦ Client access to community resources
  - ◊ Nutritional counseling
  - ◊ Client health education

LIFE SPAN CONSIDERATIONS

- ♦ Adolescent manic episodes present differently from adult episodes.
  - ◊ More psychotic features
  - ◊ Often associated with antisocial behavior
  - ◊ Often associated with substance use
  - ◊ Prodromal period of significant behavioral problems
    - School truancy
    - Failing grades

FOLLOW-UP

- Clients initially should be seen weekly to titrate medications and monitor serum blood levels of pharmacological agents.
- Treatment duration and success rates vary with individual characteristics and motivation.
- Clients and significant others should be taught symptoms of mania and depression and that the disorders are chronic illnesses.
- Relapse is common and occurs frequently.
- Relapse plans need to be developed.
- Client teaching should include risks, benefits, potential side effects, and signs and symptoms of medication toxicity.
- Educate about potential dietary and fluid intake effects on lithium level.
- Lithium and divalproex sodium are teratogenic.
    - Women of child-bearing years need effective contraceptive care while taking bipolar disorder treatment medication.
- Routine use of lab tests to monitor for therapeutic serum levels of anticonvulsants and lithium is needed.
    - Routine evaluation of CBC, renal function, and thyroid and parathyroid function (thyroid-stimulating hormone and calcium levels) is needed for clients taking lithium long term.
- Assessment for suicidality should occur during every client contact.
- All clients should be observed for the development of adverse effects of pharmacological management.
- Standardized rating scales help to monitor clinical status, establish baseline functioning, and monitor disorder course over time:
    - Young Mania Rating Scale (YMRS; Young et al., 1978)
    - A daily mood chart that tracks mood, energy, and specific information about sleep is helpful in informing both diagnosis and treatment

CYCLOTHYMIC DISORDER

DESCRIPTION

- Chronic, fluctuating mood disorder with symptoms similar to but less severe than bipolar disorder
- Numerous periods of hypomanic and dysthymic symptoms

ETIOLOGY

- Similar to that of bipolar disorder (see Bipolar Disorder Etiology, page 216)

INCIDENCE AND DEMOGRAPHICS

- Lifetime prevalence 0.4% to 1%
- Insidious onset
- Chronic course
- Begins early in life
    - 15% to 50% of persons with cyclothymic disorder subsequently develop bipolar disorder.

RISK FACTORS

- Genetic loading
- Family history
- Bipolar disorder type I
- Substance use

PREVENTION AND SCREENING

- At-risk family education
- Community education
    - Stigma reduction
    - Signs and symptoms of illness
    - Treatment potential for control of symptoms
- Early recognition, intervention, and initiation of treatment
    - Significant and protracted prodromal symptom period usually noted before full onset of illness
    - The longer the period between onset of symptoms and diagnosis, the more difficult it is to interrupt cyclicity of illness.

ASSESSMENT

Client History

- Assess for the following:
  - Fluctuating mood episodes
  - Affected people can function well during hypomanic episodes
  - May experience clinically significant distress or impaired function related to cyclicity
  - Unpredictable mood changes
  - Often regarded by others as temperamental, moody, unpredictable, inconsistent, and unreliable
  - No psychotic episodes

Physical Exam Findings

- Similar to MDD and bipolar disorder (see Bipolar Disorder Physical Exam Findings, page 220)

Mental Status Exam Findings

- Similar to MDD and bipolar disorder but with less severity of symptoms (see Bipolar Disorder Mental Status Exam Findings, page 220)

Diagnostic and Laboratory Findings

- Similar to MDD and bipolar disorder (see page 172 for Diagnostic and Laboratory Findings for MDD; see page 216 for Diagnostic and Laboratory Findings for bipolar disorder)

DIFFERENTIAL DIAGNOSIS

- Nonpsychiatric
  - Similar to MDD and bipolar disorder (see page 172 for Differential Diagnosis for MDD; see page 216 for Differential Diagnosis for bipolar disorder)
- Psychiatric
  - Bipolar disorder
  - Dysthymia
  - Substance use

CLINICAL MANAGEMENT

Pharmacological Management

- Similar to MDD and bipolar disorder (see page 172 for Pharmacological Management of MDD; see page 216 for Pharmacological Management of bipolar disorder)
- Because of increased risk for development of bipolar disorder, commonly treated with medication

Nonpharmacological Management

- Similar to MDD and bipolar disorder (see page 172 for Nonpharmacological Management of MDD; see page 216 for Nonpharmacological Management of bipolar disorder)

LIFE SPAN CONSIDERATIONS

- Usually begins in adolescence
- Onset in later life usually suggests general medical condition such as multiple sclerosis.

FOLLOW-UP

- Similar to MDD and bipolar disorder (see page 172 for Follow-up for MDD; see page 216 for Follow-up for bipolar disorder)

UNSPECIFIED MOOD DISORDER

Symptoms of a mood disorder that result in significant impairment in areas of social, occupational, or other areas of function but do not meet the full criteria of depressive or bipolar disorders are known as unspecified mood disorder. The symptoms do not clearly fit into the unspecified bipolar and related disorders or unspecified depressive disorder (APA, 2022).

CASE STUDY

A.W., a 35-year-old homemaker and mother of two children, presents to the PMHNP on referral from the primary care provider. Accompanied by her partner, the client describes worsening insomnia and poor energy. The symptoms are affecting her ability to take care of the children and the household. The partner reports that A.W. often has crying spells, is not eating, and cannot seem to concentrate. When questioned further, the partner reports that A.W. has mentioned not wanting to live and thought that "maybe A.W. was just having a bad day."

PAST PSYCHIATRIC HISTORY

- Reports depression off and on since late adolescence
- No history of treatment
- The partner adds that A.W. had "the baby blues" for several months after the births of both of their children.

PAST MEDICAL HISTORY

- Seasonal allergies and stress-induced asthma
- No significant surgical history, except for a tonsillectomy as a child
- Normal pregnancies and deliveries
- No chronic health problems identified

FAMILY HISTORY

- Significant for grandmother and father, who had "breakdowns"
- Father used alcohol excessively

SOCIAL HISTORY

A.W. is a homemaker and has two children, ages 8 and 10. The client and her partner moved to the area 6 months ago. The client does not smoke or use drugs but drinks socially. A.W. has a master's degree in English and had planned to go back to school to get a teaching certificate when the children began high school.

MENTAL STATUS EXAM

The client appears disheveled. Her hair is not combed. She appears very tired. She avoids eye contact, talks very softly, and is slow to respond to questions. She hardly moves during the interview. Her affect is constricted and sad. The client states, "I have no energy" and that her mood is "very sad." She denies hearing voices or having hallucinations. Her thoughts are appropriate and organized. The client does admit to having episodic thoughts of suicide and has a vague plan to ingest an overdose of aspirin, acetaminophen, and alcohol when the children are with her partner but has no clear timeline or planned intent. She is unable to do serial number testing, shows impaired short-term memory, exhibits a few problems with immediate recall, and has difficulty concentrating but no difficulty with abstractions. She is oriented times 3 and shows good judgment and insight. The client has above-average intelligence.

CURRENT MEDICATIONS

The client takes cetirizine for allergies and is now taking ethinyl estradiol/norgestimate contraceptive pills.

LABS

- Platelets 230/mm^3
- White blood cell (WBC) count 6,000/mm^3
- Hematocrit 40%, hemoglobin 13.0
- Na 140, K 4.0, Cl 101, CO_2 26, blood urea nitrogen (BUN) 15, creatinine 0.9, glucose 102
- Thyroid stimulating hormone (TSH) 1.1, triiodothyronine (T3) 179, thyroxine (T4) 1.3

There are several issues to consider in planning care for A.W.

1. What is the most probable diagnosis?
2. What further assessment is needed?
3. What target symptoms does the client display that are consistent with the probable diagnosis?
4. What medications would be considered?
5. If client had psychotic features with her depression, how would this change the treatment plan?

6. What nonmedication treatment would be indicated for a client with MDD with psychotic features?
7. How would the plan differ if the client had a heart condition and was taking no other medications?
8. Assume the client has started an antidepressant and returns after 2 weeks on the medication. Speech has normalized and is now more spontaneous. If the client now tells you they feel "better" and energy and motivation have improved but is still having difficulty falling and staying asleep, would your diagnosis change?
9. What further assessment should be done?
10. How would you change the treatment plan?
11. If the client returns for her follow-up appointment reporting irritable mood, racing thoughts, rapid speech, and inability to sleep, should your diagnosis and treatment plan change?

ANSWERS TO CASE STUDY DISCUSSION QUESTIONS

1. The client's most probable diagnosis is consistent with MDD.
2. Further assessment needed is to ensure that the client meets the DSM-5-TR criteria for major depression. Complete physical assessment and use of common symptom rating scale such as BDI or PHQ-9. Complete assessment for any other physical health states. The PMHNP should explore what "inability to sleep" means in specific detail.
3. The target symptoms for this client include depressed mood most of the day nearly every day, lack of energy, suicidal ideation, and mental status exam findings consistent with MDD.
4. The medications to be considered for this client are SSRIs, as this class of antidepressant medication is often considered the first-line agent for treatment of MDD.
5. If the client had psychotic symptoms, clinical management would include short-term use of an antipsychotic agent to control psychotic symptoms; an atypical antipsychotic is usually best tolerated.
6. For clients with severe MDD with psychosis, ECT might be considered.
7. If the client had cardiovascular disease, the PMHNP must look at compatibility issues to ensure that the medication choice for treatment of MDD does not have significant risk for adverse cardiac side effects. TCAs are contraindicated.
8. If the client presented for a follow-up appointment stating that she is feeling better but still has residual symptoms of sleep problems, the diagnosis would not change because the symptoms. Ms. A.W. reports are consistent with a depressive episode even though her symptoms are improving.
9. Further assessment of this client should include an assessment for mood, anhedonia, suicidal ideation, and activities over the past 2 weeks and for any indication that the antidepressant may be fueling a switch from depression to hypomania or mixed state.
10. In this client, if the treatment plan changes, monitor for further improvements. Teach A.W. about sleep hygiene measures. Discuss expected outcomes and the importance of monitoring for any significant increase in goal-directed activities, decreased need for sleep, racing thoughts, and shift in mood to euphoria or irritability. Begin psychotherapy.
11. If the client returns for a follow-up appointment reporting irritable mood, racing thoughts, rapid speech and inability to sleep, yes, the treatment plan should change. Rule out unspecified bipolar disorder, bipolar II disorder, and bipolar I disorder. The antidepressant dose should be lowered and a medication with mood stabilizing properties should be added. The client should be monitored closely and reevaluated within several days.

REFERENCES AND RESOURCES

American Psychiatric Association. (2010). Practice guidelines for the treatment of patients with major depressive disorder. https://psychiatryonline.org/pb/assets/raw/sitewide/practice_guidelines/guidelines/mdd.pdf

American Psychiatric Association. (2022). Diagnostic and statistical manual of mental disorders (5th ed., Text rev.).

American Psychiatric Nurses Association (2024). Electroconvulsive Therapy (ECT) Treatment Considerations Checklist. https://www.apna.org/electroconvulsive-therapy-ect-treatment-considerations/

Beck, A. T., Rush, A. J., Shaw, B. F., & Emery, G. (1987). Cognitive therapy of depression. Guilford Press.

Beck, A. T., Ward, C. H., Mendelson, M., Mock, J., & Erbaugh, J. (1961). An inventory for measuring depression. Archives of General Psychiatry, 4, 561–571.

Beydoun, A. (2001). Innovative treatment strategies with anticonvulsants: A focus on bipolar disorder. Primary Psychiatry, 8(6), 49–52.

Birmaher, B., Brent, D., AACAP Work Group on Quality Issues, Bernet, W., Bukstein, O., Walter, H., . . . Medicus, J. (2007). Practice parameter for the assessment and treatment of children and adolescents with depressive disorders. Journal of the American Academy of Child and Adolescent Psychiatry, 46(11), 1503–1526. https://doi.org/10.1097/chi.0b013e318145ae1c

Clewell, T. (2004). Mourning beyond melancholia: Freud's psychoanalysis of loss. Journal of the American Psychoanalytic Association, 52(1), 43–67.

Freidrich, M. (1999). Lithium: Proving its mettle for 50 years. JAMA, 281, 2271–2275.

Gilbert, P. (2006). Evolution and depression: Issues and implications. Psychological Medicine, 36(3), 287–297. https://doi.org/10.1017/S0033291705006112

Giles, D. E., Kupfer, D. J., Rush, A. J., & Roffwarg, H. P. (1998). Controlled comparison of electrophysiological sleep in families of probands with unipolar depression. American Journal of Psychiatry, 155, 192–196.

Gloaguen, V., Cottraux, J., Cucherat, M., & Blackburn, I. M. (1998). A meta-analysis of the effects of cognitive therapy in depressed patients. Journal of Affective Disorders, 49(1), 59–62.

Green, J. (2001). Helping patients understand depression and its treatment. Primary Psychiatry, 8(11), 49–53.

Hirschfeld, R., Holzer, C., Calabrese, J., Weissman, M., Reed, M., Davies, M., . . . Hazard, E. (2003). Validity of the mood disorder questionnaire: A general population study. American Journal of Psychiatry, 160, 178–180.

Hoyert, D. L., Kochanek, K. D., & Murphy, S. L. (1998). Deaths: Final data for 1997. National Vital Statistics Reports, 47(19). https://www.cdc.gov/nchs/data/nvsr/nvsr47/nvs47_19.pdf

Judd, L., Paulus, M., Schettler, P., Akiskal, H., Endicott, J., Leon, A., . . . Keller, M. (2000). Does incomplete recovery from first lifetime major depressive episode herald a chronic course of illness? American Journal of Psychiatry, 157(9), 1501–1504.

Kedzior, K. K., & Reitz, S. K. (2014). Short-term efficacy of repetitive transcranial magnetic stimulation (rTMS) in depression—Reanalysis of data from meta-analyses up to 2010. BioMedCentral Psychology, 2(1), 39.

Ketter, T. A., Miller, S., Dell'Osso, B., Calabrese, J. R., Frye, M. A., & Citrome, L. (2014). Balancing benefits and harms of treatments for acute bipolar depression. Journal of Affective Disorders, 169(Supp. 1), 24–33.

Kimrell, T., Little, R., & Dunn, T. (1999). Frequency dependence of antidepressant response to left prefrontal repetitive transcranial magnetic stimulation (rTMS) as a function of baseline cerebral glucose metabolism. Biological Psychiatry, 46, 1603–1613.

Kleimann, A., Schrader, V., Stübner, S., Greil, W., Kahl, K. G., Bleich, S., . . . Toto, S. (2016). Psychopharmacological treatment of 1650 in-patients with acute mania-data from the AMSP study. Journal of Affective Disorders, 191, 164–171. https://doi.org/10.1016/j.jad.2015.11.037

Klein, D. N., Schwartz, J. E., & Rose S. (2000). Five-year course and outcome of dysthymic disorder: A prospective, naturalistic follow-up study. American Journal of Psychiatry, 157, 931–939.

Lowe-Ponsford, F. L., & Nutt, D. J. (2001). Pathophysiology of depression. Primary Psychiatry, 8(11), 43–48.

McBride, A., & Austin, J. (1996). Psychiatric-mental health nursing: Integrating the behavioral and biological sciences. Saunders.

McClellan, J., Kowatch, R., Findling, R. L., & Work Group on Quality Issues (2007). Practice parameter for the assessment and treatment of children and adolescents with bipolar disorder. Journal of the American Academy of Child and Adolescent Psychiatry, 46(1), 107–125.

McQuade, R., & Young, A. (2000). Future therapeutic targets in mood disorders: The glucocorticoid receptor. British Journal of Psychiatry, 177, 390–395.

Monroe, S. M., Rohde, P., & Seeley, J. R. (1999). Life events and depression in adolescence: Relationship loss as a prospective risk factor for first onset of major depressive disorder. Journal of Abnormal Psychology, 108, 606–614.

Ornstein, S., Stuart, G., & Jenkins, R. (2000). Depression diagnosis and antidepressant use in primary care practices. Journal of Family Practice, 49(1), 68–71.

Sadock, B., Sadock, V., & Ruiz, P. (2017). Kaplan and Sadock's comprehensive textbook of psychiatry (10th ed.). Wolters Kluwer.

Saeed, M. (2001). Assessment and management of the suicidal patient in the managed care era. Primary Psychiatry, 8(6), 38–45.

Seligman, M. (1972). Learned helplessness. Annual Review of Medicine, 23, 407–412.

Shear, M. K., Reynolds, C .F., Simon, N. M., Zisook, S., Wang, Y., Mauro, . . . Skritskaya, N. (2016). Optimizing treatment of complicated grief: A randomized clinical trial. JAMA Psychiatry, 73(7), 685–694. https://doi.org/10.1001/jamapsychiatry.2016.0892

Shaffer, D., & Craft, L. (1999). Methods of adolescent suicide prevention. Journal of Clinical Psychiatry, 60(Suppl. 2), 70–74.

Siu, A., & U.S. Preventative Services Task Force. (2016). Screening for depression in adults. US Preventative Services Task Force recommendation statement. JAMA, 315(4), 380–387.

Stephenson, M. (2012). Finding Fairbairn-Discovery and exploration of the work of Ronald Fairbairn. Psychodynamic Practice, 18(4), 465–470. https://doi.org/10.1080/14753634.2012.721195

Stuart, G. W. (2012). Principles and practice of psychiatric nursing (10th ed.). Mosby.

Young, J. W., & Dulcis, D. (2015). Investigating the mechanism(s) underlying switching between states in bipolar disorder. European Journal of Pharmacology, 759, 151–162.

Young, R. C., Biggs, J. T., Ziegler, V. E., & Meyer, D. A. (1978). A rating scale for mania: Reliability, validity, and sensitivity. British Journal of Psychiatry, 133, 429–435.

CHAPTER 10

ANXIETY DISORDERS, OBSESSIVE–COMPULSIVE DISORDER, AND TRAUMA AND STRESSOR-RELATED DISORDERS

This chapter reviews the psychiatric-mental health nurse practitioner's (PMHNP's) evaluation of and treatment of people who have anxiety-related disorders. Anxiety disorders are among the most common of all psychiatric illnesses, and they can manifest initially as a number of physical illness states. Often only after extensive (sometimes even unnecessary) assessment and diagnostic evaluation is a client's problem correctly identified as an anxiety disorder. Because of the high degree of somatic symptomatology, it is common for clients to present to a primary care setting and thus receive initial care from a primary care provider.

Anxiety is a common and normal human emotion. PMHNPs caring for clients who present for evaluation of anxiety must be able to distinguish between normal levels of anxiety and pathological levels that are symptomatic of an underlying brain-based illness. Pathological levels of anxiety require treatment and generally will not fully abate without therapeutic intervention. Untreated high levels of anxiety predispose people to other serious health problems; therefore, pathological levels of anxiety should not go untreated (Narrow et al., 1998).

- Normal emotion of anxiety
  - Anxiety is one of the most common human emotions.
  - Anxiety exists on a continuum ranging from the absence of anxiety at one end to pathological levels that produce significant symptoms of psychiatric disorder at the other (see Table 10–1).
  - Anxiety can be a normal, healthy reaction to life stressors that motivates a person to deal with events and emotions.
  - Anxiety can be pathological if it is disproportionate to events, if it is sustained over a significant time frame, if it significantly impairs functioning, or if it is apparently unrelated to any identifiable event or situation in a person's life.
  - High pathological levels of anxiety interfere with perceptions, memory, judgment, and motor responses.

TABLE 10–1.

ASSESSING LEVELS OF ANXIETY

LEVEL OF ANXIETY	DEFINITION	PHYSIOLOGICAL SIGNS AND SYMPTOMS	PSYCHOLOGICAL SIGNS AND SYMPTOMS
Level I: Mild	Normative level experienced by all, which functions to motivate	Vital signs normal, pupils constricted, minimal increase in muscle tone	Perceptual field broadened, heightened awareness of environment
Level II: Moderate	Normative level experienced by most in response to significant stressors	Vital signs normal, mild increased heart rate, moderate increase in muscle tone	Subjective feeling of tension or worry, narrowed perceptions
Level III: Severe	Pathological level	Autonomic nervous system triggered, fight-or-flight response, pupils dilated, vital signs increased, diaphoresis, muscles rigid, hearing decreased, pain threshold increased, urinary frequency, diarrhea	Perceptual field greatly narrowed, difficulty with problem-solving, distorted perception of time, selective inattention, dissociative sensations, automatic behavior
Level IV: Panic	Pathological level	Severe symptoms markedly increased: client is pale, hypotensive, has poor eye–hand coordination, muscle pains, marked decrease in hearing, dizziness, shortness of breath	Scattered perceptions, unable to attend to environmental stimuli, illogical thinking, may exhibit hallucinations or delusions

- Cultural differences can affect behavioral manifestations of anxiety.
  - Ataques de nervios is a Latino cultural syndrome usually provoked by disruptions in family bonds and may be manifested by trembling, crying, and screaming. The attacks are usually experienced in the presence of others and the person often feels relief afterward.
  - Khyal (wind) attacks are a common manifestation among Cambodian and other Asian cultures and commonly manifest in neck soreness and tinnitus.
- Older adults often express anxiety as somatic concerns and anxiety disorders may overlap with medical conditions.

- Psychotherapy is the first-line treatment for children and adolescents who are diagnosed with an anxiety disorder.
- The role of the PMHNP in assessing anxiety is to separate normal versus pathological levels of anxiety, to intervene to lower the level of anxiety, and to improve overall functioning.

TRAUMA-INFORMED CARE

Trauma-informed care (TIC) is a concept arising in the literature after the Adverse Childhood Experiences Study in 1998 (Felitti et al., 1998). The ACE Study (1995–1997) is a joint retrospective study between the Centers for Disease Control and Prevention (CDC) and Kaiser Permanente with over 15,000 adult subjects who were questioned about their childhood experiences, and this was correlated with their long-term mental, emotional, and physical health.

The ACE questionnaire tool was a questionnaire consisting of 17 questions in 7 categories of adverse experiences (a positive score was one positive answer in a category—could score from 0 to 7; see Table 10–2).

Abuse by category

- Sexual
- Physical
- Psychological

Household dysfunction by category

- Lived with a person who had alcohol use disorder or other substance user
- Lived with a person who had mental illness issues or died by suicide
- Mother or stepmother was threatened by violence or experienced violence
- Household member in prison

Findings

- Common 52% of responders had a positive score in at least one of seven categories and 6.2% had a positive score in four or more categories
- Correlated with 10 health risk behaviors and diagnosed illnesses
- Strong dose–response relationship between experiences and health risk, pathology, and early death

These results have been replicated in numerous studies, reviews, and meta-analyses.

TABLE 10–2.
ACES STUDY—QUESTIONNAIRE CATEGORIES

ADVERSE EXPERIENCE CATEGORIES	HIGH-RISK BEHAVIORS	DIAGNOSES AND ILLNESSES
• Psychological abuse • Physical abuse • Sexual abuse • Living with drug use • Living with mental illness • Mother or stepmother threatened by violence • Household member in prison	• Smoking • Severe obesity (BMI ≥35) • Physical inactivity • Depressed mood • A attempt(s) to end their own life • Excessive alcohol use • Drug use • Parenteral drug use • Over 50 lifetime sexual partners	• Ischemic cardiac disease • Cancer • Stroke • Chronic bronchitis • Emphysema/COPD • Diabetes • Hepatitis • History of skeletal fractures (unintentional injury) • History of STI

BMI, body mass index; COPD, chronic obstructive pulmonary disease; STI, sexually transmitted infection

WHAT IS A TRAUMA-INFORMED APPROACH?

> "A program, organization, or system that is trauma-informed realizes the widespread impact of trauma and understands potential paths for recovery; recognizes the signs and symptoms of trauma in clients, families, staff, and others involved with the system; and responds by fully integrating knowledge about trauma into policies, procedures, and practices, and seeks to actively resist re-traumatization." (Substance Abuse and Mental Health Services Administration [SAMSHA], 2014)

PATHOLOGY OF CHRONIC STRESS

Chronic sustained stress in the lack of a supportive environment is toxic (Oral et al., 2016).

Stress response involves the engagement of the hypothalamus–pituitary–adrenal (HPA) axis and the sympathetic nervous system (SNS). Activation leads to cortisol secretion by the adrenals. Normally, there is a feedback loop that turns the cortisol off, but in chronic toxic stress, the cortisol levels remain high with too little cortisol over time as the HPA axis is dysregulated. This causes immune problems with increased risk of infection, chronic inflammation, decreased wound healing, and greater risk of autoimmune diseases.

THE TRAUMA-INFORMED CARE PYRAMID

> "Traumatic events (including sexual abuse, domestic violence, elder abuse, and combat trauma) are associated with long-term physical and psychological effects. These events may influence patients' health care experiences and engagement in preventative care. Although the term trauma-informed care (TIC) is widely used, it is not well understood how to apply this concept in daily health care practice. On the basis of a synthesis of a review of the literature, the TIC pyramid is a conceptual and operational framework that can help practitioners translate TIC principles into interactions with patients." (Raja et al., 2015; see Figure 10–1).

Trauma-informed interventions can work at the three levels of preventative care:

- Primary preventions: Interventions aimed at families at risk.
- Secondary prevention: Interventions for children and families following an adverse event to mitigate the impact of the event and work toward prevention.
- Tertiary prevention: Treat and reduce long-term consequences of ACEs.

The strength of TIC is the lens that the provider uses in assessments and interventions with clients.

FIGURE 10–1.
THE TRAUMA-INFORMED CARE PYRAMID

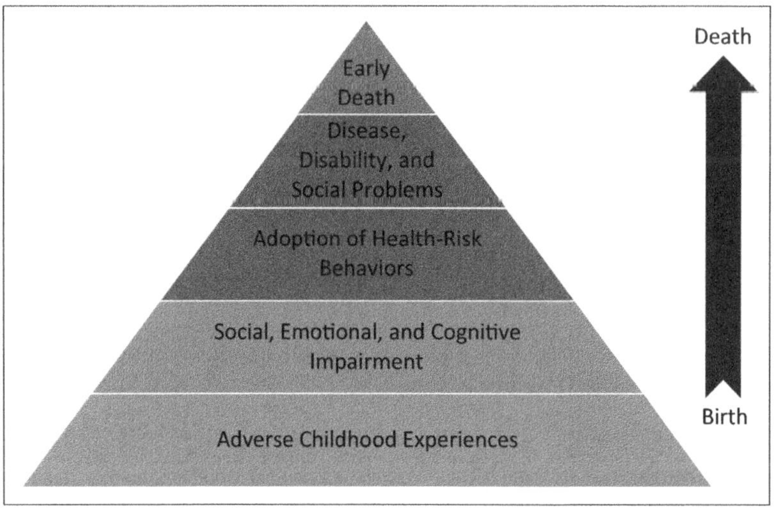

SAMSHA gives six principles that support TIC (Harris & Fallot, 2001):

- Safety: Organizations promote a sense of safety involving a conscious effort to ensure that all members and clients of an organization are physically and emotionally safe.
- Trustworthiness and transparency: Organizations must approach decisions with transparency and engender trust between staff and their clientele.
- Peer support: Peers, which include families of traumatized children as well as individuals who have lived with histories of trauma, can be critical resources for support.
- Collaboration and mutuality: All members of an organization can contribute equally to the healing of children impacted by adverse experiences.
- Empowerment, voice, and choice: Developing plans of action for clients requires client-centered approaches that empower clients.
- Cultural, historical, and gender issues: Efforts must be culturally sensitive and free of prejudices based on biases and stereotypes.

Trauma-informed interventions include the following:

- Cognitive behavioral therapy (CBT) addresses cognitive distortions and self-defeating behaviors
- Peer support
- Appropriate referrals for further care
- Dealing with behaviors using a trauma-informed lens
  - The behavior is the result of learned reactions, not bad training or habits
  - Address as a symptom, not as a "behavior problem"
- Harm reduction approaches to high-risk behaviors

RESILIENCY-INFORMED APPROACH

Trauma-informed approach asks what happened to a person so that interventions can be incorporated that recognize the affects of trauma.

The resiliency-informed approach (Miller Karas, 2023) asks questions that go beyond the trauma-informed approach and are resiliency focused such as:

  - What are your strengths?
  - What has helped you get through?
  - When did you know you were ok?
- All individuals can learn skills of well-being to build upon their strengths and improve resiliency.

ANXIETY DISORDERS

DESCRIPTION

Anxiety disorders are the most common group of psychiatric disorders and are characterized by the degree of anxiety experienced by the client, by the duration and severity of the anxiety, and by the typical behavioral manifestation of anxiety observed in the client. Anxiety ranges from acute states to chronic disorders and is accompanied by multiple somatic symptoms.

- People most often present first in primary care settings with nonspecific physical concerns.
    - Panic attacks are often confused with cardiac and respiratory disorders, so careful differential diagnostic assessment is essential.
- Frequent comorbidity exists with substance use, depression, and eating disorders.
- Symptoms significantly impair functioning and occur more days than not for a period of at least 6 months, with the person reporting little or no volitional control over the symptoms.
- Nine specific anxiety disorders are identified in the Diagnostic and Statistical Manual of Mental Disorders, Fifth Edition, Text Revision (DSM-5-TR; American Psychiatric Association, 2022; see Table 10–3)

TABLE 10–3.
DSM-5-TR ANXIETY, OBSESSIVE–COMPULSIVE DISORDER, AND TRAUMA AND STRESSOR-RELATED DISORDERS

ANXIETY DISORDERS	OBSESSIVE–COMPULSIVE AND RELATED DISORDERS	TRAUMA AND STRESSOR-RELATED DISORDERS
• Panic disorder • Agoraphobia • Specific phobia • Social anxiety (social phobia) • Selective mutism • Generalized anxiety disorder • Separation anxiety disorder • Substance or medication-induced anxiety disorder • Anxiety disorder due to another medical condition	• Obsessive compulsive disorder • Body dysmorphic disorder • Hoarding disorder • Trichotillomania (hair-pulling disorder) • Excoriation (skin-picking disorder) • Substance or medication-induced obsessive–compulsive and related disorder	• Reactive attachment disorder • Disinhibited social engagement disorder • Posttraumatic stress disorder • Acute stress disorder • Dissociative identity disorder • Dissociative amnesia • Depersonalization or derealization disorder

ETIOLOGY

- Multiple theories range from psychological to neurobiological; however, most likely there is a multifactorial etiological profile.

Psychodynamic Theory

- This theory is based on the work of Sigmund Freud (1856–1939), who believed that anxiety initially occurs in response to the stimulation of birth and the need of the infant to adapt to the changed environment.
- Subsequent anxiety results from intrapsychic conflict.
- The process of unconscious repression of sexual drive is at the core of much of the conflict.
- Conflict exists between instinctual needs of the id and the superego (conscience); anxiety signals the person of the need to deal with the id–superego conflict.
- Conflict is unconscious but anxiety is consciously perceived.
- Conflict entails fear of punishment and of doing wrong.
- Defense mechanisms are unconsciously used by the person to deal with the conflict.
- The behavioral manifestations of anxiety disorders stem from the pathological overuse of defense mechanisms.

Interpersonal Theory

- This theory is based on work of Harry Stack Sullivan (1892–1949), who believed that humans are goal directed toward attainment of satisfaction and security needs.
- Satisfaction and security needs are normally met in interpersonal interactions.
- Anxiety arises when a person's needs are unmet.
- Anxiety is first experienced in an infant's interactions with their mother.
- Subsequent anxiety arises because of interpersonal conflict.
- Conflict occurs when a person perceives their needs will not be met because of rejection, feelings of inferiority, or inability to engage with significant others.
- Sense of self becomes based on the person's perception of how others view them.

Neurobiological Theory

- Pathological levels of anxiety result from neurobiological deficits in normal brain functioning.
- Deficits are genetically mediated by and involve predominantly the limbic system, midline brainstem area, and sections of the cortex.
- Deficits predispose the person to abnormal stress responses, with hyperactivity of the autonomic nervous system causing symptoms such as increased heart rate and blood pressure, diaphoresis, papillary dilation, tremors, and increased respiratory rate.
- Problems with the HPA axis
  - Threat is perceived, and the amygdala signals the hypothalamus to secrete corticotropin-releasing hormone (CRH).
  - The amygdala also activates the SNS to initiate the fight-or-flight response.
  - The pituitary is stimulated to release adrenocorticotropic hormone (ACTH).
  - The adrenal glands are then stimulated to release cortisol, which shuts off the alarm system and restores the body to homeostasis.
- In anxiety disorders, the amygdala may not be able to shut off the response (overactive amygdala), or there may not be enough cortisol to stop the fight, flight, or freeze response.
- Neurobiological deficits result in low levels of the neurotransmitter γ-aminobutyric acid (GABA), the chemical responsible for inhibitory responses of neurons, and in the context of high levels of norepinephrine, the chemical associated with the fight, flight, or freeze response
- Neurotransmitters involved in suppressing the HPA axis are serotonin and GABA.

INCIDENCE AND DEMOGRAPHICS

- Anxiety disorders are common, with a lifetime prevalence of 28.8% among the general U.S. population.
- Except for obsessive–compulsive disorder (OCD) and social phobia, anxiety disorders are more common in girls and women than in boys and men.
- Most anxiety disorders manifest in adolescence and early adulthood (Narrow et al., 1998).
- Median age at onset is 11 years.

RISK FACTORS

- Genetic loading (National Institute of Mental Health [NIMH], Genetics Workgroup, 1998)
  - A first-degree relative of a person with panic disorder is up to 8 times more likely than the general population to develop panic disorder.
  - If a first-degree relative of a person developed panic disorder before age 20, that person is up to 20 times more likely than the general population to develop panic disorder.
- Limited range of coping skills
- History of trauma
- High levels of parental distress affect a child's ability to cope with traumatic events.

PREVENTION AND SCREENING

- At-risk family education
- Community education
  - Stigma reduction
  - Signs and symptoms of illness
  - Treatment potential for control of symptoms
- Early recognition, intervention, and initiation of treatment
  - Teach at-risk persons to recognize and manage anxiety levels.
  - Help at-risk persons reduce anxiety through improved coping activities.

ASSESSMENT

Client History

- Assess for the following:
  - Detailed history of present illness, including time frame and progression, and any associated symptoms
  - Social history, including present living situation, marital status, occupation, education level

- ◊ Medication use, including prescription, over-the-counter, alternative, supplements, and home remedies
- ◊ Clients initially may be more troubled by, and complain more often of, physical symptoms and may not identify anxiety as a concern.
- ◊ Explore the client's subjective sensations of being nervous, tense, worried, anxious, or stressed out.
- ◊ Identify current environmental stressors as experienced by the client.
- ◊ Determine if anxiety is normative or pathological.
- ◊ Pathological levels of anxiety are indicative of underlying anxiety disorder:
  - Anxiety is perceived of as distressing and out of the control of the person.
  - Anxiety is unlinked and not seen as caused by life events.
  - Anxiety is accompanied by somatic complaints, which is more uncommon in normal anxiety levels.
  - Anxiety interferes with social, occupational, and recreational activities and with activities of daily living.
    - Determine the level of the client's anxiety using the 4-point scale of mild to panic levels (1 = mild to 4 = panic; see Table 10-1).
    - Use standardized rating scales such as the Hamilton Rating Scale for Anxiety (HAM-A; Hamilton, 1959) for establishing and monitoring the client's anxiety level over time.

♦ Assess general level of health and presence of concomitant illnesses.

♦ Assess for dysfunctional coping

- ◊ Alcohol use
- ◊ Illicit substance use
- ◊ Caffeine use
- ◊ Increased nicotine use
- ◊ Misuse of anti-anxiety medications

♦ Assess for specific psychological symptoms of anxiety

- ◊ Fear of dying, losing one's mind, or a sense of unreality
- ◊ Belief that one is very ill, with no findings to support this belief
- ◊ Narrowed perceptions
- ◊ Limited eye contact

Physical Exam Findings

- Possible physical manifestations
  - Diaphoresis
  - Headaches
  - Dizziness and lightheadedness
  - Missing hair on scalp, eyebrows, or eye lashes (for trichotillomania or excoriation disorders)
  - Pupillary dilation
  - Increased muscle tone
  - Palpitations, often with tightness in chest
  - Tachycardia
  - Hypertension
  - Gastrointestinal (GI) problems such as nausea, diarrhea, or abdominal discomfort

Mental Status Exam Findings

- Appearance
  - Psychomotor restlessness
  - Tremors
  - Hand wringing
- Speech
  - Overproductive
  - Rapid
  - Distractible speech patterns
  - Thought blocking
- Mood
  - Nervous
  - Worried
- Affect
  - Anxious
  - Worried
  - Tearful

- Thought process
  - Overall organized
  - Goal-directed
  - Redirectable
- Thought content
  - Thematic for worry
  - Mild perseveration on topics of concern
- Orientation
  - Usually fully oriented
- Memory
  - Impaired short-term and immediate memory
  - Forgetful
- Concentration
  - Inattentive
  - Decreased concentration
- Abstraction
  - Abstract on proverbs and similarities
- Judgment
  - Intact
- Insight
  - Intact or limited insight

Diagnostic and Laboratory Findings

- Obtain baseline laboratory tests such as complete blood count (CBC), chemistry profile, thyroid function tests, and B_{12} level to rule out metabolic causes or unidentified conditions.
- Obtain drug toxicity screening if indicated by history.
- In some cases, clients may have laboratory results reflecting compensated respiratory alkalosis:
  - Decreased carbon dioxide levels
  - Decreased bicarbonate levels
  - Normal pH

DIFFERENTIAL DIAGNOSIS

- Many medical conditions can cause worry, fear, and normal levels of anxiety (see Table 10–4).
- Ensure that client symptoms meet criteria for anxiety disorders.

TABLE 10–4.
MEDICAL CONDITIONS THAT MAY MIMIC ANXIETY DISORDERS

GENERAL CATEGORY OF DISORDER	SPECIFIC ILLNESS
Cardiovascular	Congestive heart failure Mitral valve prolapse Myocardial infarction Arrhythmias, especially tachycardic arrhythmias Pulmonary embolism Coronary artery disease
Respiratory	Asthma Chronic obstructive pulmonary disorder Pneumonia
Endocrine	Hyperthyroidism Hyperparathyroidism Cushing's disease
Neurological	Seizure disorders Transient ischemic attacks Cerebral vascular accident Encephalitis CNS neoplasms
Metabolic	Hypoglycemia Vitamin B deficiency Porphyria
Substance use or dependency	Intoxication with CNS stimulants (e.g., cocaine, amphetamines, caffeine) Withdrawal from CNS depressants (e.g., alcohol, marijuana)

CLINICAL MANAGEMENT

- Rule out or treat any conditions that may contribute to pathological levels of anxiety.

Pharmacological Management

- Most of the medications known to improve symptoms of anxiety act directly or indirectly on the GABA system.

Selective serotonin reuptake inhibitors (SSRIs)

- Considered first-line agents for chronic anxiety disorders
- Action on serotonin system and indirectly on GABA system
- Carry no risk of dependency
- Cannot be used as needed
- Generally well tolerated
- Takes time to reach symptom control (usually 4–6 weeks)
- Best when combined with psychotherapy
- Food and Drug Administration (FDA) box warning for increased suicidality in children, adolescents, and young adults

Benzodiazepines

- Potentiate the effect of GABA
- Rapid onset of action
- Can be used as needed
- Limit to lowest possible dose and short-term use if possible because long-term use may lead to tolerance, dependence, memory impairment, and depression.
- Use should be limited to periods of excessive symptoms or high stress, or with unremitting symptoms.
- Use with extreme caution in clients with a history of substance dependence.
- Effective but carry risk for addiction, especially in persons who have a history of substance use
- The use of benzodiazepines has been associated with Alzheimer's disease.
- Benzodiazepines with longer half-lives require less-frequent dosing, have less-severe withdrawal, and have less rebound anxiety.
- Benzodiazepines with longer half-lives are more useful for continuous, moderate to severe anxiety or as bridge medications while waiting for efficacy of SSRIs:
    - Clonazepam
    - Diazepam

- Benzodiazepines with shorter half-lives require more-frequent dosing, have more-severe withdrawal, and have more rebound anxiety:
  - Alprazolam
  - Lorazepam
- Advantages of benzodiazepines with short half-lives
  - Benzodiazepines with short half-lives are often useful for intermittent or infrequent moderate to severe anxiety.
  - Less daytime sedation
  - Less drug accumulation
  - Quick onset of action
  - Useful for treatment of insomnia
- Disadvantages of benzodiazepines with short half-lives
  - Increased risk of addiction

Tricyclic antidepressants (TCAs; see page 191)

- Effective but affect multiple receptors and have problematic side-effect profiles
- Side effects often affect adherence

Non-benzodiazepine anxiolytics (see Table 10–5)

TABLE 10–5. NON-BENZODIAZEPINE ANXIOLYTICS FOR ADULTS

GENERIC	DOSAGE RANGE	SIDE EFFECTS	COMMENTS
Atenolol	25–200 mg/day	Bradycardia, hypotension, fatigue, dizziness	Used off-label
Buspirone	20–60 mg/day	Dizziness, insomnia, tremors, akathisia, stomach upset, dry mouth	Helpful adjunct for anxiety
Gabapentin	300–3600 mg/day	Ataxia, decreased coordination, sedation, disequilibrium	Used for anxiety, neuropathic pain, fibromyalgia, anti-craving Off-label use
Hydroxyzine	50–100 mg q6h p.r.n.	Xerostomia, drowsiness, dizziness, ataxia	Used for anxiety, sedation, nausea/vomiting Off-label used for insomnia
Propranolol	10–20 mg daily p.r.n.	Bradycardia, hypotension	Performance anxiety Ooff-label use

- Buspirone
  - Must be taken regularly, not as p.r.n.
- Gabapentin—off-label use
- Beta blockers (propranolol, atenolol)—off-label use
  - Usually adjunctive use with other pharmacological agent
- Hydroxyzine

Nonpharmacological Management

- Behavioral therapy
  - Systematic desensitization
  - Exposure therapy
  - Relaxation therapies
  - Biofeedback
- Cognitive behavioral therapy (CBT)
- Interpersonal therapies
- Somatic therapies
- Community self-help groups
- Alternative therapies as adjunctive treatments

COMORBIDITIES

- Anemia
- Cardiac disorders, especially in clients with dysrhythmias
- Endocrine disorders
  - Cushing's disease
  - Hyperthyroidism
  - Hypoglycemia
- Pulmonary conditions
  - Chronic obstructive pulmonary disorder
  - Asthma
  - Pulmonary embolism
  - Pneumothorax

- Adverse medication reactions
  - Caffeine
  - Nicotine
  - Anticholinergics
  - Antihistamines
  - Antipsychotics
  - Steroids
  - Bronchodilators
  - Anesthetics
- Mood disorders
- Substance use–related disorders

GENERAL HEALTH CONSIDERATIONS

- Chronic anxiety is wearing on the body; therefore, assess for effects on the cardiovascular system.
- Perform a general assessment for a healthy lifestyle.

LIFE SPAN CONSIDERATIONS

- In children, alpha-agonists are often used for anxiety.
  - Clonidine (.003–.01 mg/kg/d), off-label use
  - Guanfacine (.015–.05 mg/kg/d), off-label use

FOLLOW-UP

- General considerations
  - Clients should be seen initially weekly or biweekly to titrate medications.
  - Client teaching should include the risks, benefits, and potential side effects of medication treatment.
- If the client is taking benzodiazepines, monitor for appropriate use and potential dependence.
- If the client is taking SSRIs, monitor for common side effects and adverse effects.
  - Clients should be informed about symptoms of anxiety and that disorders are chronic illnesses; a relapse plan should be established for all clients.

- ◊ Assessment for suicidality should occur during symptom exacerbation periods.
- ◊ Because of frequent comorbidity with major depressive disorder, assess frequently for depression levels using standardized rating scales (see the following list).
- ◊ Medication should be combined with therapy to reach maximum control of symptoms.
- ◊ Clients may need encouragement to continue treatment, especially after initial symptom relief occurs.

- ♦ Standardized rating scales for anxiety disorders
  - ◊ Generalized Anxiety Disorder 7 (GAD-7; Spitzer et al., 2006)
  - ◊ Zung's Self-Rating Anxiety Scale (Zung, 1971)
  - ◊ Hamilton Rating Scale for Anxiety (HAM–A; Hamilton, 1959)
  - ◊ Yale-Brown Obsessive-Compulsive Scale (Y-BOCS; Goodman et al., 1989)
  - ◊ Screen for Child Anxiety Related Disorders (SCARED; Birmaher et al., 1977)

PANIC DISORDER

DESCRIPTION

- ♦ Panic disorder is experienced as discrete episodes or attacks with sudden onset of intense apprehension, fearfulness, or terror, often associated with sense of impending doom.
- ♦ Attacks occur without warning and in the absence of any real danger.
- ♦ Attacks build to a peak of intensity within a short, self-limiting time, usually within 10minutes of onset.
- ♦ Panic disorder is more common in women than in men.

ASSESSMENT

Client History

- ♦ Assess for the following:
  - ◊ Diagnostic criteria for panic disorder:
    - Discrete episode in which client experiences four or more of the following symptoms having a sudden onset and peaking within 10 minute of onset:
      - Chills or hot flushing
      - Fear of losing control or of going crazy

        - Fear of dying
        - Shortness of breath or smothering sensation
        - Palpitations, pounding, or accelerated heart rate
        - Chest pain, tightness, or discomfort
        - Sweating
        - Trembling or shaking
        - Nausea or abdominal distress
    - After first attack, persistent concern over having another attack, worry over the consequences of initial attack, or a significant behavioral change related to attack
    - With high somatic sensations, clients are often sensitive to new somatic experiences or perceptions.
    - Often intolerant of or concerned with common side effects of medication treatments
    - Discouraged or ashamed about "failure" to control emotions and over concern about dying when no other pathology identified
- In two-thirds of cases, major depression occurs first, followed by panic disorder symptoms.
- In one-third of cases, panic disorder symptoms precede major depression symptoms.

Physical Exam Findings

- Nonspecific, especially when client is not experiencing panic attack
- Nonspecific cardiac-related complaints during panic episodes often bring client into treatment:
    - Chest pain
    - Numbness and paresthesia
    - Shortness of breath

Mental Status Exam Findings

- General findings of anxiety as described earlier

- Findings very pronounced during panic episodes and less pronounced during nonpanic periods
- High level of anticipatory anxiety between panic episodes

Diagnostic and Laboratory Findings

No specific diagnostic or laboratory findings

DIFFERENTIAL DIAGNOSIS

- Rule out general medical conditions known to produce similar symptoms such as
    - Hyperthyroidism
    - Hyperparathyroidism
    - Pheochromocytosis
    - Vestibular dysfunction
    - Seizure disorders
    - Cardiac arrhythmias such as supraventricular tachycardia (SVT)
- Use of CNS stimulants such as
    - Cocaine
    - Amphetamines
    - Caffeine
- Another anxiety disorder such as posttraumatic stress disorder (PTSD) or phobias
- Separation anxiety disorder
- Consider general medical disorder if
    - First episode of panic attack symptoms occurs after age 45, or
    - Panic symptoms are atypical, such as
        - Vertigo,
        - Loss of consciousness,
        - Incontinence,
        - Headache,

        - Slurred speech, or
        - Amnesic pattern after attacks

- Differentiating factors from other anxiety conditions include
    - Sudden onset of attack
    - Discrete, self-limiting nature of symptoms
    - Paroxysmal symptom profile
    - Level 3–4 anxiety symptoms with somatic symptoms that are experienced as distressing and severe by the client

CLINICAL MANAGEMENT

- Follow guidelines of general clinical management of anxiety disorders.

Pharmacological Management

- SSRIs
- Benzodiazepines, usually used for short-term symptom control or "bridge" medication when starting an SSRI or other antidepressant
    - Buspar effective as an adjunct to an antidepressant
    - Other non-benzodiazepine anxiolytic meds used as adjuncts

Nonpharmacological Management

- CBT
- Individual or group therapy
- Exposure therapy
- Relaxation therapies

COMMON COMORBIDITIES

- Frequent with major depressive disorder (MDD)
- Estimated between 10% and 65% of clients with panic disorder, depending on source, also experience one of the following:

- ◊ Social phobia
- ◊ OCD
- ◊ Substance use disorders

AGORAPHOBIA

DESCRIPTION

- Agoraphobia is characterized by avoidance of places or situations from which escape may be difficult or embarrassing or in which help may not be available in the event of perceived need, such as a panic attack. Up to 50% of people meeting criteria for agoraphobia report that panic attacks or panic disorder preceded onset of agoraphobia.
- Anxiety usually leads to avoidant behavior that impairs a person's ability to travel, to work, or to carry out responsibilities of daily living.
- Differential diagnosis is assisted by the awareness that people with agoraphobia feel better and report less-significant concerns with anxiety when accompanied by a trusted companion.
- When people meet criteria for agoraphobia and panic or other anxiety disorder, both diagnoses should be assigned.

ASSESSMENT

Client History

- Assess for the following:
  - ◊ Clinical presentation meets diagnostic criteria for agoraphobia
    - Presence of agoraphobic anxiety related to fear of developing panic-like symptoms
    - Individual has never met criteria for panic disorder
    - Avoidant behavior resulting from the agoraphobic anxiety

Physical Exam Findings

- No physical exam findings specific to agoraphobia

Mental Status Exam Findings

- Consistent with finding for anxiety
- Thought content consistent with criteria for agoraphobia

Diagnostic and Laboratory Findings

- No specific diagnostic lab findings exist.

CLINICAL MANAGEMENT

- Follow guidelines of general clinical management of anxiety disorders

Pharmacological Management

- SSRIs
- Benzodiazepines for short-term use
- Beta blockers (off-label use) used for discrete episodes of social anxiety

Nonpharmacological Management

- CBT
- Supportive group therapy
- Desensitization therapy

COMMON COMORBIDITIES

- Panic disorder

SPECIFIC PHOBIAS (SIMPLE PHOBIAS)

DESCRIPTION

- In specific phobias, there is a clinically significant level of marked and persistent fear that is clearly observable and is, by client perception, clearly related to specific objects or situations.

- In adults, but not in children, exists the conscious recognition that the fear is excessive or unreasonable.
- In children, the degree of insight into the unreasonable nature of the fear increases as age increases.

RISK FACTORS

- Traumatic past exposure
  - Having been bitten by dog, having choked on food, and so forth
- Observation of another's trauma
  - Seeing others bitten by dog, seeing others choking on food, and so forth
- Excessive informational transmission
  - Repeated graphic parental warnings of dangers of certain events or situations
- Genetic loading
  - Having family member with specific phobia
  - Blood-injection-injury type is most familial
  - Subtype aggregation patterns noted within families; for example, if a person's first-degree relative has animal subtype, the risk is highest for them to develop animal subtype

ASSESSMENT

Client History

- Assess for the following:
  - The content of phobias, which can vary with culture, ethnicity, and age
  - Phobic diagnosis should occur only when accompanied by significant functional impairment, such as full avoidance of school related to fear of encountering a spider.
  - Exposure to the specific feared object or situation immediately provokes the onset of clinically significant levels of anxiety.
    - This anxiety may fit the criteria for cued panic attack.
    - The level of anxiety is related directly to the proximity of the object or situation and the degree to which escape from the object or situation is possible.
- Children manifest fear and anxiety as crying, freezing, tantrums, or excessive clinging behavior.
- Children normatively express a transient fear of animals and other natural objects.

- Person engages in avoidant behavior to prevent reaction to an object or situation or endures object or situation with dread.
  - Avoidant behavior is distressful and has implications for social, recreational, and occupational or school functioning.
- Assess for subtypes:
  - There are five common subtypes: situational, natural environment, blood-injection-injury, animal, and other.
    1. Situational type: Cued by specific situations; examples include driving, enclosed spaces, tunnels or bridges, or flying
       - Most common adult form
       - In older adults, fear of closed-in situations most common
       - Bimodal peak of onset
         - First peak, childhood
         - Second peak, mid-20s
    2. Natural environment type: Fear cued by objects in the natural environment; examples include storms, lightning, water, or heights
       - Second most common adult form
       - Onset usually during childhood
    3. Blood-injection-injury type: Cued by seeing blood or an injury or by receiving an injection or other invasive medical procedure
       - Third most common adult form
       - Strong vasovagal component that can produce other somatic sensations
         - May exacerbate underlying cardiac or respiratory disorders
         - Person often presents with fainting as chief complaint
         - Experiences paroxysmal tachycardia and hypertension followed by deceleration of heart rate and drop in blood pressure
         - Clinical presentation and disease natural history is similar to that of panic disorder with agoraphobia
    4. Animal type: Fear cued by animals or insects; examples include rats, snakes, or spiders
       - Fourth most common adult form
       - Onset usually during childhood
    5. Other type: Fear cued by range of other stimuli; examples include fear of choking, vomiting, or fear of a specific illness
       - In children, often manifests as fear of loud sounds or costumed characters

- A person can experience more than one subtype at a time.
- A phobia to one object or situation in a subclass predisposes a person to another phobia within the same subclass (e.g., fear of rats increases the risk for fear of spiders).

Physical Exam Findings

- No physical exam findings specific to specific phobias

Mental Status Exam Findings

- Consistent with finding for anxiety
- Thought content consistent with criteria for phobia

Diagnostic and Laboratory Findings

- No specific diagnostic lab findings exist.

DIFFERENTIAL DIAGNOSIS

- Avoidance behavior in PTSD, OCD, separation anxiety disorder, or psychotic disorders

CLINICAL MANAGEMENT

- Follow guidelines of general clinical management of anxiety disorders.

Pharmacological Management

- SSRIs
- TCAs
- Short term use of benzodiazepines

Nonpharmacological Management

- CBT
- Biofeedback
- Desensitization therapy

SOCIAL ANXIETY (PHOBIA) DISORDER

DESCRIPTION

- Social anxiety disorder is a marked and persistent fear of social or performance situations in which embarrassment may occur.
- Anxiety levels often are sufficient to fit criteria for a situationally bound panic attack.
- The disorder has an estimated 3% to 13% prevalence rate in the U.S. population.
- Rates are equal for the genders.

ASSESSMENT

Client History

- Onset is in the mid-teens, often following stressful or humiliating experience, and tends to remit with age.
    - Some degree of social anxiety is common and normative in adolescence.
    - Social phobia should be diagnosed only if symptoms persist for longer than 6 months.
- Differential diagnosis is assisted by awareness that people with social phobia do not feel better or experience decreased anxiety when accompanied by a trusted companion.
- Common descriptive features
    - Hypersensitivity to criticism
    - Negative self-evaluations
    - Sensitivity to rejection
    - Low self-esteem
    - Inferiority feelings
    - Lack of assertiveness

- Protracted anticipatory anxiety may occur days or weeks before the feared social situation.
- Levels of subjective distress and impaired functioning can be significant and have been associated with suicidal ideation.

Physical Exam Findings for a Person Who Is Acutely Anxious

- Sweating
- Tremors
- Palpitations
- Muscle tension
- Diarrhea
- Blushing

Mental Status Exam Findings

- Consistent for anxiety
- Thought content consistent with criteria for social anxiety

Diagnostic and Laboratory Findings

- No specific diagnostic lab findings exist

CLINICAL MANAGEMENT

- Follow guidelines of general clinical management of anxiety disorders.

Pharmacological Management

- SSRIs
- Benzodiazepines, for short-term use
- Beta blockers
  - Used for discrete episode relief
  - For example, before having to attend a scheduled social function

Nonpharmacological Management

- CBT
- Exposure therapy
- Relaxation therapy

GENERALIZED ANXIETY DISORDER

DESCRIPTION

- In generalized anxiety disorder (GAD), excessive worry, apprehension, or anxiety about events or activities occurs more days than not for a period of at least 6 months.
    - The person finds it hard to control the anxiety.
    - No clear link exists to life events or stressors.
    - Worry and anxiety interfere with activities of daily living.
    - The nature and focus of worry shift frequently.
    - A pattern of waxing and waning of symptoms exists.
- Symptoms worsen as life events stress the person.

ASSESSMENT

Client History

Assess for the following:

- In GAD, anxiety and worry are out of proportion to the actual likelihood or effect of the feared event.
- People report subjective distress caused by the constant worry but do not always describe the worry as excessive.
- Excessive anxiety and worry occurs more days than not for at least 6 months.
- The person finds it difficult to control anxiety.

Physical Exam Findings

- No physical exam findings specific to GAD
- Associated with other health states
  - Irritable bowel syndrome
  - Migraine and other headache disorders
- Physical signs of anxiety
  - Muscle tension
  - Generalized muscle ache and soreness
  - Tremors
  - Twitching
  - Subjective complaints of shakiness
  - Shortness of breath
  - Autonomic hyperarousal signs
  - Tachycardia
  - Increased respiratory rates
  - Dizziness
  - Numbness
  - Easily fatigued, often experienced as activity intolerance
  - Muscle tension and increased tone
  - Sleep disturbance

Mental Status Exam Findings

- Appearance
  - Psychomotor restlessness
- Mood
  - Anxious
  - Feeling keyed up or on edge
  - Irritability

- Concentration
  - Difficulty concentrating
- Thought content
  - Thematic for the anxiety and worry
  - Descriptive of the significant distress and impairment in daily functioning caused by GAD

Diagnostic and Laboratory Findings

- No specific diagnostic lab findings exist

DIFFERENTIAL DIAGNOSIS

- PTSD
- Adjustment disorder with anxiety
- Obsessions in OCD
- Anxiety associated with another disorder such as hypochondriasis or social phobia

CLINICAL MANAGEMENT

Pharmacological Management

- SSRIs
- Buspar
- Benzodiazepines as p.r.n. agents

Nonpharmacological Management

- Good candidates for therapy as single-treatment modality
- CBT
- Relaxation therapies

- Stress management
- Supportive counseling

COMMON COMORBIDITIES

- Mood disorders
- Other anxiety disorders
- Substance-related disorders

LIFE SPAN CONSIDERATIONS

- Children
  - Anxiety is common in children, but it is important to assess normal versus pathological levels.
  - Anxiety is manifested in excessive worry over competence or quality of performance in school, work, sports, or other activities.
  - Common worry often manifests as anxiety over punctuality or catastrophes such as earthquakes or war.
  - Often accompanied by the following:
    - Overly conforming behavior
    - Perfectionist self-expectations
    - Excessive seeking of approval of others
    - Need for frequent reassurance about performance

SEPARATION ANXIETY DISORDER

- Developmentally inappropriate and excessive distress occurring after the age of 4 when faced with separation from a major attachment figure
- Refer to Chapter 15: Disorders of Childhood and Adolescence
- May persist into adulthood and in the DSM-5-TR it can be diagnosed in adulthood

OBSESSIVE–COMPULSIVE DISORDER

DESCRIPTION

- Obsessive-compulsive disorder (OCD) is the presence of anxiety-provoking obsessions or compulsions that function to reduce the person's subjective anxiety level.
    - Obsession
        - Defined as recurrent and persistent thoughts, impulses, or images that are experienced and cause anxiety and distress
        - Experienced as intrusive and inappropriate
        - Ego-dystonic experience in which a person feels the content of obsession is alien to their belief structure and not the kind of common thought, impulse, or image they usually experience
    - Compulsion
        - Defined as repetitive behaviors or mental actions that a person feels driven to perform in response to an obsession.

RISK FACTORS

- Genetic predisposition
    - Familial transmission pattern
        - Disease rates are higher in people with a first-degree relative who has OCD than in the general population.
        - Rates are also higher in people with a first-degree relative who has Tourette's syndrome than in the general population.
- PANDAS (pediatric autoimmune neuropsychiatric disorders associated with streptococcal infections) should be considered in all children with sudden-onset OCD symptoms.

ASSESSMENT

Client History

- Assess for the following:
    - Diagnostic criteria
        - Presence of either obsessions or compulsions

        - The person recognizing that the obsession or compulsion is excessive or unreasonable
        - The obsession or compulsion is causing marked distress, is time consuming, or interferes with normal daily activity.

Obsessions

- Common obsessions include the following:
    - Repeated thoughts about contamination, dirt, or germs
    - Repeated doubts, such as having hit someone with a car or having left an oven on, without evidence
    - Need to have things in a specific order, with marked distress when that order is disturbed
    - Aggressive or horrific thoughts
        - May occur in pregnancy and postpartum periods and manifest as intrusive thoughts about something happening to their baby or doing something to their baby; the thoughts are highly ego-dystonic
        - Sexual imagery
- Obsessions usually do not involve real-world worries such as concern over finances.
- The person recognizes that the thoughts, impulses, or images are a product of their own mind.
- The person attempts to ignore or suppress thoughts, impulses, or images or to override them with other thoughts or actions.
- People often avoid situations in which the content of obsession may be encountered (e.g., avoiding public restrooms to avoid contamination).

Compulsions

- Common compulsions include repetitive actions, usually behavioral, and are often called rituals:
    - Handwashing
    - Excessive cleaning
    - Checking to see, for example, if the lights are turned off, the stove is turned off, or the doors are locked
    - Needing to place objects in certain order
    - Common mental actions include the following:
        - Counting
        - Silently repeating words
        - Praying

- Behaviors or mental acts are not experienced as pleasurable and are intended to prevent or reduce distress and subjective anxiety.
    - If the person resists the compulsion, the anxiety and subjective tension usually increase.
    - Some people believe that the compulsion can prevent some dreaded event or situation that is experienced as an obsession, such as sexual or horrific images.

Physical Exam Findings

- No physical exam findings specific to OCD
- Dermatitis may be present related to excessive handwashing or overuse of caustic cleaning agents.
- Hypochondriasis and somatic fixation common

Mental Status Exam Findings

- Consistent with finding for anxiety
- Thought content dominated by obsessions
- Behavioral manifestations of rituals may be noted

Diagnostic and Laboratory Findings

- No specific diagnostic lab findings exist.

DIFFERENTIAL DIAGNOSIS

- Body dysmorphic disorder
- Eating disorders
- Trichotillomania
- Hypochondriasis
- Obsessive–compulsive personality disorder
- Tic or stereotypic movement disorder

CLINICAL MANAGEMENT

- Follow guidelines of general clinical management of anxiety disorders.

Pharmacological Management

- SSRIs (clients often need higher dosing range for adequate symptom control)
- TCAs (clomipramine)
- Second-generation antipsychotics such as risperidone are off label but have data supporting their adjunctive use with SSRI medication

Nonpharmacological Management

- CBT
- Exposure therapy

COMMON COMORBIDITIES

- Major depression
- Eating disorders
- Other anxiety disorders

LIFE SPAN CONSIDERATIONS

- Children
  - Common in childhood, usually with prepubertal onset
  - More common in boys than in girls
  - Washing, checking, and ordering are the most common behavioral manifestations.
  - Common comorbidities in children include the following:
    - Learning disorders
    - Disruptive behavioral disorders
    - Tourette's syndrome
  - Associated in children with group A beta-hemolytic streptococcal infections (e.g., scarlet fever, strep throat)

- Older adults
  - More obsessions than compulsions are usually present
  - Obsessive content characteristically about dying
  - Compulsions characteristically about washing and cleaning

POSTTRAUMATIC STRESS DISORDER

DESCRIPTION

- Posttraumatic stress disorder (PTSD) is the reexperiencing of an extremely traumatic event accompanied by symptoms of increased arousal and avoidance of stimuli associated with the trauma.
- The traumatic event can be experienced directly or witnessed.
  - Common experienced trauma includes
    - Military combat
    - Violent personal assault such as robbery or rape
    - Kidnapping or hostage situation
    - Terrorist attack
    - Torture
    - Prolonged sexual abuse
    - Natural or human-made disasters
  - Common witnessed trauma includes
    - Observing the death of or significant injury to another
    - Unexpectedly witnessing of any of the aforementioned traumas
    - Learning of the sudden or unexpected death of or significant injury to family member or close friend
- A relationship exists between the person's physical proximity to the traumatic event and the likelihood of symptom onset.

RISK FACTORS

- Experienced or witnessed trauma
- Genetic predisposition
  - Assumed to have strong genetic etiological component and tends to run in families

- ◊ History of major depression in first-degree relative related to increased risk of developing PTSD

ASSESSMENT

Client History

- ♦ Assess for the following:
  - ◊ Symptoms cannot predate exposure to trauma.
  - ◊ Presenting symptoms and history can be delineated as one of three subtypes:
    - Acute: Duration of symptoms less than 3 months
    - Chronic: Symptoms lasting 3 months or longer
    - Delayed onset: At least 6 months between traumatic event and the onset of symptoms

Physical Exam Findings

- ♦ No physical exam findings specific to PTSD
- ♦ Increased rates of somatic complaints
- ♦ Insomnia is frequently the chief complaint on presentation for evaluation.
- ♦ Distractibility in motor tasks
- ♦ Measurable increased autonomic symptoms
  - ◊ Tachycardia
  - ◊ Diaphoresis
  - ◊ Increased respiratory rates
  - ◊ Pupillary dilation
  - ◊ Increased startle response

Mental Status Exam Findings

- ♦ Consistent with finding for anxiety
- ♦ Thought content consistent with criteria for PTSD and often dominated by traumatic experience
- ♦ May demonstrate some psychotic findings during flashback episodes

Diagnostic and Laboratory Findings

- Diagnostic criteria (symptoms for 1 month or longer)
    - Exposure to a traumatic event
        - The person experienced, witnessed, or was confronted with an event involving the actual or threatened death or serious injury, and the person's response involved intense fear, helplessness, or horror.
    - The traumatic event is persistently reexperienced in one or more of the following ways:
        - Recurrent and intrusive, distressing recollection of the event, including images, thoughts, and perceptions
        - May be experienced as flashbacks
        - Rare cases involve dissociative states lasting hours to days
        - Recurrent distressing dreams about the event
        - Acting or feeling as if the traumatic event were reoccurring
        - Intense psychological distress at exposure to cues that symbolize or resemble aspects of the traumatic event
        - Physiological reactivity on exposure to cues that symbolize or resemble aspects of the traumatic event
    - Three or more avoidance symptoms
        - Persistent avoidance of stimuli associated with the traumatic event and numbing of responsiveness
        - Efforts to avoid talking about or thinking about traumatic event
        - Avoidance of activities, places, or people that arouse recollections of traumatic event
        - Inability to recall important aspects of event
        - Marked decreased interest or participation in activities
        - Feelings of detachment or estrangement from others
        - Restricted range of affect
        - Sense of foreboding and of shortened future, premature death, or no expectation for success or happiness
    - Two or more increased arousal symptoms
        - Persistent symptoms of increased arousal
        - Difficulty falling asleep
        - Irritability or outburst of anger
        - Difficulty concentrating

        - Hypervigilance
        - Exaggerated startle response
    - ◊ Symptoms causing significant distress or impairment in activities of daily functioning
- Symptoms usually occur within 3 months of trauma
- Duration of symptoms highly variable
- Symptoms remit within 3 months in one-half of cases
- Common waxing and waning of symptoms related to internal and external cues that resemble the trauma

Diagnostic and Laboratory Findings

- No specific diagnostic lab findings exist.

DIFFERENTIAL DIAGNOSIS

- Adjustment disorder
- Brief psychotic disorder
- Acute stress disorder
- Intrusive thoughts in OCD

CLINICAL MANAGEMENT

- Follow guidelines of general clinical management of anxiety disorders.

Pharmacological Management

- SSRIs
- TCAs
- Benzodiazepines are not recommended in the treatment of PTSD
- Antipsychotics may be useful during episodes of flashbacks.
- Alpha antagonists (e.g., prazosin) may be used for treating nightmares (off-label use).

Nonpharmacological Management

- CBT
- Exposure therapy with response prevention (ERP)
- Supportive group therapy
- Relaxation therapies
- Eye movement desensitization and reprocessing (EMDR)

COMMON COMORBIDITIES

- Major depression
- Dysthymia
- Substance use or dependence

LIFE SPAN CONSIDERATIONS

- Can occur at any age, including childhood
  - Children
    - Expression of fear and horror occurs in disorganized or agitated behavior.
    - Repetitive play behaviors show themes or aspects of trauma.
    - Frightening dreams, but without recognized content, are common.
    - In young children, learning that a traumatic event occurred to a parent or a caregiver may be the precipitating factor.

DISSOCIATIVE DISORDERS

- Dissociative amnesia, depersonalization or derealization, and dissociative identity disorder (DID)
- Dissociation is a defense mechanism that protects a person from overwhelming anxiety by emotionally separating.
  - Dissociation causes gaps or interruption in the person's memory.
- Depersonalization or derealization: A persistent feeling of oneself not being real, or the environment not being real; reality testing remains intact

- ◊ Depersonalization and derealization are generally perceived as uncomfortable.
- ◊ Etiology of depersonalization and derealization can be physical or psychological.
- ◊ Physical causes are seizures, migraine headaches, psychedelic drugs, and alcohol.
- ◊ Psychological causes are severe anxiety and traumatic stress.

- DID is characterized by two or more distinct personality states ("alters").
  - ◊ Personality states are generally split off from one another, leading to gaps in recall of everyday events.
  - ◊ Symptoms cause significant distress and impaired functioning.
  - ◊ Comorbid with PTSD
  - ◊ Etiology is a history of severe physical or sexual trauma, or both, in childhood.

BODY DYSMORPHIC DISORDER

- Preoccupation with one or more perceived defects or flaws in physical appearance
- Engages in repetitive behaviors (checking mirror, reassurance-seeking, and so on) in response to appearance concerns
- Preoccupation causes considerable distress
- Insight ranges from good to poor to absent (fixed delusion)

HOARDING DISORDER

- Persistent difficulty discarding possessions, regardless of actual value
- Experiences marked distress in response to pressure to discard
- Results in accumulation of possessions that compromise living space or ability to function, including maintaining a safe environment for self or others
- Insight ranges from good to poor to absent (fixed delusion)

TRICHOTILLOMANIA

- Recurrent pulling out of one's hair despite repeated attempts to stop
- Causes significant distress or impairment in functioning
- Hair-pulling is not an attempt to improve a perceived defect or flaw

EXCORIATION DISORDER

- Recurrent skin picking that results in lesions despite attempts to stop
- Results in significant distress or impairment
- Behavior not better explained by physiologic response to substance (e.g., methamphetamine use) or intentional attempt at self-harm

CASE STUDY

R.E. is a 47-year-old school custodian with a long history of feeling nervous, having difficulty controlling worry, and being restless. R.E. reports doing well until about 4 weeks ago when traveling overseas with the church group for a caring mission in South America. R.E. noted feeling "depressed by seeing all the poverty and despair in those places" and began to have difficulty falling and staying asleep. Reported experiencing disturbing dreams about "the poverty and despair." The sleep disturbances persisted upon returning home and R.E. started feeling anxious and could not concentrate during the workday.

One week ago, R.E. began to feel overwhelmed by worry and was unable to go to work. Describes experiencing discrete "attacks" of rapid heart rate, sweating, and difficulty breathing and went to a local emergency department several times, was evaluated, and each time was given "a shot" and sent home. The emergency department doctor also suggested he contact a therapist. R.E. was not convinced that the distress was due to anxiety. On the third visit to the emergency department, R.E. was given a prescription for alprazolam 0.5 mg #30 with the directions "take as needed for anxiety" and was referred back to the primary care provider. Although the client initially felt the medication was helping, R.E. has continued to have difficulty falling and staying asleep and has continued to have "bad dreams." Reports needing 4 tablets of alprazolam yesterday before finally falling asleep until this morning and now believes "the medicine isn't working."

The client states, "there is something really wrong with me and nobody believes me. Everyone thinks it's all in my head. I know I'm anxious, but what if there's also something wrong with my heart? Doctors miss things all the time. . . ." The client now presents to the PMHNP at the hospital-based outpatient psychiatry department.

MENTAL STATUS EXAM

- Appearance: Well-nourished, well-dressed
- Motor: Some motor restlessness
- Speech: Some pressure
- Affect: Anxious
- Mood: Depressed
- Thought process and content: Thematic for fear of serious cardiac etiology not being adequately assessed or treated. There is no evidence of an overt delusional process.
- Abstractive on proverbs
- Memory: Impaired
- Concentration: Impaired

SOCIAL HISTORY

- Married and has three children
- Works as a high school custodian
- Overweight at 280 lbs., with sedentary lifestyle
- Smokes two packs a day
- Does not drink alcohol for religious reasons
- Partner very concerned and supportive

PAST PSYCHIATRIC HISTORY

- Hospitalized in 1998 for "nerves"
- At that time started on paroxetine 20 mg/d
- After 3 months, the dose was raised to 40 mg q.d. and remained on that dose for the next 18 months, when the medication was tapered off under his primary care provider's supervision.
- Has had no significant exacerbation of symptoms since initial treatment

PAST MEDICAL HISTORY

- History of seizure disorder since childhood; well-controlled with levetiracetam

CURRENT MEDICATIONS

- Alprazolam 0.5 mg, p.o. p.r.n. q4h.

LABS

- Electrocardiography (ECG), CBC, thyroid function tests, and chemistry panel done in emergency department and all within normal limits

SCREENING TOOLS

- Current level of anxiety: moderate–severe

IN PLANNING CARE FOR THIS CLIENT, THE PMHNP HAS MANY ISSUES TO CONSIDER

1. What is the most likely diagnosis?
2. How will the PMHNP separate comorbidity from complications of current diagnosis?
3. What medication adjustments would the PMHNP make?
4. How will the PMHNP address the family issues?
5. How often will the PMHNP plan to see the client?

   Given the level of initial distress, the PMHNP decides to restart paroxetine and continue using alprazolam as a bridge medication while waiting for a therapeutic response to the antidepressant.

6. What considerations should be given to using a benzodiazepine in a client with panic disorder?

   The client has now been taking paroxetine 20 mg for the past 2 weeks and has not had a panic attack since beginning treatment with the scheduled dose of benzodiazepine that was started with the re-initiation of paroxetine.

   The client no longer worries that he has a heart condition and falls asleep quickly, but continues to have some mild middle-phase insomnia that lasts up to 1 hour. The client is able to eventually fall back to sleep but wakes up feeling anxious. The client is tearful at times during the day and worries that the panic attacks will recur if the benzodiazepine is stopped.

7. How should the PMHNP adjust the treatment plan?
8. The client has been taking paroxetine 40 mg q.d. for the past month and is now taking clonazepam 0.5 mg q.a.m. and q.h.s. for the past 2 weeks after experiencing sedation while taking 0.5 mg q.a.m. and 1.0 mg q.h.s. The client continues to experience mild–moderate anxiety periodically most days. How should the PMHNP alter the treatment plan?
9. At what point should the PMHNP begin to taper the client off the clonazepam?

ANSWERS TO CASE STUDY DISCUSSION QUESTIONS

1. The client meets criteria for panic disorder. It is not unusual for people who have panic attacks to misinterpret the symptoms as cardiac or other etiology. The PMHNP must also assess for a mood disorder as symptoms anxiety and mood symptoms often overlap.
2. The PMHNP should perform a complete assessment, which includes a physical examination, mental status examination, and lab studies. The client's current medications should be evaluated, and the chronology of symptoms should be compared to any changes in his health status.
3. After assessing the efficacy of the treatment history, the PMHNP should consider restarting paroxetine.
4. Several approaches might be appropriate, including using psychoeducation for the family, providing supportive counseling, or involving the family in family therapy.
5. The client should be seen frequently until symptoms are stable. Weekly appointments during the initial phase of treatment would be ideal.
6. Before starting a benzodiazepine, the PMHNP should assess the client's history of recent and remote substance use. Potential risks versus benefits of short-term use must also be discussed along with the expectation that the medication will be tapered once the antidepressant is therapeutic. The PMHNP should discuss the expected therapeutic outcome of using an SSRI or other antidepressant. When using a benzodiazepine, consider using scheduled dosing to prevent the onset of panic symptoms. Clients who have severe anxiety often underdose or overdose medications to address their symptoms. Discuss expectations that the client will not adjust his dose of medication without direction. Short-acting benzodiazepines require dosing more frequently than long-acting benzodiazepines and may contribute to the client connecting the feeling of being anxious with taking a pill.
7. The PMHNP should consider switching to a long-acting benzodiazepine that may be scheduled in the a.m. and h.s. to provide better nighttime and early morning coverage. The PMHNP should discuss the expected outcome of each medication with the client. The PMHNP should increase the paroxetine dose in increments back to the dose that was previously therapeutic (40 mg).
8. As long as the client is not having considerable side effects, increase the paroxetine to 50 mg q.d. Continue weekly psychotherapy. Continue clonazepam.
9. Although benzodiazepines should be used for as brief a period as possible, discontinuing the medication too quickly may result in relapse. Unless otherwise indicated by side effects, benzodiazepine taper should begin after the client is at an adequate dose of antidepressant and he is no longer having significant anxiety symptoms

REFERENCES AND RESOURCES

American Nurses Association, American Psychiatric Nurses Association, & International Society of Psychiatric-Mental Health Nursing (2022). Psychiatric-mental health nursing: Scope and standards of practice (3rd ed.). American Nurses Association.

American Psychiatric Association. (2022). Diagnostic and statistical manual of mental disorders (5th ed., Text rev.).

Birmaher, B., Khetarpal, S., Brent, D., Cully, M., Balach, L., Kaufman, J., & McKenzie Neer, S. (1997). The Screen for Child Anxiety Related Emotional Disorders (SCARED): Scale construction and psychometric characteristics. Journal of the American Academy of Child & Adolescent Psychiatry, 36(4), 545–553.

Cohen, J. A., & Mannarino, A. P. (2015). Trauma-focused cognitive behavior therapy for traumatized children and families. Child and Adolescent Psychiatric clinics of North America, 24(3), 557–570. https://doi.org/10.1016/j.chc.2015.02.005

Davidson, J. R. (2000). Trauma: The impact of post-traumatic stress disorder. Journal of Psychopharmacology, 14(Suppl. 1), 5–12.

Felitti, V. J., Anda, R. F., Nordenberg, D., Williamson, D. F., Spitz, A. M., Edwards, V., Koss, M. P., & Marks, J. S. (1998). Relationship of childhood abuse and household dysfunction to many of the leading causes of death in adults. The Adverse Childhood Experiences (ACE) Study. American Journal of Preventive Medicine, 14(4), 245–258. https://doi.org/10.1016/s0749-3797(98)00017-8

Fernandez-Lewis, R., Hinton, D., Laria A., Patterson, E., Hofmann, S., Craske, M. G., . . . Liao, B. (2010). Culture and the anxiety disorders: Recommendations for DSM-V. Depression and Anxiety, 27, 212–229.

Goodman, W. K., Price, L. H., Rasmussen, S. A., Mazure, C., Fleischmann, R. L., Hill, C. L., Heninger, G. R., & Charney, D. S. (1989). The Yale-Brown Obsessive Compulsive Scale. I. Development, use, and reliability. Archives of general psychiatry, 46(11), 1006–1011. https://doi.org/10.1001/archpsyc.1989.01810110048007

Grant, J. E., Fineberg, N., van Ameringen, M., Cath, D., Visser, H., Carmi, L., . . . van Balkom, A. J. (2016). New treatment models for compulsive disorders. European Neuropsychopharmacology, 26(5), 877–884. https://doi.org/10.1016/j.euroneuro.2015.11.008

Guess K. F. (2006). Posttraumatic stress disorder: early detection is key. The Nurse practitioner, 31(3), 26–35. https://doi.org/10.1097/00006205-200603000-00008

Hamilton, M. (1959). The assessment of anxiety states by rating. British Journal of Medical Psychology, 32(1), 50–55.

Harris, M., & Fallot, R. D. (2001). Envisioning a trauma-informed service system: A vital paradigm shift. New Directions for Mental Health Services, (89), 3–22. https://doi.org/10.1002/yd.23320018903

Hembree, E. (2002). Psychosocial treatment of post-traumatic stress disorder. Primary Psychiatry, 9(2), 49–52.

Hoskins, M., Pearce, J., Bethell, A., Dankova, L., Barbui, C., Tol, W. A., . . . Bisson, J. I. (2015). Pharmacotherapy for post-traumatic stress disorder: Systematic review and meta-analysis. The British Journal of Psychiatry, 206(2), 93–100. https://doi.org/10.1192/bjp.bp.114.148551

Kessler, R. C., Chin, W. T., Merikangas, K. R., Demler, O. M., & Walters, E. E. (2005). Prevalence, severity and comorbidity of 12-month DSM-IV disorders in the National Comorbidity Survey Replication. Archives of General Psychiatry, 62, 617–627.

Lopez, I., Rivera, F., Ramirez, R., Guarnaccia, P., Canino, G., & Bird, H. (2009). Ataques de Nervios and their psychiatric correlates in Puerto Rican children from two different contexts. Journal of Nervous and Mental Disease, 197(12), 923–929.

Margolin, G., & Gordis, E. B. (2000). The effects of family and community violence on children. Annual Review of Psychology, 51, 445–479.

Meredith, P. V., & Horan, N. M. (2000). Adult primary care. Saunders.

Miller-Karas, E. (2023). Building resilience to trauma the trauma and community resiliency models (2nd ed.). Routledge.

Narrow, W. E., Rae, D. S., & Regier, D. A. (1998). NIMH epidemiology note: Prevalence of anxiety disorders. One-year prevalence best estimates calculated from ECA and NCS data. National Institute of Mental Health.

National Institute of Mental Health, Genetics Workgroup. (1998). Genetics and mental disorders.

Oral, R., Ramirez, M., Coohey, C., Nakada, S., Walz, A., Kuntz, A., Benoit, J., & Peek-Asa, C. (2016). Adverse childhood experiences and trauma informed care: The future of health care. Pediatric Research, 79(1-2), 227–233. https://doi.org/10.1038/pr.2015.197

Raines, A. M., Allan, N. P., Oglesby, M. E. & Short, N. A. (2015). Specific and general facets of hoarding: A bifactor model. Journal of Anxiety Disorders, (34), 100–106.

Raja, S., Hasnain, M., Hoersch, M., Gove-Yin, S., Rajagopalan, C. (2015). Trauma informed care in medicine: Current knowledge and future research directions. Family Community Health, 38(3), 216–226.

Regier, D. A., Rae, D. S., & Narrow, W. E. (1998). Prevalence of anxiety disorders and their comorbidity with mood and addictive disorders. British Journal of Psychiatry, (Suppl. 34), 24–28.

Spitzer, R.L., Kroenke, K., Williams, J. and Lowe, B. (2006). A brief measure for assessing generalized anxiety disorder: The GAD-7. Archives of Internal Medicine, 166(10), 1092–1097.

Stark, E. A., Parsons, E. E., Van Hartevelt, T. J., Charquero-Ballester, M., McManners, H., Ehlers, A., . . . Kriingelbach, M. L. (2015). Post-traumatic stress influences the brain even in the absence of symptoms: A systematic, quantitative meta-analysis of neuroimaging studies. Neuroscience and Biobehavioral Reviews, 56, 207–221.

Substance Abuse and Mental Health Services Administration. (2014). Concept of trauma and guidance for a trauma-informed approach. U.S. Department of Health and Human Services. https://ncsacw.acf.hhs.gov/userfiles/files/SAMHSA_Trauma.pdf

Substance Abuse and Mental Health Services Administration. (2017). Trauma-informed approach and trauma-specific interventions. U.S. Department of Health and Human Services. http://www.samhsa.gov/nctic/trauma-interventions

Yehuda, R. (1999). Biological factors associated with susceptibility to posttraumatic stress disorder. Canadian Journal of Psychiatry, 44(1), 34–39.

Yehuda, R. (2000). Biology of posttraumatic stress disorder. Journal of Clinical Psychiatry, 61(Suppl. 7), 14–21.

Zung, W. W. K. (1971). A rating instrument for anxiety disorders. Psychometrics, 12, 371–379.

CHAPTER 11

SCHIZOPHRENIA SPECTRUM AND OTHER PSYCHOTIC DISORDERS

This chapter describes a category of severe mental illnesses that have a researched biological basis to the disorders. Schizophrenia, the prototypic disorder of this category of illnesses, is multifaceted and affects a person's ability to function in many spheres of daily life. Of the psychotic disorders, schizophrenia is the illness that has been heavily researched and the one we know the most about.

The other disorders that comprise this category of illnesses are presented after an in-depth discussion of schizophrenia. Almost all the information provided for schizophrenia and for the clinical management of this disorder will pertain to the other psychotic disorders presented in this chapter.

GENERAL DESCRIPTION OF PSYCHOTIC DISORDERS

- These brain-based psychiatric disorders are grouped together because of similarity in frequent psychotic symptoms. Each disorder has a different etiology.
- Psychotic disorders are some of the most debilitating classes of psychiatric disorders, as determined by the degree of functional impairment and financial burden of severe mental illness.
- Psychotic implies an inability to test reality.
    - Manifests in symptoms (see Table 11–1) such as the following:
        - Hallucinations
        - Delusions
        - Disorganized thinking and speech
        - Referential thinking
        - Abnormal motor behavior
        - Negative symptoms
- Psychotic disorders are generally known to have a strong genetic component.

TABLE 11–1.
SYMPTOMS OF PSYCHOSIS

CLINICAL MANIFESTATION	DEFINITION	TYPE (ARRANGED IN ORDER OF COMMONALITY)
Hallucinations	False sensory experience without stimuli being present	Auditory visual Tactile Olfactory Gustatory Note: Hypnogogic* and hypnopompic* experiences are considered normative and do not fall under the true definition of hallucinations.
Delusions	A false belief firmly maintained despite evidence to the contrary	Persecutory Religious Grandiose Somatic Jealous Erotomanic
Disorganized thinking (often referred to as formal thought disturbance or disorder)	Problems with information organization and interpretation that is best assessed in the speech patterns of clients	Loose association Derailment Speaks tangentially Word salad
Disorganized behavior	Unusual behavior ranging from childlike silliness to anger	Silliness Unpredictable anger Difficulties with activities of daily living Disheveled Odd or unusual dress Inappropriate sexual activity Stereotypic motor activities
Referential thinking and delusions of control	Belief that events, actions, or situations in the environment hold special significance or meaning	Thought insertion Thought withdrawal Thought control Thought broadcasting
Illusional	Misperception of actual environmental stimuli	Auditory Visual Tactile Olfactory Gustatory

* Hypnopompic hallucination = a false perception that occurs when one is waking up; hypnogogic hallucination = a false perception that occurs when one is falling asleep; both are not considered pathological hallucinations.

SCHIZOPHRENIA

DESCRIPTION

- Schizophrenia causes significant disturbance in many areas of functioning:
  - Cognition
  - Perception
  - Emotion
  - Behavior
  - Eye movement
  - Socialization

ETIOLOGY

- Theories exist, ranging from psychological to neurobiological.
- The etiological profile is probably multifactorial.

Neurobiological Theory

- Multiple th profile is probably multifactorial.
- Implicates three areas of neurobiological functioning: genetics, neurodevelopment, and neurobiological defects
  - Genetics
    - Studies of twins have identified schizophrenia as having a strong genetic component.
      - Incidence increases from 1% risk of illness in general population to 50% risk in monozygotic twin of a person with schizophrenia.
      - 15% risk in dizygotic twin of a person with schizophrenia.
    - 40% risk in children if both parents have schizophrenia.
    - Specific gene has not yet been identified.
    - Numerous single nucleotide polymorphism (SNP) a genetic factor for susceptibility have been linked to schizophrenia.
    - Chromosomes 6p24–22 have been implicated (Sadock et al., 2017).

- Neurodevelopment
  - Genetic defects are believed to cause abnormal neuronal cell development, connection, organization, and migration.
    - These include inadequate synapse formation, excessive pruning of synapses, and excitotoxic death of neurons.
  - Intrauterine insults may contribute to the etiological picture:
    - Prenatal exposure to toxins, including viral agents
    - Oxygen deprivation
    - Maternal malnutrition, substance use, or other illness
- Neurobiological defect
  - Several abnormal brain structures have been identified in people with schizophrenia:
    - Enlarged ventricles
    - Smaller frontal and temporal lobes
    - Reduced symmetry in temporal, frontal, and occipital lobes
    - Cortical atrophy
    - Decreased cerebral blood flow
    - Hippocampal and amygdala reduction (Sadock et al., 2017)
  - Abnormalities lead to suspected impaired neuronal communication.
  - Suspected alterations in chemical neuronal signal transmission
    - Excess dopamine in mesolimbic pathway
    - Decreased dopamine in the mesocortical pathway
    - Excess glutamate
    - Decreased γ-aminobutyric acid (GABA)
    - Decreased serotonin

INCIDENCE AND DEMOGRAPHICS

- Geographic and historical variations in incidence give insight into etiological factors; higher rates seen in the following factors:
  - Urban-born
  - First-born

- ◊ Lower socioeconomic status
- ◊ Born in winter and early spring

- ♦ Schizophrenia tends to occur less often in women than in men.
  - ◊ Men: Onset ages 18–25 years
    - Tend to have more negative symptoms than women
    - Tend to have poorer prognosis, more hospitalizations, and less responsiveness to medications than women
  - ◊ Women: Onset ages 25–35 years
    - Usually have less premorbid dysfunction than men
    - Usually experience more dysphoria than men
    - Tend to have paranoid delusions and more hallucinations than men
    - Age of onset has pathophysiological and prognostic significance
  - ◊ Earlier age of onset
    - Tend to be men
    - Have poorer premorbid functioning
    - Have more evidence of structural brain abnormalities
    - Have more prominent negative symptoms
    - Have more cognitive impairment
    - Have poorer prognosis
  - ◊ Later age at onset
    - Tend to be women
    - Have less evidence of structural abnormalities
    - Have less cognitive impairment
    - Have better prognosis

POSSIBLE RISK FACTORS

- ♦ Genetic loading
  - ◊ First-degree relative with schizophrenia
- ♦ Prenatal exposure to flu or virus
- ♦ Prenatal malnutrition
- ♦ Obstetrical complications
- ♦ Central nervous system (CNS) infection in early childhood

PREVENTION AND SCREENING

- At-risk family education
- Community education
  - Stigma reduction
  - Signs and symptoms of illness
  - Treatment potential for control of symptoms
- Early recognition, intervention, and initiation of treatment
  - Significant and protracted prodromal symptom period usually noted before full onset of illness
  - Usually mild manifestations of criteria symptoms
  - Odd or unusual beliefs but not to delusional proportion
  - Feel unliked or picked on but not to delusional proportion
  - Odd speech patterns but not illogical
    - Digressions
    - Tangentiality
  - Overly concrete or abstractive
  - Odd behavior but not disorganized
  - Collects odd or worthless items
  - Mumbles to self
  - Isolates self and avoids interaction with others

ASSESSMENT

Client History

- There exists no single pathognomonic symptom of schizophrenia, but rather a constellation of symptoms.
- Schizophrenia is a disease of information processing.
- The symptoms are behavioral and cognitive.
- The illness is associated with marked impairment in social or occupational functioning.

- Prominent dysfunctions exist in many spheres of daily living.
  - Interpersonal relationships
    - 60% to 70% of clients do not marry
  - Social or occupational functioning
    - "Downdrift" functionality is noted over time.
    - Lower academic achievement compared to unaffected siblings
    - Difficulty holding a job
    - Underemployed relative to intellectual capacity
  - Self-care deficits
    - Poor hygiene
    - Difficulty with financial management
    - Limited independent living skills
- Characteristic symptom clusters for the illness (see Table 11–2) include the following:
  - Positive symptom cluster
  - Negative symptom cluster
  - Associated symptoms
- Diagnostic and Statistical Manual of Mental Disorders, Fifth Edition, Text Revision (DSM-5-TR; American Psychiatric Association, 2022) diagnostic criteria for schizophrenia includes the following:
  - Two or more of the following are frequently present during a 1-month period and at least one must be delusions, hallucinations, or disorganized speech:
    - Delusions: Bizarre and unorganized type; examples include delusions that manifest as loss of control over mind or body:
      - Thought withdrawal
      - Thought insertion
    - Hallucinations: Bizarre and unorganized type; examples include hallucinations that are improbable or readily apparent as not likely to have occurred
    - Disorganized speech
    - Grossly disorganized behavior
    - Negative symptoms
    - Significant impairment usually is evident by social or occupational dysfunction.
    - Duration of symptoms lasts for at least 6 months

TABLE 11–2.
POSITIVE AND NEGATIVE SYMPTOM CLUSTERS OF SCHIZOPHRENIA

SYMPTOM CLUSTER	EXPLANATION	CLINICAL MANIFESTATIONS
Positive symptoms	Symptoms that respond positively to and that can be controlled by antipsychotic medications Reflect excesses or distortions of normal brain functioning Caused by increased dopamine in the mesolimbic pathway	Hallucinations, delusions Referential thinking Disorganized behavior Hostility Grandiosity Mania Suspiciousness
Negative symptoms	Symptoms less responsive to antipsychotic medications but respond better to atypical antipsychotic medications Represent a decrease or loss of normal functioning Caused by decreased dopamine in the mesocortical pathway	Affective flattening Alogia or poverty of speech Avolition Apathy Abstract-thinking problems Anhedonia Attention deficits
Associated symptoms	Symptoms not required to be present to diagnose the disorder but often are present and a focus of treatment	Inappropriate affect Dysphoric mood Depersonalization Derealization High anxiety

- The course of illness is variable.
- Many clients have a fairly stable illness course.
- Some clients have clear episodic remissions and exacerbation periods.
- Negative symptoms tend to appear first as the illness develops.
- Positive symptoms appear to decrease over time, but negative symptoms persist.
- Negative symptoms are more debilitating.

- Factors predictive of good prognosis
  - High level of premorbid functioning
  - Acute onset
  - Later age at onset
  - Clear precipitating event
  - Married or partnered
  - Good support system
  - Positive symptoms
  - Short interval between treatment and onset of first symptoms
- The sooner the client is treated, the better the prognosis.
- A longer untreated premorbid period is associated with a poorer prognosis.
  - Absence of structural brain abnormalities
  - Family history of mood disorders
  - No family history of schizophrenia
- Subtype identification is of limited clinical value because illness course, response to treatment, and prognosis appear unrelated to subtype (see Table 11–3).

TABLE 11–3.
SUBTYPES OF SCHIZOPHRENIA*

SUBTYPE	CHARACTERISTIC
Paranoid	Prominent delusions or auditory hallucinations Lack of prominence of disorganized speech or behavior
Disorganized	Prominence of disorganized speech, behavior, and flat or inappropriate affect
Catatonic	Prominence of motor symptoms, including immobility as evidenced by catalepsy or stupor, excessive motor movement that is purposeless and not influenced by environmental stimuli, extreme negativity, mutism, oddities of posturing, echolalia,* and echopraxia*
Undifferentiated	Presence of symptoms consistent with schizophrenia but not a prominence of symptoms consistent with any of the other subtypes
Residual	Absence of prominent delusions, hallucinations, disorganized speech, and disorganized or catatonic behavior, and the continued presence of disturbance as indicated by presence of negative symptoms

*Subtypes are no longer diagnosed in the DSM-5-TR. Echolalia = repetition of the last-heard words of other people; echopraxia = imitation of observed behavior or movements.

Physical Exam Findings

- Abnormal smooth pursuit eye movements
- Abnormal saccadic eye movement
- Poor eye–hand coordination
    - Client identified as "clumsy" or "awkward"
- Presence of neurological nonlocalizing "soft signs" such as the following:
    - Astereognosis: Loss of ability to judge the form of an object by touch
    - Twitches, tics, or rapid eye blinking
    - Dysdiadochokinesia: Impairment of the ability to perform rapidly alternating movements
    - Impaired fine-motor movement
    - Left–right confusion
    - Mirroring
- Presence of neurological localizing "hard signs" such as the following:
    - Weakness
    - Decreased reflexes
- Other abnormalities that may be noted include the following:
    - Highly arched palate
    - Narrow or wide-set eyes
    - Subtle malformations of the ears

Mental Status Exam Findings

- Appearance
    - Odd
    - Unusual
    - Peculiar
- Speech
    - Bizarre content
    - Disorganized

    - ◊ Tangential
    - ◊ Loose association
- ♦ Affect
    - ◊ Blunted
    - ◊ Flat
    - ◊ Inappropriate
- ♦ Mood
    - ◊ Blandness
    - ◊ Impoverished
- ♦ Thought process
    - ◊ Psychotic
    - ◊ Hallucination
    - ◊ Delusion
    - ◊ Referential
    - ◊ Thought control, insertion, or withdrawal
    - ◊ Thought content
    - ◊ Thematically matched to psychotic content
    - ◊ May be impoverished
- ♦ Cognition
    - ◊ Illogical
    - ◊ Disorganized
- ♦ Orientation
    - ◊ Usually intact
- ♦ Memory
    - ◊ May have impaired short-term
- ♦ Concentration
    - ◊ Impaired during acute episodes
- ♦ Abstraction
    - ◊ Concrete on formal testing
- ♦ Judgment
    - ◊ Impaired for self-welfare

Diagnostic and Laboratory Findings

- No specific diagnostic lab findings exist.
- Abnormalities noted in structural studies
  - Enlargement of lateral ventricles
  - Widened cortical sulci
  - Diffuse decrease in volume of white and gray matter
  - Decreased volume of temporal lobe
  - Decreased volume in hippocampus, amygdala, and thalamus (Sadock et al., 2017)
- Abnormalities noted in functional studies
  - Hypofrontality
  - Decreased cerebral blood flow and metabolism
  - Diffuse hypometabolic action in cortical–subcortical circuitry

DIFFERENTIAL DIAGNOSIS

- Nonpsychiatric disorders
  - Epilepsy
  - CNS neoplasm
  - AIDS
  - Acute intermittent porphyria
  - B12 deficiency
  - Heavy-metal poisoning
  - Huntington's disease
  - Neurosyphilis
  - Systemic lupus erythematosus
  - Wernicke–Korsakoff syndrome
  - Wilson's disease
- Psychiatric disorders
  - Bipolar affective disorder
  - Substance-induced psychotic disorder
    - Amphetamines
    - Hallucinogens
    - Alcoholic hallucinosis

    - Barbiturate withdrawal
    - Cocaine
    - PCP (phencyclidine or angel dust)
  - ◊ Mood disorders with psychotic features (see Chapter 9)
  - ◊ Schizoaffective disorder (see page 323)
  - ◊ Schizophreniform disorder (see page 320)
  - ◊ Brief psychotic disorder (see page 328)
  - ◊ Delusional disorder (see page 325)
  - ◊ Schizotypal personality disorder (see Chapter 14)
  - ◊ Schizoid personality disorder (see Chapter 14)
  - ◊ Paranoid personality disorder (see Chapter 14)

CLINICAL MANAGEMENT

- ♦ Assess for acuity level
  - ◊ During acute psychotic episodes, client may require brief hospitalization to
    - Ensure client safety,
    - Rapidly stabilize client's symptom level in a controlled environment, and/or
    - Monitor treatment adherence with the goal of stabilization and recovery.
- ♦ Clinical management during nonacute episodes occurs most often in community settings.

Pharmacological Management

- ♦ Pharmacological therapy is the primary treatment modality, augmented by nonpharmacological treatments.
- ♦ Most clients will require lifelong medication.
- ♦ Client and family education is important for treatment adherence.
- ♦ Adjunctive medications may be used to achieve full symptom control:
  - ◊ Antidepressants
  - ◊ Anxiolytics
  - ◊ Anticonvulsants
- ♦ Atypical antipsychotics (see Table 11–4)
  - ◊ Primary first-line treatment agents
  - ◊ First introduced in the 1990s

TABLE 11–4.
ATYPICAL ANTIPSYCHOTICS

AGENT	DOSAGE	SIDE EFFECTS	COMMENTS
Aripiprazole	5–30 mg/day injection (acute agitation); 5.25–15 mg IM, (long acting) or 200–400 mg IM monthly	Headache, agitation, anxiety, insomnia, somnolence, akathisia, GI problems	Partial agonist of D2 receptors Monitor weight, BMI, waist circumference Monitor serum lipids and glucose Assess family and personal history of cardiovascular disease
Asenapine	5–10 mg p.o. b.i.d. sublingual	Akathisia, somnolence	Monitor weight, BMI, waist circumference Monitor serum lipids and glucose Assess family and personal history of cardiovascular disease
Brexpiprazole	2–4 mg p.o. q.d.	Akathisia, weight gain	Monitor serum lipids and glucose Assess family and personal history of cardiovascular disease
Cariprazine	1.5–6 mg p.o. q.d.	EPSE, akathisia, GI upset, restlessness, somnolence	Monitor serum lipids and glucose Assess family and personal history of cardiovascular disease
Clozapine	25–900 mg/day	Common: Tachycardia, dizziness, drowsiness hypersalivation (sialorrhea), weight gain, hyperlipidemia Rare: Agranulocytosis, myocarditis, neuroleptic malignant syndrome, agranulocytosis, myocarditis, neuroleptic malignant syndrome	Only drug for treatment-resistant schizophrenia Must be enrolled in a clozapine REMS program Risk for neutropenia is monitored by the ANC only, not in conjunction with the WBC count During first 6 months: weekly; during second 6 months: every 2 weeks; then monthly if ANC normal If ANC levels less than 500/μL suspend drug Clients can be rechallenged if the prescriber determines benefits outweigh the risks; monitor for myocarditis

(Continued)

TABLE 11–4. (CONTINUED)

AGENT	DOSAGE	SIDE EFFECTS	COMMENTS
Clozapine (continued)			Dose-related seizure risk Significant weight gain and risk of diabetes Rare hyperprolactinemia Monitor weight, BMI, waist circumference Monitor serum lipids and glucose Assess family and personal history of cardiovascular disease
Iloperidone	12–24 mg/day in divided doses	Orthostatic hypotension, sedation, dizziness	Titrate slowly due to the alpha 1 antagonist properties Might be helpful for posttraumatic stress disorder Hyperarousal symptoms due to alpha 1 blocking Monitor weight, BMI, waist circumference Monitor serum lipids and glucose Assess family and personal history of cardiovascular disease
Lumateperone	42 mg/day	Somnolence, headache, dyslipidemia, nausea	Fasting lipid panel, weight at baseline, then periodically; CBC w/ diff initial treatment. Discontinue if ANC <1000; consider discontinuing if unexplained decrease in WBC
Lurasidone	40–160 mg/day	Akathisia, sedation, and nausea	Should be taken with food to increase absorption Use with caution at lower doses in clients with renal and hepatic impairment Monitor weight, BMI, waist circumference Monitor serum lipids and glucose Assess family and personal history of cardiovascular disease
Olanzapine	Tablet and intramuscular injection (acute): 5–20 mg/day	Sedation, weight gain, hyperlipidemia, elevated glucose, elevated liver function tests, mild prolactin elevation	Significant weight gain Monitor weight, BMI, waist circumference Monitor serum lipids and glucose Assess family and personal history of cardiovascular disease

(Continued)

TABLE 11–4. (CONTINUED)

AGENT	DOSAGE	SIDE EFFECTS	COMMENTS
Olanzapine (continued)	Injection: 150–405 mg every 2–4 weeks	Long-acting preparation (Zyprexa, Relprevv) requires that clients be monitored for 3 hours post-injection due to risk of post-injection delirium sedation syndrome	
Paliperidone	Tablets: 3–12 mg/day Injection: 39–234 mg IM Injection every 3 months: 273 mg, 410 mg, 546 mg, or 819 mg IM	Orthostatic hypotension, hyperprolactinemia, GI upset, dizziness, headache	Extended-release risperidone Greatest prolactin elevation among atypical psychotics Monitor weight, BMI, waist circumference Monitor serum lipids and glucose Assess family and personal history of cardiovascular disease
Primavanserin	34 mg/day	Peripheral edema, nausea, confusion, constipation	Not approved for use with clients with dementia experiencing psychosis unless related to Parkinson diagnosis. Increases mortality risk in the older adults taking antipsychotic treatment for dementia-related psychosis.
Risperidone	Tablet, liquid, and orally disintegrated tablets: 2–8 mg	Hypotension, galactorrhea, nausea, insomnia	Doses >6 mg associated with a higher incidence of extrapyramidal symptoms; less weight gain than with clozapine or olanzapine Greatest prolactin elevation among atypical psychotics Monitor weight, BMI, waist circumference Monitor serum lipids and glucose Assess family and personal history of cardiovascular disease

(Continued)

TABLE 11–4. (CONTINUED)

AGENT	DOSAGE	SIDE EFFECTS	COMMENTS
Quetiapine	Tablet; 50–800 mg/day	Common: Tachycardia, dizziness, hypersalivation (sialorrhea), weight gain, hyperlipidemia Rare: Agranulocytosis, myocarditis, neuroleptic malignant syndrome	Transient and asymptomatic elevated liver function tests Monitor for cataract development Divided doses: b.i.d. or t.i.d. No prolactin elevation Monitor weight, BMI, waist circumference Monitor serum lipids and glucose Assess family and personal history of cardiovascular disease
Ziprasidone	Tablets: 40–200 mg/day Injectable: 10–20 mg IM (acute treatment)	Hypotension, sedation, dizziness Rare: Prolongation of QTc interval, skin reaction, DRESS	Requires QTc monitoring Avoid co-administration with other drugs known to prolong QTc Taking with food increases absorption to twice the usual rate Use caution when administering with clients at risk for hypokalemia, hypomagnesemia, after myocardial infarction, or with congestive heart failure Monitor weight, BMI, waist circumference Monitor serum lipids and glucose Assess family and personal history of cardiovascular disease

ANC, absolute neutrophil count; BMI, body mas index; CBC, complete blood count; DRESS, drug reaction with eosinophilia and systemic symptoms; EPSE, extrapyramidal side effects; GI, gastrointenstial; REMS, risk evaluation and management strategy; QTc, corrected QT (interval); WBC, white blood cell

Note. All atypical antipsychotic medications have a FDA box stating an increase in mortality exists when used in older adults with dementia-related psychosis. Must be used with caution.

- ◊ Have fewer significant neurological side effects compared to typical antipsychotic medication
- ◊ Effectively treat positive and negative symptoms
- ◊ Expensive (some generics now available)
- ◊ Fewer clinically significant side effects related to extrapyramidal symptoms (EPS) and tardive dyskinesia (TD) compared to typical antipsychotics
- ◊ Can cause extrapyramidal side effects (EPSE; see five common types in Table 11–5) but with lower risk compared to typical antipsychotics
- ◊ Lower incidence of TD (see the following sections).
- ◊ Improved compliance
- ◊ Function as serotonin–dopamine antagonists (SDAs)
- ◊ D2 and 5-HT2A blockade
- ◊ Mode of action
    - In addition to the dopaminergic blockade found in first-generation antipsychotics, second-generation drugs capitalize on the interplay between dopamine and serotonin. Serotonin binds to 5HT2a heteroreceptors. On dopamine neurons, thus further shutting off release of dopamine. By antagonizing (blocking) the 5-HT2A heteroreceptors on dopamine neurons, dopamine release in the nigrostriatal, tuberoinfundibular, and mesocortical pathways is enhanced.
        - Dopamine pathways: These explain both the therapeutic effects and the side effects of atypical antipsychotics.
        - Mesolimbic pathway: SDAs block dopamine in this pathway, causing decreased positive symptoms.
        - Mesocortical pathway: SDAs increase dopamine in this pathway, causing decreased negative symptoms.
        - Nigrostriatal pathway: Dopamine has a reciprocal relationship with acetylcholine (Ach). When serotonin is blocked by the SDA, dopamine increases; therefore, Ach decreases, which causes decreased EPSE. (EPSE is caused by increased Ach.)
        - Tuberoinfundibular pathway: Dopamine inhibits prolactin. The blockade of dopamine by SDAs causes prolactin to increase, causing galactorrhea and gynecomastia.

- ♦ Typical antipsychotics (first-generation; see Table 11–6)
    - ◊ First introduced in the 1950s
    - ◊ Generic (inexpensive)

TABLE 11–5.
EXTRAPYRAMIDAL SIDE EFFECTS (EPSE)

SIDE EFFECT	DEFINITION
Akathisia	Motor restlessness; inability to remain still; rocking, pacing, or constant motion of unilateral limb; also can manifest as a subjective sense of restlessness without objective finding Note: Often mistaken for increasing anxiety
Akinesia	Absence of movement, difficulty initiating motion, subjective feeling of lack of motivation to move Note: Often mistaken for laziness or lack of interest
Dystonia	Muscle spasm; spasticity of muscle group, especially back or neck muscles; subjectively painful Note: Often mistaken for agitation or unusual, stereotypic movements characteristic of schizophrenia
Pseudo-Parkinson's	Presence of symptoms of Parkinson's disease produced by D2 blockade; includes shuffling gait, motor slowing, mask-like facial expression, pill rolling, tremors, and muscle rigidity Note: Mask-like facial expression often confused as affective blunting or flattening
Tardive dyskinesia	Involuntary abnormal muscle movement of the mouth, tongue, face, and jaw that may progress to limbs; can be irreversible; can occur as an acute process at initiation of medications or as a chronic condition at any point in treatment

- ◊ Cross-classified as neuroleptics because of significant side effects
- ◊ High client teaching needs
- ◊ Therapeutic effect related primarily to D2 receptor blockade
    - Useful for treating positive symptoms by blocking dopamine in the mesolimbic pathway
    - Can make negative symptoms worse by blocking dopamine in the mesocortical pathway
- ◊ Can be used as sustained-released injectable agents
- ◊ Decanoate—long-acting injectable dose forms of typical antipsychotics:
    - Fluphenazine decanoate (limited availability due to low production)
    - Haloperidol decanoate

TABLE 11–6.
TYPICAL ANTIPSYCHOTICS

AGENT	DOSAGE	SIDE EFFECTS	COMMENTS
Chlorpromazine	50–2,000 mg/day	High: Sedation, hypotension Moderate: EPSE, anticholinergic	Allergic dermatitis Photosensitivity ECG changes: QTc monitoring
Fluphenazine	2–40 mg/day	Very high: EPSE Low: Anticholinergic, sedation, hypotension	Monitor LFTs, CBC with differential if pre-existing or history of leukopenia; BUN/Cr, ophthalmologic exam if prolonged use
Haloperidol	2–40 mg/day oral; 50–300 mg IM/month	Very high: EPSE High: Anticholinergic, sedation Low: Hypotension	In older adults monitor for oculogyric crisis and pneumonia
Loxapine	20–250 mg/day	High: EPSE Moderate: Sedation, Hypotension Low: Anticholinergic	Monitor LFTs, CBC with differential, ophthalmic exam with prolonged use
Perphenazine	8–64 mg/day	High: EPSE Low: Anticholinergic, sedation, hypotension	Monitor BUN/Cr, LFTs, CBC with differential, ophthalmologic exam if prolonged treatment
Thioridazine	50–800 mg/day	High: Anticholinergic, sedation, hypotension, prolonged QT interval Low: EPS	ECG changes: QTc Monitoring irreversible retinal pigmentation at doses >800 mg/day Decreased libido Retrograde ejaculation
Thiothixene	60 mg/day	High: Neuroleptic, malignant syndrome tardive dyskinesia, extrapyramidal symptoms, seizures Low: Anticholinergic, sedation, hypotension	Monitor CBC with differential if pre-existing or history of pyramidal seizure, tardive leukopenia/dyskinesia, dystonia neutropenia, ophthalmologic exam if prolonged use
Trifluoperazine	40 mg/day	High: Neuroleptic malignant syndrome, tardive dyskinesia, extrapyramidal symptoms, seizure Low: Anticholingeric, sedation, hypotension	Monitor CBC with differential if pre-existing or history of leukopenia/neutropenia, ophthalmologic exam if prolonged use

BUN/CR, blood urea nitrogen/creatinine; CBC, complete blood count; ECG, electrocardiogram; EPS, extrapyramidal symptoms; EPSE, extrapyramidal side effects; LFT, liver function tests; QTc, corrected QT (interval)

- ◊ High potency: Have a greater risk of EPSE but lower risk of sedation and anticholinergic symptoms
- ◊ Low potency: Have a greater risk of sedation and anticholinergic side effects but lower risk of EPSE
- ◊ Caffeine and nicotine cause diminished antipsychotic effect; an increased dose may be needed.
- ◊ Because of multiple clinically significant side effects, are not considered first-line treatment agents
- ◊ Side effects leading to poor adherence

- ♦ Hyperprolactinemia associated with the antipsychotics may cause sexual problems, galactorrhea, amenorrhea, gynecomastia, and bone demineralization in postmenopausal women not taking estrogen.
- ♦ EPSE most common side effect (see Table 11-6)
  - ◊ Caused by D_2 receptor antagonism. (When dopamine receptors are blocked, Ach increases, which causes EPSE; a reciprocal relationship exists between Ach and dopamine.)
  - ◊ Medications to treat EPSE
    - First line—anticholinergic/antihistamine
    - Second line—dopamine agonist/beta-adrenergic antagonists/beta-adrenergic agonists
    - Third line—Vesicular MonoamineTransporter 2 (VMAT2) inhibitors
    - Fourth line and use with care—benzodiazepine
- ♦ Tardive dyskinesia (TD)
  - ◊ TD is a potentially irreversible movement disorder that may occur in people who are treated for more than 1 year with typical antipsychotics.
  - ◊ Symptoms consist of abnormal, involuntary movements such as lip smacking, chewing, tongue protrusion, or twisting movements of the trunk or limbs.
  - ◊ Perioral movements are most common.
  - ◊ Treatment involves discontinuation of the offending agent and often starting an atypical antipsychotic.
  - ◊ Clients taking typical antipsychotics should have routine abnormal involuntary muscle movement screening every 6 months.
    - Assessment of abnormal movement rating scales
      - Abnormal Involuntary Movement Scale (AIMS)
      - Dyskinesia Identification System Condensed User Scale (DISCUS)
      - Simpson–Angus Rating Scale (SAS)

- ◊ Client and family education on the detection of early signs and symptoms of abnormal movements
- ◊ If abnormal movements are noted, consider reducing the dose or switching to an atypical antipsychotic.
- ◊ Risk factors include
  - Long-term treatment with neuroleptics
  - Older age
  - Female sex
  - Presence of mood or cognitive disorder
- ◊ Neuroleptic malignant syndrome (NMS)
  - Rare but potentially life-threatening
  - Can occur at any point during treatment
  - Most common with typical but has been reported with atypical antipsychotics
  - Risk factors include the following:
    - Rapid dose escalation
    - Use of high-potency typical antipsychotic
    - Parenteral administration of antipsychotics
  - Assess for the following abnormal labs:
    - Elevated CPK (creatine phosphokinase)
    - Elevated WBC (white blood cell) count
    - Elevated LFTs (liver function tests)
  - Assess for symptoms known to occur first:
    - Altered sensorium
    - Hyperthermia
    - Hyperreflexia
  - Assess for symptoms of autonomic instability:
    - Hypotension
    - Extreme muscular rigidity
    - Hyperthermia
    - Tachycardia

        - Diaphoresis
        - Tachypnea
        - Coma and potentially death
    - Treatment
        - Seek immediate medical care for treatment
        - Discontinue antipsychotic medication(s)
        - Administration of Dantrium (dantrolene) or Parlodel (bromocriptine) for antipsychotic-induced dopamine receptor blockade
        - Antipyretic (acetaminophen) and cooling blanket for hyperthermia
        - Intravenous hydration
        - Benzodiazepine for muscular rigidity (catatonic symptoms)

◇ Other common side effects related to effects on receptors other than dopamine

- Alpha adrenergic blockade
    - Cardiovascular side effects
    - Orthostatic hypotension
- Muscarinic cholinergic blockade
    - Dry mouth
    - Blurred vision
    - Constipation
    - Urinary retention
- Endocrine side effects
    - Weight gain
    - Increased prolactin levels
- Neurological side effects
    - Lowering of seizure threshold
- Other side effects
    - Photosensitivity
    - Agranulocytosis

Nonpharmacological Management

- Individual therapy
  - Usually supportive rather than insight oriented
  - Focuses on establishing reality testing
  - Builds daily life skills
  - Assists client in establishing and meeting life goals
  - Cognitive behavioral therapy (CBT) for management of hallucinations and delusions
- Group therapy
  - Focuses on problem-solving
  - Focuses on education
- Medication groups
- Life skills groups
- Proactive crisis management planning to deal with potential relapse needs
  - Identify symptom triggers.
  - Identify symptoms that indicate relapse.
  - Identify past pattern of relapse to help predict future relapses.
  - Identify self-care interventions.
  - Identify point at which professional intervention is required.
  - Identify support network of family and friends.
  - Identify other resources to be mobilized when symptom level increases.
- Assertive community treatment (ACT)
  - Evidence-based case management program
  - Multidisciplinary treatment team
- Illness management recovery (IMR)
  - Evidence-based recovery program
- Education modules
  - Recovery strategies, information on mental illness, building supports, using medication, drugs and alcohol, coping, reducing relapse, mental health system, advocacy, and stress-vulnerability model (Whitley et al., 2009)
- Milieu therapy
  - Provides for structure and safety needs

  - ◊ Provides socialization and interpersonal support
  - ◊ Encourages independency
- ♦ Client and family education
  - ◊ Explain underlying pathology of illness.
  - ◊ Discuss signs and symptoms.
  - ◊ Assist in identifying strategies for living with illness.
  - ◊ Assist in understanding and making decisions about care options.
  - ◊ Develop relapse prevention plan.
  - ◊ Promote overall health.

COMMON COMORBIDITIES

- ♦ Rates of substance use and misuse are high.
  - ◊ 20% to 40% comorbidity
- ♦ Nicotine dependence is especially high.
  - ◊ 80% to 90% comorbidity
  - ◊ Tend to use cigarettes with highest nicotine content
- ♦ Drug interaction with antipsychotic medications
  - ◊ May need to reduce doses when client quits or cuts back.
- ♦ Other common psychiatric comorbidities are anxiety disorders (see Chapter 10), especially panic disorder, and obsessive–compulsive disorder (OCD).

GENERAL HEALTH CONSIDERATIONS

- ♦ Schizophrenia is significantly associated with shorter-than-expected life span when compared to the general population.
- ♦ Persons with a severe mental illness (SMI) prematurely lose 10 to 25 years of life compared to the general population.
  - ◊ Reasons are unclear but may include overall general lack of routine health care and high levels of comorbidity (see the following sections)
- ♦ Suicide
  - ◊ Suicide rates are high; assess for suicidal ideations at every visit.
  - ◊ 10% die by suicide.

  - 20% to 40% attempt to end their own life by suicide.
  - Known risk factors for suicide include the following:
    - Male sex
    - Ages 45 or younger
    - Presence of depressive symptoms
    - Hopelessness
    - Unemployed
    - Treatment resistant
    - Recent hospitalization
    - Post-psychotic period
    - Comorbid substance use
- General medical illnesses
  - Clients need access to ongoing primary care.
  - High rates of cardiometabolic illnesses
  - Monitor client for development of metabolic syndrome, diabetes, hypertension, hyperlipidemia, respiratory illnesses, and cardiac illnesses.
- Monitor weight gain, lipids, and blood glucose.
- Provide weight management and nutritional assistance.
- Use the body mass index (BMI) as the accepted standard for determining if a client's weight places them at risk of developing serious health problems.
- BMI categories
  - Underweight: BMI 18.5 or less
  - Normal weight: BMI 18.5–24.9
  - Overweight: BMI 25.0–29.9
  - Obese: BMI 30.0–39.9
  - Severely obese: BMI 40 and higher.
- Risks related to BMI
  - Clients who are overweight to obese as determined by BMI have
    - 2.9 times increased risk for diabetes
    - 2.9 times increased risk for hypertension
    - 2.1 times increased risk of coronary artery disease
    - 3.0 times increased risk for endometrial cancer
    - 2.7 times increased risk for colon cancer

LIFE SPAN CONSIDERATIONS

- Children
  - Hallucinatory and delusional content less rich, elaborate, and bizarre
  - Visual hallucinations more common than auditory
- Older adults
  - More women than men with rare late onset
  - Although exhibiting prodromal social isolation, are more often married
  - Prognosis usually better; more responsive to medications due to dominance of positive symptom cluster (see the following sections)
  - FDA box warning on all atypical antipsychotic medications warns of an increase in mortality in older adults with dementia-related psychosis
  - Risk factors
    - Postmenopausal states
    - Presence of human leukocyte antigen
    - Positive family history
  - Symptoms
    - Predominance of positive symptoms
    - High levels of persecutory delusions and hallucinations
    - Lower levels of disorganized behavior
    - Preservation of social and occupational interest
    - Fewer negative symptoms

FOLLOW-UP

- Chronic illness
  - Usually requires lifelong treatment
  - Case management necessary to coordinate aspects of care
- Relapse periods
  - Develop relapse plan with client and family.
- Multiple health needs
  - Perform frequent assessment of general health status.
  - Address comorbid nicotine addiction.

- Preventative care
  - Monitor routine labs to screen for complications of treatment:
    - Serum glucose and lipid panels
    - Weight, BMI, and waist-to-hip ratio
    - Liver and kidney function (based on medication)
    - Complete blood count
    - See American Diabetes Association, American Psychiatric Association, American Association of Clinical Endocrinologists, & North American Association for the Study of Obesity Guidelines (2004)
  - Perform annual eye exam if on typical antipsychotic agent or Seroquel (quetiapine)
- Clinical outcome measures
  - Standardized rating scales include the following:
    - Positive and Negative Syndrome Scale (PANNS)
    - Brief Psychiatric Rating Scale (BPRS)
    - Scale for Assessment of Positive Symptoms (SAPS)
    - Scale for Assessment of Negative Symptoms (SANS)

SCHIZOPHRENIFORM DISORDER

DESCRIPTION

- Closely resembles schizophrenia
- Two differences from schizophrenia
  - Total duration of the illness is at least 1 month but less than 6 months, including prodrome, active illness period, and residual symptom phase
  - Does not require impaired social or occupational functioning for diagnosis, although these may be present

ETIOLOGY

- Similar to schizophrenia (see Schizophrenia Etiology, page 295)

DEMOGRAPHICS

- Little is known
- Fivefold increase in men
- Lifetime prevalence rate of 0.11%

RISK FACTORS

- Similar to schizophrenia (see Schizophrenia Risk Factors, page 297)

PREVENTION AND SCREENING

- Identification of individuals at high risk and monitoring
- Relative with schizophrenia and bipolar disorder

ASSESSMENT

Client History

- Assess for the following:
  - Two or more of the following frequently present during a 1-month period
    - Delusions
    - Hallucinations
    - Disorganized speech
    - Grossly disorganized behavior
    - Presence of negative symptoms
  - Duration of symptoms for at least 1 month and for no longer than 6 months
  - Almost all information provided for schizophrenia pertains to this disorder, except for the following:
    - Occurs much less often than schizophrenia; incidence is 0.03% of general U.S. population
    - Approximately one-third recover completely within 6 months
    - Remaining two-thirds develop schizophrenia or schizoaffective disorder (see page 323)

Physical Exam Findings

- Similar to schizophrenia (see Schizophrenia Physical Exam Findings, page 301)

Mental Status Exam Findings

- Similar to schizophrenia (see Schizophrenia Mental Status Exam Findings, page 302)

Diagnostic and Laboratory Findings

- Similar to schizophrenia (see Schizophrenia Diagnostic and Laboratory Findings, page 304)

CLINICAL MANAGEMENT

- Similar to schizophrenia (see Schizophrenia Clinical Management, page 305)
- Assess for acuity level.
- During acute psychotic or affective episodes, client may require brief hospitalization to
  - Ensure client safety;
  - Rapidly stabilize client's symptom level in a controlled environment; and
  - Ensure client compliance with treatment to reach stabilization.
- Clinical management during nonacute episodes occurs most often in community settings.

Pharmacological Management

- Similar to schizophrenia (see Schizophrenia Pharmacological Management, page 305)

Nonpharmacological Management

- Similar to schizophrenia (see Schizophrenia Nonpharmacological Management, page 316)

FOLLOW-UP

- Similar to schizophrenia (see Schizophrenia Follow-Up, page 319)

SCHIZOAFFECTIVE DISORDER

DESCRIPTION

- An uninterrupted period of illness in which the person experiences psychotic symptoms similar to those seen in schizophrenia as well as mood symptoms similar to major depressive disorder (MDD) or bipolar disorder (see Schizophrenia, page 295; MDD, page 172; and Bipolar Disorder, page 216).

ETIOLOGY

- Cause is unknown
- The disorder may be a psychotic spectrum disorder, mood spectrum disorder, or both.

PREVALENCE AND DEMOGRAPHICS

- Less than 1%
- Equal number males and females.
- Depressed type of the disorder is more common in older persons
- Men with the disorder tend to exhibit more antisocial behaviors.

RISK FACTORS

- Family history of schizophrenia or bipolar disorder

PREVENTION AND SCREENING

- Screening persons with a positive family history

ASSESSMENT

Client History

- Assess for the following:
  - Symptoms of schizophrenia—two or more of the following frequently present during a 1-month period:
    - Delusions
    - Hallucinations
    - Disorganized speech
    - Grossly disorganized behavior
    - Presence of negative symptoms but usually less severe than those in schizophrenia
  - Symptoms of one or more mood disorders (see Chapter 9):
    - Major depressive episode
    - Manic episode
    - Mixed-mood episode
  - Presence of delusions or hallucinations for at least 2 weeks in the absence of prominent mood symptoms
  - Two subtypes differentiated by type of mood-related symptoms
    - Depressive: When prominent mood symptoms are of the depressive type only
    - Bipolar: When predominant mood symptoms are manic or mixed type

Physical Exam Findings

- Similar to schizophrenia (see Schizophrenia Physical Exam Findings, page 301)

Mental Status Exam Findings

- Similar to schizophrenia (see Schizophrenia Mental Status Exam Findings, page 302)

Diagnostic and Laboratory Findings

- Similar to schizophrenia (see Schizophrenia Diagnostic and Laboratory Findings, page 304)

CLINICAL MANAGEMENT

Pharmacological Management

- Similar to schizophrenia (see Schizophrenia Pharmacological Management, page 305)
- Similar to MDD or bipolar disorder (see MDD, page 172 and Bipolar Disorder, page 216)

Nonpharmacological Management

- Similar to schizophrenia (see Schizophrenia Nonpharmacological Management, page 316)
- Similar to MDD or bipolar disorder (see MDD, page 172 and Bipolar Disorder, page 216)

FOLLOW-UP

- Similar to schizophrenia (See Schizophrenia Follow-Up, page 319)
- Similar to MDD or bipolar disorder (see Schizophrenia Nonpharmacological Management, page 316)

DELUSIONAL DISORDER

DESCRIPTION

- Presence of one or more non-bizarre delusions lasting for at least 1 month
- Psychosocial functioning and daily behavior not at all impaired except as they surround content of delusion
- Seldom any other symptoms; in rare cases may have hallucinations or mood disturbances

ETIOLOGY

- Cause is unknown

PREVALENCE AND DEMOGRAPHICS

- 0.2% to 0.3% of population in the United States
- Mean onset is ~40 years of age
- Men are more likely to have paranoid delusions
- Women are more likely to have delusions of erotomania

RISK FACTORS

- Person with disorders of the limbic system and basal ganglia

PREVENTION AND SCREENING

- Unknown

ASSESSMENT

Client History

- Assess for the following:
    - Presence of delusions
        - Well-organized and potentially believable
        - Any unusual behavior is explainable if content of delusion understood
- Subtypes (categorized by thematic content of delusion)
    - Erotomanic
        - Delusional content focused on false belief that another person is in love with the client
        - Usually focused on idealized or spiritual love and only infrequently has strong sexual content
        - Focus of love is usually a famous or powerful person who does not usually know the client
            - In rare cases, the person may know client
        - Leads to obsessive behaviors such as surveillance or stalking
    - Grandiose
        - Delusional content focuses on the client having some great talent, skill, or knowledge

        - May have a strong religious component, such as prophecy or deity connections (special connection to God)
    - Jealous
        - Delusional content focuses on false belief that client's spouse or partner is being unfaithful with someone else
            - Belief has no connection with realistic evidence
            - Usually seen in men
        - Client may try to control behavior of spouse or partner in an attempt to prevent imagined infidelities
    - Persecutory
        - Delusional content focuses on clients' belief that others are out to spy on them, or otherwise do them harm
            - Often angry and hostile at perceived persecution
    - Somatic
        - Delusional content focuses on bodily functions and sensations
        - Often belief that a body part is infected, absent, emits a strange odor, or is misshapen or malformed
    - Mixed
        - No clear predominant theme for the delusional content
        - Related symptoms that can be present but are not required for diagnosis include
- May become depressed over protracted problems with thematic content
- May become involved in legal difficulties related to behaviors based on delusional content
- May be subjected to or request unnecessary medical tests and procedures

Physical Exam Findings

- No physical exam findings specific to delusional disorder

Mental Status Exam Findings

- Normal except for delusions
    - Abstraction
        - May be concrete on proverbs during delusional episodes

- ◊ Thought process
  - Presence of delusions
  - Perseveration on topics related to delusion
- ◊ Thought content
  - Thematic for type of delusion

Diagnostic and Laboratory Findings

- ♦ No specific diagnostic lab findings exist.

CLINICAL MANAGEMENT

Pharmacological Management

- ♦ Similar to schizophrenia (see Schizophrenia Pharmacological Management, page 305)

Nonpharmacological Management

- ♦ Similar to schizophrenia (see Schizophrenia Nonpharmacological Management, page 316)

BRIEF PSYCHOTIC DISORDER

DESCRIPTION

- ♦ Disorder with sudden onset of psychotic symptoms lasting at least 1 day but less than 1 month

ETIOLOGY

- ♦ Unknown cause

INCIDENCE AND DEMOGRAPHICS

- Unknown incidence
- Occurs more in younger clients (20 to 30 years of age)

RISK FACTORS

- Family history of psychotic disorder

PREVENTION AND SCREENING

- Unknown

ASSESSMENT

Client History

- Assess for the following:
  - Onset in adolescence or early adulthood
  - Positive-type psychotic symptoms
    - Delusions
    - Hallucinations
    - Grossly disorganized behavior
    - Disorganized speech
  - Can occur with or without identified stressor
  - Person always returns to premorbid level of functioning

Physical Exam Findings

- No physical exam findings specific to brief psychotic disorder

Mental Status Exam Findings

- Similar to schizophrenia (see Schizophrenia Mental Status Exam Findings, page 324)

Diagnostic and Laboratory Findings

- No specific diagnostic lab findings exist.

CLINICAL MANAGEMENT

Pharmacological Management

- Similar to schizophrenia (see Schizophrenia Pharmacological Management, page 325)

Nonpharmacological Management

- Similar to schizophrenia (See Schizophrenia Nonpharmacological Management, page 316)
- Acute episode requires frequent monitoring for safety needs because of the following:
  - Confusion
  - Rapid shifting in emotions
  - Impaired judgment
  - Inability to meet nutritional and hygiene needs

SHARED PSYCHOTIC DISORDER (FOLIE Á DEUX)

DESCRIPTION

- Characterized by development of a delusion in a client who has a close relationship with another person who already has a psychotic disorder with a prominent delusion

ETIOLOGY

- Cause is unknown

INCIDENCE AND DEMOGRAPHICS

- Unknown

RISK FACTORS

- Unknown

PREVENTION AND SCREENING

- Unknown

ASSESSMENT

Client History

- Assess for the following:
  - Client in close contact with a person who already has a delusion and
    - That person usually has schizophrenia.
    - That person usually is the dominant person in the relationship.
    - That person gradually imposes their delusion on the client.
    - Usually the relationship is long term and very close.
  - Aside from the delusional content, the client's behavior is otherwise normal.

Physical Exam Findings

- No physical exam findings specific to shared psychotic disorder

Mental Status Exam Findings

- Similar to schizophrenia (see Schizophrenia Mental Status Exam Findings, page 302)

Diagnostic and Laboratory Findings

- No specific diagnostic lab findings exist.

CLINICAL MANAGEMENT

Pharmacological Management

- Similar to schizophrenia (see Schizophrenia Pharmacological Management, page 305)

Nonpharmacological Management

- Similar to schizophrenia (see Schizophrenia Nonpharmacological Management, page 316)
- Chronic disease course
- Poor prognosis if relationship continues, especially if person with delusion goes untreated
- Good prognosis if the client can be separated from person with the delusion

CASE STUDY

C.V., a 23-year-old client who has been recently diagnosed with schizophrenia experienced the first psychotic break at age 22 while serving in the military. The client lives at home with their parents and is reluctant to accept the diagnosis, stating "I got bad weed in the service and I will be fine once the weed leaves my body." C.V. has been adherent with appointments but only intermittently takes the prescribed risperidone (3 mg p.o. b.i.d.). The parents are threatening to kick C.V. out of the house if treatment is not consistent.

C.V. has a history of juvenile-onset diabetes and has struggled to maintain a diabetic diet and to control weight. When asked to identify current goals, the client wishes to find a good partner, have children, and settle down to a normal life. There are many issues to consider in planning care with this client.

1. What is the top priority for the psychiatric-mental health nurse practitioner (PMHNP)?
2. What medications changes would the PMHNP consider?
3. What is the relationship between diabetes and schizophrenia?
4. How will the comorbid illness affect the PMHNP's care planning?
5. What routine ongoing monitoring will he require?

ANSWERS TO CASE STUDY DISCUSSION QUESTIONS

1. The top priority for the PMHNP is to build a therapeutic alliance with the client.
2. Medication changes appropriate for this client include switching to an alternative atypical antipsychotic medication that has a lower risk for weight gain and elevated glucose levels.
3. The relationship between diabetes and schizophrenia is that individuals with schizophrenia have a twofold increase of developing diabetes, which is considered an independent risk factor.
4. Because clients with schizophrenia are at high risk for developing cardiometabolic illness as comorbidities, the care plan must address both physical health, specifically diabetes management, and mental health.
5. Routine monitoring for clients taking atypical antipsychotics includes ongoing surveillance of serum glucose, A1c, lipid profile, complete blood count, weight, height, and body mass index.

REFERENCES AND RESOURCES

American Diabetes Association, American Psychiatric Association, American Association of Clinical Endocrinologists, & North American Association for the Study of Obesity. (2004). Consensus development conference on antipsychotic drugs and obesity and diabetes. Diabetes Care, 27(2), 596–601.

American Psychiatric Association. (2022). Diagnostic and statistical manual of mental disorders (5th ed., Text rev.).

Fontanella, C. A., Campo, J. V., Phillips, G. S., Hiance-Steelesmith, D. L., Sweeney, H. A., Tam, K., . . . Hurst, M. (2016). Benzodiazepine use and risk of mortality among patients with schizophrenia: A retrospective longitudinal study. Journal of Clinical Psychiatry, 77(5), 661.

Rector, N. A., & Beck, A. (2002). A clinical review of cognitive therapy for schizophrenia. Current Psychiatric Reports, 4, 284–292.

Richardson, C., Faulkner, G., McDevitt, J., Skrinar, G., Hutchinson, D., & Piette, J. (2005). Integrating physical activity into mental health services for persons with serious mental illness. Psychiatric Services, 56(3), 324–331.

Sable, J. A. (2002). Antipsychotic treatment for late-life schizophrenia. Current Psychiatric Reports, 4, 299–306.

Sadock, B. J., Sadock, V. A., & Ruiz, P. (2017). Kaplan & Sadock's comprehensive textbook of psychiatry. (10th ed.). Wolters Kluwer.

Staal, W. G., Hulshoff Pol, H., Schnack, G., van Haren, N. E., Seifert, N., & Kahn, R. (2001). Structural brain abnormalities in chronic schizophrenia at the extremes of the outcome spectrum. American Journal of Psychiatry, 158, 1140–1142.

Stahl, S. M. (2020). Stahl's essential psychopharmacology: Prescriber's guide. (7th ed.). Cambridge University Press.

Tamminga, C. (2001). Treating schizophrenia now and developing strategies for the next decade. CNS Spectrums, 6, 987–991.

Tandon, R., & Jibson, M. D. (2001). Pharmacologic treatment of schizophrenia: What the future holds. CNS Spectrums, 6, 980–986.

Tiihonen, J., Mittendorfer-Rutz, E., Torniainen, M., Alexanderson, K., & Tanskanen, A. (2016). Mortality and cumulative exposure to antipsychotics, antidepressants, and benzodiazepines in patients ate schizophrenia: An observational follow-up study. American Journal of Psychiatry, 173(6), 600–606. https://doi.org/10.1176/appi.ajp.2015.15050618

U.S. Food and Drug Administration. (2013). FDA Drug Safety Communication: FDA is investigating two deaths following injection of long-acting antipsychotic Zyprexa Relprevv (olanzapine pamoate). https://www.fda.gov/drugs/drug-safety-and-availability/fda-drug-safety-communication-fda-review-study-sheds-light-two-deaths-associated-injectable

Whitley, R., Gingerich, S., Lutz, W., & Mueser, K. (2009). Implementing the illness management and recovery program in community mental health settings: Facilitators and barriers. Psychiatric Services, 60(2), 202–209.

CHAPTER 12

NEUROCOGNITIVE DISORDERS

Cognitive disorders often are thought of as disorders of older adults. Although most common in this population, cognitive disorders can occur at any age. Very young or very old people with cognitive disorders have multiple health needs. Older adult clients usually have more than one chronic illness, and psychiatric disorders can be accompanied by other comorbidities.

Psychiatric-mental health nurse practitioners (PMHNPs) must approach clients with cognitive disorders by conducting a multisystem assessment.

COGNITIVE DISORDERS

DESCRIPTION

- Cognitive disorders cause a clinically significant deficit in cognition that represents a major change from the person's previous baseline level of functioning.
- Two common disorders
  - Delirium
  - Dementia

ETIOLOGY

- Cognitive disorders are a complex general medical condition resulting in changes in multiple domains including memory, interpersonal relationships, and behavior.
- Cognitive disorders can result from injury, medical condition, substance use or misuse, a reaction to medications or other ingested agents, or a combination of some or all these factors.

DELIRIUM

DESCRIPTION

- Delirium is a syndrome and not a disease, with an acute onset that causes short-term changes in cognition.
- The hallmark symptom is a disturbance of consciousness accompanied by changes in cognition.
- Subtypes of delirium
    - Hyperactive: Agitated, restless, hyperalert
    - Hypoactive: Lethargic, slowed, apathetic
    - Mixed: Cycles between hyperactive and hypoactive

ETIOLOGY

- Occurs due to changes in one of the following:
    - General medical condition
    - Substance induced
    - Multiple physical health problems
    - Medication, sleep deprivation, or other causes

INCIDENCE AND DEMOGRAPHICS

- Common, especially in older adults
- Often overlooked and mistaken for other medical conditions or dementia
- In persons with psychiatric disorders, often mistaken for worsening of psychotic symptoms instead of a distinct condition
- Prevalence varies based on age, client setting, and sample
    - Highest in hospitalized older adults
    - 0.4% in general U.S. population ages 18 years or older
    - 1% to 2% in persons ages 65 or older
    - 6% to 56% of hospitalized clients
    - 15% to 53% in postoperative older adults
    - 70% to 87% of older adults in the intensive care unit
    - 60% in nursing home clients

- 25% in clients with cancer
- 80% in terminal clients nearing death
- Poor prognosis
  - 1 year mortality rate of clients with delirium is up to 40%

RISK FACTORS

- Advancing age
- Multisystem medical illness
  - The more physically ill the client, the higher the risk.
- Substance use
- Visual or hearing impairment
- Past episode of delirium or preexisting brain disorder or cognitive impairment

PREVENTION AND SCREENING

- At-risk family education
- Community education
  - Stigma reduction
  - Signs and symptoms of illness
  - Treatment potential for control of symptoms
- Use of the Confusion Assessment Method (CAM) instrument
- Early recognition, intervention, and initiation of treatment
  - Whenever a client's clinical presentation changes rapidly from baseline, consider delirium as one possible differential diagnosis.

ASSESSMENT

Client History

- Assess for the following:
  - Key findings
    - Disturbance of consciousness develops over a short time, usually hours to days.
    - This disturbance tends to fluctuate during the day.

- Sleep–rest cycle disturbances
  - Reversal of the sleep–wake cycle is common: clients are awake at night and sleep during the day.
- Impaired recent and intermediate memory
- Psychomotor agitation
  - The client exhibits purposeless, random actions.

- Course of illness may resolve within hours to days
- The more quickly the underlying physiological disturbance is recognized and treated, the more rapidly the delirium will resolve.
- Symptoms, when unrecognized, may persist for months.
- Most symptoms resolve within 3 to 6 months.

Physical Exam Findings

- Evidence that significant clinical symptoms are a consequence of direct physiological processes, substance use or misuse, or general medical condition
- Usually nonspecific neurological abnormalities
  - Tremors
  - Incoordination
  - Urinary incontinence
  - Myoclonus
  - Nystagmus
  - Asterixis—a flapping motion of the wrists
  - Increased muscle tone and reflex

Mental Status Exam Findings

- Appearance
  - Unconcerned with appearance
  - Disheveled
  - Highly inattentive
- Speech
  - Impaired

    - Disorganized
    - Rambling
    - Incoherent
    - Slurred
- Affect
    - Rapid, unpredictable shifts in affective state without known precipitation
    - Lethargic
    - Agitated
- Mood
    - Difficult to elicit from client
- Thought process
    - Disorganized
    - Distractible
    - Perceptual disturbances
        - Illusions most common
        - Hallucinations are typically visual and accompanied by illusions
- Thought content
    - Disorganized, distorted thought
    - Delusions and hallucinations are common.
- Orientation
    - Disorientation is usually the first symptom to appear.
    - Client usually disoriented to time and place
- Memory
    - Impaired recent and immediate memory
- Concentration
    - Grossly impaired
- Abstraction
    - Grossly impaired
- Judgment
    - Grossly impaired

Diagnostic and Laboratory Findings

- Findings consistent with underlying physiological etiology
- Workup includes standard tests
  - Blood chemistry
  - Complete blood count (CBC)
  - Thyroid function tests
  - Syphilis
  - Human immunodeficiency virus (HIV) antibody test
  - Urinalysis
  - Chest radiograph
  - Serum or urine drug screen
- Electroencephalogram (EEG) abnormalities
  - Generalized slowing
  - Generalized increased activity if delirium is related to alcohol withdrawal

DIFFERENTIAL DIAGNOSIS

- Dementia (see the following section)
- Substance intoxication or withdrawal (see Chapter 13)
- Schizophrenia (see Chapter 11)
- Schizophreniform disorder (see Chapter 11)
- Mood disorders with psychotic features (see Chapter 9)

CLINICAL MANAGEMENT

- Undertake treatment of the underlying condition or disorder.
- Avoid the use of new medications whenever possible, because using them can cloud the diagnostic picture.

Pharmacological Management

- Symptomatic treatment

- Agitation and psychotic symptoms
  - Antipsychotic agents
    - Haloperidol (Haldol)
    - Atypical antipsychotic agents
    - Anxiolytic agents for insomnia

Nonpharmacological Management

- Monitor for safety needs.
- Determine reality orientation frequently.
- Pay attention to basic needs:
  - Hydration
  - Nutrition
- Client should be neither sensory-deprived nor overstimulated.
- It is helpful to have in the client's room familiar people; familiar pictures or decorations; a clock or calendar; and regular orientation to person, place, or time.

GENERAL HEALTH CONSIDERATIONS

- Delirium is associated with high morbidity and mortality.
- High morbidity results from injury or its associated problems related to inactivity:
  - Pneumonia
  - Hydration and nutritional deficits
- Safety concerns exist.
- Mnemonic: DELIRIUM (Dick & Morency, 2011)
  - Drugs
  - Electrolyte abnormality
  - Low oxygen saturation
  - Infection
  - Reduced sensory input
  - Intracranial
  - Urinary or renal retention
  - Myocardial

LIFE SPAN CONSIDERATIONS

- Children
    - Especially susceptible
    - Related to immature brain development
    - Often mistaken for uncooperative behavior
    - If a child is not soothed by common methods (e.g., parental presence), delirium is suspected.
    - Most common in febrile states
    - Medications known to affect cognition
        - Especially common with anticholinergic medications
- Older adults
    - Susceptibility related to physiological changes of aging
    - Older men more prone than older women for unknown reasons

DEMENTIA

DESCRIPTION

- Dementia is a group of disorders characterized by gradual development of multiple cognitive deficits:
    - Impaired executive functioning
    - Impaired global intellect with preservation of level of consciousness
    - Impaired problem-solving
    - Impaired organizational skills
    - Altered memory
- Various forms of dementia share common symptoms but have different underlying pathologies.
    - Dementia of Alzheimer's type (DAT)
        - Most common type
        - Gradual onset and progressive decline without focal neurological deficits
        - Hallmark amyloid deposits and neurofibrillary tangles
    - Vascular dementia (VD)
        - Second most common type

- Formerly called multi-infarct dementia
- Primarily caused by cardiovascular disease and characterized by step-type declines
- Most common in men with preexisting high blood pressure and cardiovascular risk factors
- Hallmarks: Carotid bruits, funduscopic abnormalities, and enlarged cardiac chambers

◊ Dementia due to HIV disease

- Classified as a subcortical dementia
- Parenchymal abnormalities visualized on magnetic resonance imaging (MRI) scan
- HIV-associated neurocognitive disorder or HIV encephalopathy are less severe forms.
- HIV can cause many psychiatric symptoms.
- Manifests by progressive cognitive decline, motor abnormalities, and behavioral abnormalities
- Co-occurs with obsessive–compulsive disorder, posttraumatic stress disorder, generalized anxiety disorder, depression, and mania
- Development of dementia in client with HIV is an indicator of poor prognosis; death usually occurs within 6 months.
- Psychotic symptoms usually occur in late-stage infection.
- Clinical signs of late-stage HIV-related dementia include cognitive, motor, behavioral, and affective impairment:
    - Global cognitive impairment
    - Mutism
    - Seizures
    - Hallucinations
    - Delusions
    - Apathy
    - Mania
- Antiretrovirals and protease inhibitors can interact with psychotropic medications because many are metabolized by the cytochrome P450 (CYP) system or are CYP3A4 inhibitors. Therefore, prescribing psychotropic medications in this client population should be done with caution while monitoring for drug interactions.

- ◇ Pick's disease
  - Also known as frontotemporal dementia
  - Neuronal loss, gliosis, and Pick's bodies present
  - More common in men
  - Personality and behavioral changes in early stage
  - Cognitive changes in later stages
  - Kluver-Bucy syndrome: Hypersexuality, hyperorality, and placidity
- ◇ Creutzfeldt-Jakob disease
  - Fatal and rapidly progressive disorder
  - Occurs mainly in adults in middle age or older
  - Initially manifests with fatigue, flulike symptoms, and cognitive impairment
  - Later manifests with aphasia, apraxia, emotional lability, depression, mania, psychosis, marked personality changes, and dementia
  - Death usually occurs within 6 months.
- ◇ Huntington's disease
  - Subcortical type of dementia
  - Characterized mostly by motor abnormalities (e.g., choreoathetoid movements)
  - Psychomotor slowing and difficulty with complex tasks
  - Memory, language, and insight usually intact until late stages
  - High incidence of depression and psychosis
- ◇ Lewy body disease
  - Caused by Lewy inclusion bodies in the cortex
  - Presents with recurrent visual hallucinations
  - Parkinson features (bradykinesia, cogwheel rigidity, tremor)
  - Adversely react to antipsychotics

ETIOLOGY

- ◆ Multiple theories ranging from psychological to neurobiological
  - ◇ Probable multifactorial etiological profile
- ◆ Primary cause mostly unknown
- ◆ General medical condition, result of substance use, reaction to medications or other ingested agents, or combination of some or all of these factors

- Diffuse cerebral atrophy and enlarged ventricles in DAT
- Decreased acetylcholine (Ach) and norepinephrine in DAT
- Genetic loading
  - Genes on chromosomes 1, 14, and 21 have been identified in families with a history of DAT.
  - Autosomal dominant trait
  - Inherited alleles for apolipoprotein ε4 (APOE ε4) on chromosome 19 are suspected to be related to late-onset dementia.

INCIDENCE AND DEMOGRAPHICS

- Often misdiagnosed or unrecognized, especially in early stages and in young clients
- Prevalence of 1.6% for people in the United States ages 65 or older
  - 16% to 25% in people ages 85 or older
- DAT the most common
  - Affects an estimated 4 million in the United States
  - Duration of illness averages 8 to 10 years

RISK FACTORS

- Age
- Multisystem medical illnesses
- Genetic loading
  - Family history of dementia in a first-order relative
- History of substance use or misuse

PREVENTION AND SCREENING

- At-risk family education
- Community education
  - Stigma reduction
  - Signs and symptoms of illness
  - Treatment potential for control of symptoms

- Early recognition, intervention, and initiation of treatment
    - Allows for ruling out of age-related memory changes or unidentified conditions
    - Cognitive and functional evaluation at least every 3 years for people ages 65 or older
    - Baseline and regular cognitive evaluation to monitor cognitive decline and treatment response to medications in persons diagnosed with dementia
- The U.S. Preventive Services Task Force concluded that there is insufficient evidence to determine if the benefits of routine screening outweigh the harms (U.S. Preventive Services Task Force [USPSTF], 2014).

ASSESSMENT

Client History

- Assess for the following:
    - Detailed history of present illness, including time frame, progression, and associated symptoms
    - Past medical history of hypertension, strokes, head trauma, and psychiatric illness
    - Psychiatric history of depression, anxiety, and schizophrenia
    - Social history, including present living situation; marital status; occupation; education; and alcohol, tobacco, or illicit drug use
    - Medications, including prescription, over-the-counter, herbals, supplements, and home remedies
    - Initial and periodic functional history and assessment
    - Validate history with family or caregiver.
    - Memory impairment—immediate and intermediate
        - Most prominent feature of disorder
        - Usually earliest symptom
        - Produces multiple deficits in daily functioning
        - Unable to learn new information
        - Forgets past information
        - Loses valuables
        - Forgets daily activities such as eating and dressing
        - Becomes easily lost
        - Has other cognitive deficits such as impaired executive functioning

- ◊ Instruments for assessing level of impairment
    - Not in public domain
        - Mini-Mental State Examination (MMSE)
    - In public domain
        - Montreal Cognitive Assessment (MoCA)
        - Mini-Cog
        - St. Louis University Mental Status Examination (SLUMS)
- ◊ Remember to always consider visual, sensory, language, and physical disabilities as well as level of education when administering mental status tests.

Physical Exam Findings

- Amaurosis fugax: Unilateral transient vision loss, described as "curtain over eye"
- Unilateral focal–motor weakness
- Asymmetrical reflexes

Mental Status Exam Findings

- Appearance
    - ◊ Apraxia
    - ◊ Decreased self-care activities of daily living
- Speech
    - ◊ Deterioration of language skills
    - ◊ Aphasia
    - ◊ Circumlocutory phrases
    - ◊ Indefinite object recognition (such as calling items "things" and being unable to find discrete name)
    - ◊ In advanced stages are
        - Mutism
        - Echolalia
        - Affect
    - ◊ Lability

- Mood
  - Depressed
  - Often difficult to elicit from client
- Thought process
  - Agnosia
- Thought content
  - Difficult to elicit from client
- Orientation
  - Disoriented to time and place
  - Disoriented to person in late stages of disorder
- Memory
  - Impaired in many dimensions of memory
    - Word registration
    - Recall
    - Retention
    - Recognition
    - Concentration
  - Distractible
- Abstraction
  - Concrete on proverb testing
- Judgment
  - Grossly impaired for self and social judgment

Diagnostic and Laboratory Findings

- CBC, chemistry profile, thyroid function tests, B_{12} level, and folate level to rule out metabolic causes or unidentified conditions
- Syphilis drug toxicity screening if indicated by history
- Alcohol and illicit drug screen if suspected or indicated
- Urinalysis if urinary tract infection suspected
- Arterial oxygen or pulse oximetry if hypoxemia suspected

- Computed tomography (CT) or MRI not routinely used
- EEG not useful
- Neuropsychological testing recommended to complete diagnostic assessment

DIFFERENTIAL DIAGNOSIS

- Nonpsychiatric
  - Parkinson's disease
  - Hearing loss
  - B_{12} and folate deficiencies
  - Trauma, especially with history of falls
  - Hypothyroidism
  - Infection
  - Cerebrovascular accident
  - Polypharmacy
  - Alcohol intoxication
- Psychiatric
  - Mood disorders (see Chapter 9)
  - Delirium (see previous section)
  - Anxiety disorders (see Chapter 10)

CLINICAL MANAGEMENT

General Considerations

- Rule out or treat any conditions that may contribute to cognitive impairment.
- Discontinue unnecessary medications, especially sedatives and hypnotics.

Pharmacological Management

- Cognitive symptoms
  - N-methyl-D-aspartate (NMDA) glutamate receptor antagonists

- Prevent overexcitation of glutamate receptors and stabilize the neurodegenerative process
- Memantine (maximum dose 20 mg/day IR, 28 mg/day ER)
  - Moderate to severe dementia
  - May slow the degenerative process
  - Promotes synaptic plasticity
  - May be used in combination with cholinesterase inhibitors
  - Memantine/donepezil (maximum dose 28 mg ER/10 mg IR q.d. combination medication)
  - Cholinesterase inhibitors
- May be initiated for mild to moderate Alzheimer's disease
- Can lead to modest clinical improvement in some clients, with studies showing 2- to 3-point improvement in MMSE testing
- Treat only symptoms, slow loss of function, and may improve agitated behaviors
- Do not prevent pathological progression of disease
- Not effective in severe, end-stage disease
- Should stop if side effects, usually nausea and vomiting, develop
- Commonly used agents
  - Donepezil (maximum dose 23 mg/day)
    - Approved for mild, moderate, and severe Alzheimer's disease
    - Nausea, diarrhea, vomiting, appetite and weight loss, abnormal dreams, insomnia, dizziness common
  - Rivastigmine tartrate (maximum dose 12 mg/day)
    - Indicated for mild to moderate Alzheimer's disease and Parkinson's disease dementia
    - Transdermal: 9.5 or 13.3 mg/24 hours
    - Re-titrate if a lapse in treatment occurs
- Psychosis and agitation
  - Try nonpharmacological therapies first.
  - Use antipsychotic agents for agitation or psychotic symptoms regularly.
  - Use lowest effective dose and attempt to wean periodically.
  - Antipsychotics may cause many side effects of significance in the older adult:
    - Extrapyramidal symptoms

        - Sedation
        - Postural hypotension
        - Anticholinergic side effects
    - Benzodiazepines may be used for treating anxiety or infrequent agitation.
- Depression
    - Treat clients with depressive symptoms:
        - Depressed mood
        - Insomnia
        - Fatigue
        - Irritability
        - Appetite loss
    - Use lowest effective dose.
    - Treat for 6 to 12 months and then attempt to taper; depression may reoccur and need to be treated as a chronic condition.
    - Clients may have less depression as the dementia progresses and they become less aware of their circumstances.

Nonpharmacological Management

- Educate client and family about the illness, treatment, and community resources.
- Assist with long-term planning, including financial, legal, and advanced directives.
- Assess home and driving safety.
- Use behavioral therapy to identify causes of problem behaviors and changes to the environment to reduce the behavior.
- Use recreational therapy, art, and pet therapy to reduce agitation and promote normalized behavior.
- Use reminiscence therapy or life review to process through any unresolved issues and recollect the past.
- Maintain a simple daily routine for bathing, dressing, eating, toileting, and bedtime.
- Integrate cultural beliefs into the management of all clients with dementia.
- Psychotherapeutic approaches for HIV-related dementia
    - Major psychodynamic themes for people with HIV-related dementia are issues of guilt, self-esteem, and fear of dying.

- ◊ Because the client may not be able to give a complete and accurate history, family or friends should be questioned about any unusual behavior or mental status changes.
- ◊ Changes in the level of activity, in interest in other people, or in personality are clues to an acute central nervous system disturbance.
- ◊ Some changes are directly due to brain dysfunction, whereas other changes are due to psychological distress of a systemic problem—anxiety that the person is dying.
- ◊ The spectrum of neuropsychiatric and neurological manifestations depends on the severity of immunosuppression.
- ◊ Psychiatric disorders may preexist or result from HIV.
- ◊ Even subtle neurocognitive impairment can affect psychological coping.
- ◊ Neuropsychiatric disorders are much more prevalent in late-stage illness.

LIFE SPAN CONSIDERATIONS

- ♦ Primarily a disease of older adults but can occur in children
  - ◊ Diagnosis based on impaired cognition; diagnoses not applicable until ages 4 to 6 years, when cognition can be fully assessed
  - ◊ Dementia in children usually presents as deterioration in functioning, such as school performance or delay in normal development.

MAJOR OR MINOR NEUROCOGNITIVE DISORDER DUE TO TRAUMATIC BRAIN INJURY

DESCRIPTION

- ♦ Diagnostic and Statistical Manual of Mental Disorders, Fifth Edition, Text Revision (DSM-5-TR; American Psychiatric Association [APA], 2022) diagnostic criteria are not met for a major or minor neurocognitive disorder.
- ♦ The disorder includes evidence of a traumatic brain injury (TBI)—an impact to the head or other mechanism of rapid movement or displacement of the brain within the skull—with one or more of the following:
  - ◊ Loss of consciousness
  - ◊ Posttraumatic amnesia
  - ◊ Disorientation and confusion

    - ◇ Neurological signs (neuroimaging demonstrating an injury; new onset of seizures; worsening seizure disorder; visual field cuts; hemiparesis; anosmia)

- ♦ The neurocognitive disorder presents immediately after the occurrence of the traumatic brain injury or immediately after recovery of consciousness and persists past the acute postinjury period.

ETIOLOGY

- ♦ Brain injury resulting when the head is hit or violently shaken, such as from a blast or explosion

INCIDENCE AND DEMOGRAPHICS

- ♦ About 2% of the population and estimated 30% of returning soldiers

RISK FACTORS

- ♦ Combat duty exposing personnel to improvised explosive devices (IEDs) used by opposing factions

PREVENTION AND SCREENING FOR MILITARY PERSONNEL

- ♦ Mandatory post-deployment screening for all veterans returning from combat assignment
- ♦ TBI screening
    - ◇ Exposure to events (such as blasts, vehicle accidents, falls) that may have caused brain injury
    - ◇ Immediate symptoms (such as loss of consciousness, feeling dazed, head injury, amnesia of event)
    - ◇ Onset or worsening of problems (such as with memory, balance, headaches, dizziness, irritability, sensitivity to bright light, sleep problems) that may indicate brain injury
    - ◇ Presence of symptoms in past week

- Four factors complicate recovery from combat-related concussions compared with mild TBI acquired in civilian settings.
  1. The physically and emotionally traumatic environment in which they occur
  2. The potentially repetitive and cumulative nature of concussions sustained over a tour (or multiple tours) of combat duty
  3. The high incidence of comorbid mental health conditions
  4. The difficulty in following typical recommendations for post-concussion care, such as rest (U.S. Department of Veteran Affairs, 2022)

ASSESSMENT

Physical Findings and Mental Status

- Symptoms of TBI (see Table 12–1)
- Risk for suicide
  - Factors increasing risk for suicide attempt with TBI
    - Male sex
    - Ages 18 and 19
    - Psychiatric disorder
    - Aggressive behavior
    - Substance use

Diagnostic and Laboratory Findings

- No current diagnostic test can retrospectively diagnose mild TBI or determine that current symptoms or problems are due to a past mild TBI. Conventional structural neuroimaging studies are typically normal in mild TBI.

DIFFERENTIAL DIAGNOSIS

- Posttraumatic stress disorder (PTSD)
- Depression
- Anxiety
- Other mental health diagnosis

TABLE 12–1.
SYMPTOMS OF TRAUMATIC BRAIN INJURY

MILD TBI	**MENTAL STATUS CHANGES**

	• Acute symptoms
	  • Dazed and confused
	• Other mental status changes
	  • Poor concentration
	  • Memory difficulty
	  • Intellectual impairment
	  • Irritability
	  • Depression
	  • Anxiety

	PHYSICAL FINDINGS
	• Dizziness • Balance problems • Headaches • Tinnitus • Numbness and tingling • Vison changes • Sensitivity to light • Sensitivity to sound • Extreme fatigue • Sleep problems
MODERATE TO SEVERE TBI	**INCLUDES MENTAL STATUS CHANGES AND PHYSICAL FINDINGS FROM MILD TBI AND:**
	• Chronic, worsening headaches • Repeated nausea and vomiting • Seizures • Difficult to arouse from sleep • Slurred speech • Unequal pupils • Confusion • Restlessness and agitation • Extreme weakness or numbness • Loss of coordination

TBI, tramatic brain injury

CLINICAL MANAGEMENT

Pharmacological Management

- No specific medications for TBI
- Treat related symptoms according to current evidence-based standards.

- Increased sensitivity to side effects of medication (secondary to head injury)
    - Sedation
    - Anticholinergic side effects (decrease memory)
    - Seizures with tricyclic antidepressants (TCAs), bupropion, and amantadine (lower seizure threshold)
    - Extrapyramidal symptoms, neuroleptic malignant syndrome, tardive dyskinesia
    - Neuroleptics: Decrease neuronal recovery
    - Benzodiazepines: Decrease memory, increase confusion, decrease coordination, misuse potential
- Cognitive disorders recommendations
    - Methylphenidate: Increase attention, processing speed, general cognitive function, learning, and memory
    - Dextroamphetamine: Increase attention, processing speed
    - Bromocriptine (off label, possibly helpful): Increase executive function
    - Amantadine (off label, possibly helpful): Increase general cognitive function, attention, concentration
- When using medications, start low and go slow.

Nonpharmacological Management

- Treat comorbidities. (Military personnel with TBI frequently have PTSD, which makes treatment of TBI more difficult.)
- Safety plan for suicide risk; limit availability of means.
- Teach family to identify signs of risk for suicide.
- Follow up for 1 year after anyone with TBI makes an attempt to end their own life.
- Treat vestibular dysfunction with physical therapy to reduce dizziness.
- Treat traumatic vision syndrome with occupational therapy; scanning and accommodation difficulties lead to headaches, irritability, and fatigue.
- Treat memory impairment with occupational therapy to teach memory improvement skills.
- Teach about symptoms and implications for relationships, employment, and so on.
- Avoid alcohol.
- Neuropsychological testing

- Psychotherapy
  - Supportive
  - Cognitive behavioral therapy (CBT)
- Increase understanding of relationships between cognition and emotion
- Target adjustment or development of new beliefs and assumptions (see Table 12–2)
  - Behavioral therapy
  - Family therapy
- Behavioral, affective, and personality changes are most difficult for families to adjust to.
- Tips for families include the following:
  - If concentration is an issue, ask the TBI survivor for one thing at a time. Use of white noise machines may reduce distractions. It may take longer to complete tasks.
  - If memory is an issue, keep note pads near the phone for messages and in other places throughout the house. Keep a "memory book." Make a calendar and keep it in a central location.
  - If anger or irritability is an issue, leave the situation if possible and wait for the TBI survivor to calm down. Use a soft, calm voice. Keep your distance and give the TBI survivor space.
  - Resources
  - Military Health System and Defense Health Agency: https://health.mil/Military-Health-Topics/Centers-of-Excellence/Traumatic-Brain-Injury-Center-of-Excellence
    - Brain Injury Association of America: http://www.biausa.org
    - U.S. Department of Veterans Affairs: www.va.gov
- Tips for the PMHNP for therapy with the client with TBI:
  - Determine what having a TBI means to the client.
  - Focus on "real life" difficulties in the here-and-now.

TABLE 12–2.
COGNITIVE IMPAIRMENT AND ASSOCIATED CORE FEATURES OF COGNITIVE BEHAVIORAL THERAPY

COGNITIVE IMPAIRMENT	THERAPY CORE FEATURE
Impulsivity	"Stop–think–reflect"
Decreased awareness, encoding, and recall	Monitoring problems and successes
Memory	Use of audiotapes of sessions
Executive impairment	Develop independent problem-solving for everyday difficulties

- ◊ Monitor speed and complexity of comments.
- ◊ Adjust session length according to level of attention and fatigue.
- ◊ Reestablish an acceptable sense of self.
- ◊ Instill hope without making predictions of a successful rehabilitation outcome.

LIFE SPAN CONSIDERATIONS

- ♦ Mild TBI
  - ◊ Most clients achieve full recovery within 3 months; if residual symptoms continue, 80% to 85% will clear within 6 months

FOLLOW-UP

- ♦ Symptoms may occur immediately but may also appear much later, which underscores the importance of screening for TBI
- ♦ Resource for guidelines, conditions and concerns: Psychological Health Center of Excellence: www.airforcemedicine.af.mil/News/Display/Article/1353398/deployment-health-clinical-center-is-now-the-psychological-health-center-of-exc/

STIMULANT-INDUCED MILD NEUROCOGNITIVE DISORDER

DESCRIPTION

- ♦ Stimulant-induced mild neurocognitive disorder was added to the existing substance-induced mild neurocognitive disorders in the DSM-5-TR (APA, 2022).
- ♦ DSM-5-TR diagnostic criteria are not met for a major or minor neurocognitive disorder.
- ♦ Neurocognitive impairments cannot be contributed to an episode of delirium and last longer than the period of intoxication and acute withdrawal.
- ♦ The stimulant is capable of causing neurocognitive impairments.
- ♦ Neurocognitive impairments remain stable or improve over time with discontinuation of the stimulant.
- ♦ Cannot be better explained by another medical condition or mental health disorder.

NEUROLOGICAL SIGNS

- Learning difficulty
- Memory deficits
- Executive dysfunction
- Determine if the deficits were present prior to stimulant use.

INCIDENCE AND DEMOGRAPHICS

- The prevalence is not well known.

RISK FACTORS

- Substance use disorder

ASSESSMENT

Physical Findings and Mental Status

- Determine if symptoms were present prior to stimulant use.
  - Impulse control and executive dysfunction can result in substance use/misuse.
- Risk for suicide
- Rebound depression
- Hypersomnia
- Apathy
- Substance use

Diagnostic and Laboratory Findings

- No current diagnostic test can retrospectively diagnose

DIFFERENTIAL DIAGNOSIS

- TBI
- Infections associated with substance use disorders such as HIV, hepatitis C virus, syphilis
- Substance use
- Substance withdrawal

CLINICAL MANAGEMENT

Pharmacological Management

- No specific medications
- Treat related symptoms according to current evidence-based standards.

Nonpharmacological Management

- Motivational interviewing
- Cognitive behavioral therapy
- Contingency management
- Community reinforcement approach

FOLLOW-UP

- Determined by severity of symptoms.

CASE STUDY

W.K., a 59-year-old homemaker with a positive family history for Alzheimer's disease, has been very worried lately because, "I believe I am losing my memory." The client has hesitated to go for an evaluation because of this concern and is very upset as this belief is shared with the PMHNP. W.K. gives a social history of being happily married for the past 35 years and of having several children and two new grandchildren, has had no recent stressors, has felt a slow decline in memory for the past 2 years, and believes no one else has noticed, but recently it is harder to hide her deficit from the family.

W.K. has been employed as a nurse for the past 25 years at the local hospital but has begun to notice a decline in the ability to keep track of all of the information needed to do the job well. The client has a history of asthma and periodically uses a rescue inhaler and steroids to manage her asthma, routinely takes one aspirin a day, and uses over-the-counter kava kava when feeling stressed. She has been taking pravastatin 20 mg/day for cholesterol level for the past 2 years. No significant physical findings are evident on physical examination, but she does show mild impairment in short-term memory testing during the mental status examination. There are many issues to consider in planning care with this client:

1. What is the probable diagnosis at this time?
2. What further assessment is needed?
3. What does the PMHNP need to take into account when considering medication for this client?
4. Would the PMHNP include the family in care planning at this time?
5. Are medications indicated at this time?

ANSWERS TO CASE STUDY DISCUSSION QUESTIONS

1. The correct diagnosis in this case is unspecified neurocognitive disorder.
2. Additional assessment information needed is to refer client for a complete medical examination.
3. Before starting the client on medication, the PMHNP needs to understand the correct diagnosis for the client's symptoms and the stage of their illness and to discuss the client's preference for treatment.
4. In this case, yes, family should be involved as early as possible.
5. For this client, medication is not indicated at this time.

REFERENCES AND RESOURCES

American Psychiatric Association. (2022). Diagnostic and statistical manual of mental disorders (5th ed., text rev.).

Bickley, L. S. (2023). Bates' guide to physical examination and history taking (13th ed.). LWW.

Borson, S., Scanlan, J., Brush, M., Vitaliano, P., & Dokmak A. (2000). The mini-cog: A cognitive 'vital signs' measure for dementia screening in multilingual elderly. International Journal of Geriatric Psychiatry, 15, 1021–1027.

Burke, M., & Laramie, J. A. (2003). Primary care of older adults (2nd ed.). Mosby.

De Lange, E., Verhaak, P. F., & van der Meer, K. (2013). Prevalence, presentation and prognosis of delirium in older people in the population, at home and in long term care: A review. International Journal of Geriatric Psychiatry, 28(2), 127–134.

Dick, K., & Morency, C. R. (2011). Delirium. In K. Devereaux & S. Crock (Eds.), Geropsychiatric and mental health nursing (2nd ed., pp. 255–272). Jones & Bartlett Learning.

Doornbos, M. M. (2002). Family caregivers and the mental health care system: Reality and dreams. Archives of Psychiatric Nursing, 15(4), 39–46.

Harper, M. G., Lyons, W. L., & Potter, J. F. (Eds.) (2022). Geriatric review syllabus. American Geriatrics Society.

Jacobson, S. (2014). Clinical manual of geriatric psychopharmacology (2nd ed.). American Psychiatric Publishing.

Melillo Devereaux, K., & Houde Crocker, S. (2011). Geropsychiatric and mental health nursing (2nd ed.). Jones & Bartlett Learning.

Pfeiffer, E. (1975). A short portable mental status questionnaire for the assessment of organic brain deficit in elderly patients. Journal of American Geriatric Society, 23, 433–441.

Sadock, B., Sadock, V., & Ruiz, P. (2017). Kaplan and Sadock's comprehensive textbook of psychiatry (10th ed.). Wolters Kluwer.

Stahl, S. M. (2020). Stahl's essential psychopharmacology: Prescriber's guide (7th ed.). Cambridge University Press.

Steffens, D., Blazer, D., & Thakur, M. (2015). Textbook of geriatric psychiatry (5th ed.). American Psychiatric Publishing.

U.S. Department of Veterans Affairs. (2022). Polytrauma/TBI system of care. http://www.polytrauma.va.gov/understanding-tbi/

U.S. Preventive Services Task Force. (2003). Screening for dementia: Recommendations and rationale. http://www.acpjournals.org/doi/full/10.7326/0003-4819-138-11-200306030-00014

CHAPTER 13

SUBSTANCE-RELATED AND ADDICTIVE DISORDERS

One of the most common but least well-addressed classes of disorders is substance use disorders. Psychiatric-mental health nurse practitioners (PMHNPs) who work in primary psychiatric settings or integrated primary care settings commonly treat clients with substance-related disorders. These disorders can stand alone or be part of a complex co-occurring illness with either general medical conditions or psychiatric disorders.

Many substances can be used and misused. No matter what the substance, the continuum of use can range from mild to severe. Although the specific substances of misuse will determine many of the physical, behavioral, and cognitive symptoms exhibited by the client, some commonalities exist for all substances.

This chapter focuses on the PMHNP role in determining the severity of substance use and the available clinical management and treatments. It also emphasizes alcohol use disorders as a primary example. Alcohol is discussed because it is the most commonly misused substance, it is well researched, and PMHNPs will most often encounter people in clinical settings with an alcohol use disorder. Much of what is known about disorders of alcohol use is believed to be transferable to other substances.

SUBSTANCE-RELATED DISORDERS

DESCRIPTION

- Substance use disorders are a cluster of disorders in which cognitive, behavioral, and physiological symptoms indicate that a person continues using a substance despite significant substance-related problems (American Psychiatric Association [APA], 2022).
- Psychiatric symptom clusters may be related to substance use, discontinuation of substance use, or withdrawal from habitual substance use.
- Substance use disorders lead to changes in brain circuits and physiological functions that lead to a need for detoxification and a possible need for long-term treatment.
- The word substance can describe a drug of misuse, a medication, or a toxin that produces psychoactivation and alters cognitive, behavioral, and affective perceptions.

- Dependence: Repeated use of a substance with or without physical dependence
- Harmful use: Use that is inconsistent with social pattern use
- Misuse: Usually applies to a prescribed substance
- Intoxication: Reversible syndrome caused by a specific substance affecting memory, judgment, behavior, or social or occupational functioning
- Withdrawal: Substance-specific symptoms that occur after stopping or reducing use
- Tolerance: Needing more of the substance to get the desired effect

ETIOLOGY

- Multiple theories ranging from psychological to neurobiological
- Probable multifactorial etiological profile
- Two common types of theories: psychodynamic and biological
- Psychodynamic theory
  - Behaviors of harmful use are seated in oral-stage fixation.
  - A person seeks gratification through oral behaviors.
  - Maladaptive regressive behaviors can become overlearned, fixed, and reinforced through dysfunctional family patterns.
  - Sociocultural factors attempt to explain population-based differences in substance use rates.
- Biological theory
  - Genetic loading
    - People with a strong genetic vulnerability to addiction are thought to have defects in the working of the reward center of the brain, which predisposes them to stronger-than-normal positive rewards that draw them to substance use.
  - Gender differences
  - Racial/ethnic differences
  - A person is predisposed to stronger-than-normal negative rewards, making it more difficult to stop substance use once it has begun.
  - Involves two neurobiological processes:
    1. Reinforcement
       - Brain-based changes in structure and function can lead to addictive behavior.

- The process of positive and negative rewards is physiologically linked to memory function.
- Changes appear to occur with any substance of misuse.
- Reinforcement results in "feel good" sensations when a substance of misuse is used and in "feel bad" sensations when the substance exits the body.
- Positive rewards of reinforcement result in the social rewards commonly associated with substance use, such as disinhibition, euphoric mood, and anxiety reduction.
  - Mediated by dopamine pathways
- Negative rewards are aversive, such as increased anxiety and dysphoria.
  - Mediated by the γ-aminobutyric acid (GABA) pathways
- Reinforcement occurs in the ventral tegmental area and the nucleus accumbens of the brain, collectively called the reward center.
- Dopamine release within the reward center is enhanced further by the release of natural morphine-like neurotransmitters called neuropeptides (enkephalins, beta-endorphins).
- Neuropeptides further enhance the reinforcing pleasure experienced by the person.
- With repeated substance use, the dopamine system becomes increasingly sensitized.
- Eventually, associated substance use stimuli (e.g., pictures of drug paraphernalia) can cause dopamine release, leading to reinforcement of use and often to increased substance use.

2. Neuroadaptation
   - Brain-based changes in structure and function can lead to tolerance and withdrawal.
   - Drug-specific alterations in the normal level and function of neurotransmitters occur as the body adapts to the chronic presence of the substance of misuse.
   - Neuroadaptive processes become significant when the person stops substance use.
   - These processes become the basis for withdrawal symptoms because adaptive responses are unopposed when the substance is no longer present.

- Neuroadaptive changes may be more enduring in some persons, possibly lasting for years, thus increasing the potential for relapse.
- This concept helps to explain why, after a long period of sobriety, a person who returns to substance use often picks up at the same level of tolerance and physical impact as experienced before sobriety.

INCIDENCE AND DEMOGRAPHICS

- Persons ages 18 to 24 years of age have high prevalence rates for using most substances.
- The United States has higher rates of substance use than any other developed country.
- More than 50% of U.S. clients with a psychiatric disorder have a comorbid substance use disorder.
    - Persons with schizophrenia are 4 times more likely to have a substance use comorbidity than the general population.
    - Persons with bipolar affective disorder are 5 times more likely to have a substance use comorbidity than the general population.
- More than 2 million admissions annually are made to inpatient substance use treatment facilities.
    - Although now legal in some states, marijuana is the most commonly misused illegal substance.
- Alcohol is the most commonly misused legal substance.
    - Rates are higher in men than in women.
    - 90% of men have used alcohol.
    - 70% of women have used alcohol.
    - Rates are highest in African Americans, Hispanic Americans, and Native Americans; rates are lowest in Asian Americans.
    - 55% of fatal driving accidents in the United States occur with a driver under the influence of alcohol.
    - 50% of crimes in the United Stated are committed under the influence of alcohol.
    - The lifetime risk for alcohol use disorder is 15% in the general U.S. population.
- Opioids
    - In 2017, among 70,237 drug overdose deaths, 47,600 (67.8%) involved opioids; this increases across age groups, racial/ethnic groups, county urbanization levels, and in multiple states.

- ◇ In 2021 synthetic opioid-involved overdose death rates increased 51% to 66% of overdose deaths (The Commonwealth Fund, 2023).
- ◇ Diagnostic and Statistical Manual of Mental Disorders, Fifth Edition, Text Revision (DSM-5-TR; APA, 2022) diagnostic criteria for opioid use disorder (OUD)
    - A problematic pattern of opioid use leading to clinically significant impairment or distress is manifested by two or more of the following within a 12-month period:
        - Opioids are often taken in larger amounts or over a longer period than was intended
        - A persistent desire or unsuccessful efforts to cut down or control opioid use
        - A great deal of time is spent in activities necessary to obtain the opioid, use the opioid, or recover from its effects;Craving or a strong desire or urge to use opioids
        - Recurrent opioid use resulting in a failure to fulfill major role obligations at work, school, or home
        - Continued opioid use despite having persistent or recurrent social or interpersonal problems caused or exacerbated by the effects of opioids
        - Important social, occupational, or recreational activities are given up or reduced because of opioid use
        - Recurrent opioid use in situations in which it is physically hazardous
        - Continued opioid use despite knowledge of having a persistent or recurrent physical or psychological problem that is likely to have been caused or exacerbated by the substance
        - Tolerance*
        - Withdrawal*

*Experiencing these symptoms while taking opioids solely under appropriate medical supervision is an exception to (i.e., does not meet) these criteria for OUD.

RISK FACTORS

- ♦ Genetic loading
    - ◇ Family history of substance use or major depressive disorder (MDD)
- ♦ Association with peer structure with heavy substance use
- ♦ Co-occurring psychiatric disorder

- Age and sex (younger, males)
- Existence of chronic pain
- Untreated chronic pathological-level anxiety

PREVENTION AND SCREENING

- At-risk family education
  - Stigma reduction
  - Signs and symptoms of illness
  - Treatment potential for control of symptoms
- Early recognition, intervention, and initiation of treatment to prevent disease development of complications of disorder
- Implications of alcohol and other drug use during pregnancy:
  - Fetal alcohol syndrome (FAS)
    - Prevalence: one third of all infants born to girls or women with alcohol use disorder
    - Signs: low birth weight and height, microphthalmia, short palpebral fissure, midface hypoplasia, smooth or short philtrum, thin upper lip
  - Birth defects
- Acute alcohol intoxication in nontolerant persons such as teenagers
  - Coma
  - Respiratory depression
  - Death
- CAGE Screening Test (Substance Abuse and Mental Health Services Administration [SAMSHA], 2016)
  - Most commonly used screening tool for alcohol misuse
  - Administered by asking the client four questions
  - Each positive answer scored as 1 point; negative answers receive no score
  - The more positive answers, the greater the likelihood of an alcohol use disorder.
  - Clients scoring 2 or greater are at mild to moderate risk for alcohol dependency, and the score is considered clinically significant
  - Clients scoring 3 to 4 are considered at high risk for alcohol dependency

CAGE Screening Test

C: Have you ever felt the need to cut down on your drinking?

A: Have people annoyed you by mentioning your drinking?

G: Have you ever felt bad or guilty about your drinking?

E: Have you ever had a drink the first thing in the morning to steady your nerves or get rid of a hangover (eye-opener)?

- Other screening tools
  - AUDIT: Alcohol Use Disorders Identification Test: A 10-item validated screening tool developed by the World Health Organization (WHO) to assess alcohol consumption, drinking behaviors, and problems related to alcohol use. A clinician version and self-report are included. A chart of equivalents for alcoholic beverages is included (SAMSHA, 2023).
    - A score of 1–7 is low-risk.
    - A score of 8–14 indicates harmful use.
    - A score of 15 or more indicates alcohol dependence.
  - DAST: Drug Abuse Screening Test: Originally developed as a 28-item, self-report or interview to access the degree of problems related to drug use other than alcohol or tobacco in the past 12 months. The DAST has been condensed and can be used in a variety of settings.
    - DAST-20 (adult)
      - A score of 1–5 is low risk.
      - A score of 6–10 is intermediate risk.
      - A score of 11–15 is substantial risk.
      - A score of 16–20 is severe risk.
    - DAST-10 (adult)
      - A score of 1–2 is low risk.
      - A score of 3–5 is intermediate risk.
      - A score of 6–8 is substantial risk.
      - A score of 9–10 is severe risk.
    - DAST-A (adolescent)
      - A score of 6 or more indicates a substance use problem.

- ◊ S-MAST: Short Michigan Alcoholism Screening Test (or Geriatric Version)
- ◊ CRAFFT: Children and adolescents younger than 21 years of age
- ◊ Opiate ingestion symptoms last in relation to the half-life of the injected opiate.

- ♦ Withdrawal precipitated by medication (i.e., naloxone, naltrexone) is more abrupt and severe, and reports of life-threatening autonomic instability and delirium have been reported in the literature.
- ♦ Withdrawal may be inadvertent (given Narcan, ran out of opioid, person hospitalized with an undisclosed heroin habit), required by setting (i.e., incarceration), or supervised withdrawal (detoxification) as part of a treatment program.
- ♦ Use of a validated tool to quantify symptoms of opiate withdrawal
  - ◊ COWS (Clinical Opiate Withdrawal Scale; Wesson & Ling, 2003): A scale of 11 items that quantifies symptoms of withdrawal; clinician administered inpatient or outpatient and assesses the following symptoms:
    - Resting pulse rate
    - Sweating
    - Restlessness
    - Pupil size
    - Bone or joint aches
    - Runny nose or tearing
    - Gastrointestinal upset
    - Tremor
    - Yawning
    - Anxiety, irritability
    - Gooseflesh
    - The scores indicate severity of withdrawal and physical dependence:
      - A score of 5–12 is mild.
      - A score of 13–24 is moderate.
      - A score of 25–36 is moderately severe.
      - A score of 36 or greater indicates severe withdrawal.

ASSESSMENT

Client History

- ♦ Assess for the following:
  - ◊ Detailed history of present illness, including time frame, progression, and associated symptoms

    - ◊ Social history, including present living situation, relationship status, education, occupation, spirituality, and substance use/misuse history to include tobacco, alcohol, prescription, and illicit substances
    - ◊ Medication use, including prescription, over-the-counter, alternative, supplements, and home remedies
    - ◊ Initial and periodic functional history and assessment
    - ◊ Validate history with a family member
    - ◊ Identify the category of substance used by the client.

- ♦ Knowing category allows for anticipation of physical impact of substance and to predict potential symptoms of withdrawal
- ♦ Clients often misuse substances from categories with similar pharmacological properties.
- ♦ Categories of misused substances
    - ◊ Alcohol
    - ◊ Amphetamines or similar sympathomimetics
    - ◊ Caffeine
    - ◊ Cannabis
    - ◊ Cocaine
    - ◊ Hallucinogens
    - ◊ Inhalants
    - ◊ Nicotine
    - ◊ Opioids
    - ◊ Phencyclidine (PCP) or similar arylcyclohexylamines
    - ◊ Sedatives
    - ◊ Hypnotics
    - ◊ Anxiolytics
- ♦ Assess for presence of substance use
    - ◊ Maladaptive pattern of substance use manifested by recurrent and significant adverse consequences related to repeated use of a substance
    - ◊ Specific criteria needed to identify substance use disorder
        - Maladaptive pattern of use occurring for at least a 12-month period of sustained use
        - Must be accompanied by repeated failure to fulfill major role obligation

        - Must be accompanied by use in situation that presents as physically hazardous, such as drinking and driving
        - Use continues despite multiple problems related to substance use patterns, such as legal, interpersonal, or social problems

- Assess for presence of substance use disorder
    - Cluster of cognitive, behavioral, and physiological symptoms indicating that the person continues use of a substance despite significant substance related problems
    - Synonymous with addiction
    - Pattern of repeated use that leads to clinically significant impairment or distress with two or more of the following symptoms within a 12-month period:
        - Tolerance
        - Withdrawal
        - Using larger amounts than intended
        - Persistent craving or unsuccessful attempts to cut down
        - Large amount of time spent obtaining substance, using substance, or recovering from its effects
        - Activities decreased or given up because of use
        - Using despite consequences
- Physiological dependence implies tolerance and withdrawal
- Degree of tolerance and withdrawal symptoms are substance specific.
    - Can be physical, psychological, or both, depending on the substance
    - Withdrawal symptoms are almost always the opposite of the acute action of the substance.
    - Categories of substances with pronounced, obvious withdrawal symptoms:
        - Alcohol
        - Opioids
        - Sedatives
        - Hypnotics
        - Anxiolytics
    - Categories of substances with less pronounced, less obvious withdrawal symptoms:
        - Stimulants
        - Nicotine
        - Cannabis

- ◊ Categories of substances with little to no pronounced, obvious withdrawal symptoms:
    - Hallucinogens
    - PCP

♦ Assess for the presence of substance withdrawal or intoxication

- ◊ Clients misusing or harmfully using substances present for assessment either under the influence of the substance (intoxication) or experiencing problems related to cessation of substance use (withdrawal)
- ◊ Intoxication: Reversible substance-specific syndrome caused by recent ingestion of a psychoactivating substance. Signs and symptoms include the following:
    - Altered mental status—from euphoria to lethargy to coma
    - Miotic pupils (pinpoint)
    - Slowed bowel sounds
    - Normal to low heart rate and blood pressure
    - Hypoventilation/respiratory depression
- ◊ Withdrawal: Potentially nonreversible substance-specific syndrome caused by cessation or significant reduction in heavy, prolonged use of a substance. Signs and symptoms include the following:
    - Gastrointestinal (GI) distress: Abdominal cramps, diarrhea, nausea, and/or vomiting
    - Flulike symptoms: Lacrimation, rhinorrhea, diaphoresis, shivering, and piloerection (goosebumps)
    - Sympathetic nerve and central nervous system (CNS) arousal: Mydriatic pupils (dilated), mild hypertension and tachycardia, anxiety and irritability, insomnia, agitation, restless leg syndrome, general restlessness, tremor, and, less frequently, low-grade temperature and tactile sensitivity
    - Yawning, sneezing, anorexia, dizziness, myalgias/arthralgias, and leg cramps (Farrell, 1994)
- ◊ Use a validated tool to quantify symptoms of alcohol withdrawal:
    - CIWA (Clinical Institute Withdrawal Assessment Alcohol Scale; Sullivan et al., 1989): A scale of 10 items that quantifies symptoms of alcohol withdrawal using objective and subjective assessment.
    - Assesses the following symptoms:
        - Nausea and vomiting
        - Tremor
        - Paroxysmal sweats
        - Anxiety
        - Agitation

        - Tactile disturbance
        - Auditory disturbance
        - Visual disturbance
        - Headache, fullness in head
        - Orientation, clouding of sensorium
    - The score quantifies the severity of symptoms:
        - A score of less than 10, no pharmacological treatment is indicated.
        - A score of 10–20, clinical judgement is required to determine treatment
        - A score of greater than 20, severe alcohol withdrawal
  - ◊ Blood alcohol levels determine presence of alcohol in the body
    - Tolerant persons often have higher blood levels with less impairment than nontolerant persons.
    - Must interpret blood alcohol levels of a client based on their degree of tolerance
  - ◊ Diagnostic criteria for substance withdrawal include the following:
    - Cessation or reduction in substance use that has been heavy or prolonged
    - Two or more of the following symptoms within several hours or days of reduction or cessation of the substance:
        - Hand tremor
        - Insomnia
        - Autonomic hyperactivity (sweating, increased heart rate, and increased blood pressure)
        - Nausea or vomiting
        - Hallucinations or illusions
        - Psychomotor agitation
        - Anxiety
        - Seizures
- ♦ Structured interview allows for assessment of the use patterns and consequences of a person's substance use
  - ◊ Assess for all dimensions of the impact of substance use or dependence in the person.
    - Current use
    - Pattern of use
    - Consequences (interpersonal, occupational, legal)
    - Physical health consequences

Physical Exam Findings

- Substance use or dependence produces many physical symptoms.
  - Usually a result of sequelae of use or misuse rather than findings specific to misuse or dependence
- Generally nonspecific when viewed in isolation
- Must be considered as a cluster of symptoms that raise an index of suspicion of substance use disorder potential
  - Abdominal pain and tenderness
  - Nausea
  - Weight loss
  - Gastrointestinal bleeding
  - Hypertension
  - Anxiety
  - First-episode seizure in adult
- Physical findings related to alcohol use disorders (Domino et al., 2015; National Institute on Alcohol Abuse and Alcoholism [NIAAA], 2016).
  - Brain: Mood changes, behavior changes
  - Head, eyes, ears, nose, throat (HEENT): Poor oral health
  - Cardiovascular: Hypertension, cardiomyopathy, tachycardia
  - Gastrointestinal: Liver disease, cirrhosis, peptic ulcer, esophageal malignancies
  - Neurologic: Tremor, cognitive deficits, peripheral neuropathy, Wernicke-Korsakoff syndrome
  - Metabolic: Hyperlipidemia

Mental Status Exam Findings

- Nature of findings depends heavily on whether the client is experiencing substance intoxication or withdrawal or is substance-free at the time of assessment.
  - Index of suspicion for substance-related disorder should be raised if client presents differently during different periods of assessment (Sadock et al., 2017).
- Stimulants: Agitation, anxiety, irritability, mood swings, elevated mood
- Opioids: Mood swings, aggression, disinhibition, impaired cognition, slurred speech, psychomotor slowing
- Hallucinogens: Mood swings, hallucinations, paranoia, flashbacks, panic, impaired judgement

- Cannabis: Confusion, paranoia, panic
- Inhalants: Agitation, irritability, confusion, hallucinations

Diagnostic and Laboratory Findings

- Complete blood count (CBC), chemistry profile, thyroid function tests, and B_{12} level to rule out metabolic causes or unidentified conditions
- Drug toxicity screening, if indicated by history
- Alcohol dependence and misuse produce biomarkers include the following:
  - 300 mg/dl or greater indicates excessive alcohol misuse
  - 150 mg/dl or greater indicates intoxication and possible excessive alcohol misuse
  - 100 mg/dl on routine exam or greater indicates an increased possibility of excessive alcohol use
  - Aspartate transaminase (AST)/alanine transaminase (ALT) ration >2.0
  - Elevated: Glutamyl transferase, mean corpuscular volume, prothrombin time, uric acid, total cholesterol, and triglycerides
  - Decreased: Magnesium, calcium, potassium, blood urea nitrogen, hemoglobin, hematocrit, platelet count and albumin (Domino et al., 2015).

DIFFERENTIAL DIAGNOSIS

- Endocrine disorders
  - Cushing's disease
- Neurological disorders
  - Seizure disorders
- Cardiovascular disorders
  - Myocardial infarction
- Mood disorders
  - MDD
  - Bipolar disorder
- Anxiety disorders
- Personality disorders

- Differential diagnostic consideration for acute alcohol withdrawal
  - Many acute general health conditions can mimic symptoms of alcohol withdrawal.

CLINICAL MANAGEMENT

- Rule out or treat any conditions that may contribute to clinical findings.
- Note: 80% to 90% of people who have an alcohol use disorder do not receive treatment.
  - Common reasons for failure to receive needed treatment
    - Lack of diagnosis
    - Lack of referral
    - Lack of access to services
    - Resistance to treatment
- The genetics of substance use disorder vulnerability are becoming better known, which allows for preventative and early intervention treatments.
- The knowledge base of the pathophysiology of dependence has promoted new somatic interventions.
- Psychopharmacology offers the promise of a new era in the treatment of addictions.
- Clinical management differs depending on the substance-related syndrome exhibited by the person.
  - Acute withdrawal
  - Acute intoxication
  - Long-term sobriety maintenance
  - Relapse prevention
- Alcohol withdrawal carries a high risk of mortality.
- Clinical management of alcohol withdrawal is a specialized treatment that requires specific experience in this type of care.
- Some clinical findings may assist in identification of clients at risk for severe alcohol withdrawal:
  - Agitation
  - Decreased short-term memory
  - Disorientation

  - ◊ Hallucinations
  - ◊ Irregular pulse
  - ◊ Ophthalmoplegia
- ♦ CIWA Scale
  - ◊ Used to determine the likelihood of withdrawal and delirium tremens (DTs), which usually occur within the first 24 to 72 hours after cessation of alcohol.
  - ◊ Assesses 10 common withdrawal symptoms:
    - Nausea and vomiting
    - Tremors
    - Paroxysmal sweats
    - Anxiety
    - Agitation
    - Tactile disturbances
    - Auditory disturbances
    - Visual disturbances
    - Headaches
    - Altered sensorium
  - ◊ Each symptom is graded on a 0- to 7-point scale, with the exception of orientation and sensorium, which are graded on a 0- to 4-point scale. The higher the total score (maximum = 67), the more likely the person will experience severe withdrawal and DTs: 0–9 = absent or very mild withdrawal, 10–15 = mild withdrawal, 16–20 = moderate withdrawal, and 21–67 = severe withdrawal and possible DTs.
- ♦ Medically assisted detoxification as a bridge to medically assisted treatment is the best treatment for pregnant women during pregnancy, as withdrawal and use of cycles can result in preterm labor, fetal distress, or placental abruption. An infant born to a mother taking opioids for medical or illicit purposes, or who is being treated with buprenorphine or methadone, will go through withdrawal after birth. Neonatal abstinence syndrome is treated to reduce the withdrawal symptoms, and the infant is monitored and assisted through withdrawal (American College of Obstetricians and Gynecologists [ACOG], 2012).
- ♦ Opioid medications for treatment of withdrawal (these medications are also used in Medication for Substance Use Disorders [MSUD] training and require an addendum to the Drug Enforcement Administration [DEA] license to be prescribed)
- ♦ The goal is to bridge the client through withdrawal and continue the opioid treatment in a treatment program:

- ◊ Buprenorphine (Subutex, Suboxone [with naloxone]): A partial mu-opioid agonist and kappa-receptor antagonist with a long half-life. Naloxone is added to the sublingual formulation as a deterrent to diversion and intravenous use; the naloxone is not absorbed through the buccal membranes.
- ◊ Buprenorphine has the advantage that it can be prescribed and administered through an outpatient program.
- ◊ Because of the mechanism of action, to allow for successful transition, the person needs to be in moderate withdrawal before the buprenorphine is started.
- ◊ Methadone: Long-acting full mu-receptor agonist. Lethal in overdose related to cardiac arrhythmia; therefore it is only given in supervised settings. In the United States, methadone supervised withdrawal to treatment must be in a designated opioid treatment program or in an inpatient hospital (only if the person is hospitalized for another reason than opioid withdrawal).
- ◊ The literature shows that both methadone and buprenorphine are effective for treatment of withdrawal symptoms and are superior to clonidine (alpha agonist) in keeping clients off illicit opioids. However, use of these medications means that the person remains opioid dependent.

Pharmacological Management

- Pharmacological treatments are symptom-specific.
- Clinical management of acute withdrawal
    - ◊ Detoxification (detox) agents replace uncontrolled use of substance with slow tapering of controlled substance to minimize neuroadaptive rebound.
- Multiple daily doses of benzodiazepines are used according to a fixed schedule and gradually tapered over several days.
- Examples include the following:
    - ◊ Lorazepam
    - ◊ Chlordiazepoxide
    - ◊ Diazepam
    - ◊ Oxazepam
- Polytherapy is a newer approach that matches drugs required for safe and effective withdrawal with neurotransmitter deficits created by substance use.
    - ◊ Selective serotonin reuptake inhibitors (SSRIs)
    - ◊ Opioid antagonists nalmefene hydrochloride, naltrexone, or naltrexone for extended-release injectable suspension
    - ◊ N-methyl-D-aspartate (NMDA) agonists

- Antiseizure medications such as carbamazepine and valproic acid are sometimes used to decrease the potential for seizures.
- Adrenergic medications are sometimes used to decrease blood pressure and pulse rate associated with withdrawal.
  - Clinical management of craving (see Table 13–1)
- Use anti-craving medication such as naltrexone, acamprosate, ondansetron, or buprenorphine.
- Use behavior treatment to help client learn substitute behaviors.
  - Clinical management and maintenance of sobriety (see Table 13–1)
- Person may require ongoing treatment for comorbid psychiatric disorder.
- May use aversion treatment to avoid alcohol in persons with alcohol dependence.
  - Disulfiram
  - Do not administer until the person has been alcohol-free for at least 12 hours.
- Advise client to refrain from using anything that contains alcohol (e.g., vinegar, aftershave lotion, perfumes, mouthwash, cough medication) while taking disulfiram and up to 2 weeks after discontinuing disulfiram.

TABLE 13–1.
PHARMACOLOGICAL AGENTS USEFUL IN TREATING CRAVING AND MAINTAINING

PHARMACOLOGICAL AGENT	CHEMICAL CATEGORY	ACTION EFFECT
Acamprosate	Homotaurine	Decrease craving
Buprenorphine	Opioid partial agonist, opioid antagonist	Decrease craving
Buprenorphine/naloxone	Opioid partial agonist, opioid antagonist	Decrease craving and blocks effects of opioids
Citalopram	Selective serotonin reuptake inhibitor	Decrease desire
Disulfiram	Aldehyde dehydrogenase inhibitor	Aversion therapy
Methadone	Narcotic analgesic	Suppresses withdrawal
Nalmefene	Opioid antagonist	Increases abstinence
Naloxone	Opioid antagonist	Blocks effects of opioids

Note. Adapted from Goldberg, J. F., & Stahl, S. (2021). Practical psychopharmacology. Cambridge University Press.

- Disulfiram can elevate liver function test (LFT) results; monitor LFTs. It may potentially induce mania in clients with bipolar disorder.
  - General health maintenance medication to treat vitamin deficiencies in persons with alcohol dependence include thiamine, folic acid, and B-complex vitamins.
- Clonidine (alpha-2 adrenergic receptor agonist)
  - This medication can be used in combination with an opioid treatment, as a primary agent with or without other adjunct medication. It is most effective with opioid treatments; however, it is used where opioid treatments are undesirable (e.g., prison) or unavailable (they require a specific program and DEA license).
  - Clonidine is most effective against the autonomic symptoms of sweating, diarrhea, intestinal cramps, nausea, anxiety, and irritability. It is less effective against myalgias, restlessness, insomnia, and craving.
- Emergency treatment of overdose: Naloxone and respiratory support
  - Naloxone is a pure opioid antagonist that replaces opioids at the receptor sites:
    - Available in intravenous (IV), intramuscular (IM), and intranasal forms. The intranasal response is slower and a larger dose is required.
    - Kits and cartridges are available in some states without a prescription.
    - Dosing depends on clinical presentation—usually 0.4 up to 5–10 mg.
    - Larger doses will push person into profound withdrawal.
    - Goal of naloxone is adequate ventilation, not mental status normalization.
    - Depending on the opioid half-life, the drug may outlast naloxone, be aware of a return to hypoventilation.

Other Adjunct Medications Targeting Withdrawal Symptoms

- Anxiety, irritability, restlessness
  - Diphenhydramine: 50 to 100 mg orally every 4 to 6 hours as needed (maximum 300 mg daily)
    - May also treat nausea
    - Use reduced dose in hepatic impairment
    - IV and IM administration are available
  - Hydroxyzine: 25 to 100 mg orally every 6 to 8 hours as needed (maximum 400 mg daily)
    - May also treat lacrimation and rhinorrhea
    - Use reduced dose (50%) in renal or hepatic impairment
    - The availability of IM administration of benzodiazepines

- ◊ Although benzodiazepines are effective medications for anxiety, they are also controlled substances with a high potential for misuse and may not be allowed in some settings.
    - Clonazepam: 0.5 to 1.5 mg orally every 6 to 8 hours as needed (maximum 6 mg daily). Use with caution and reduce dose in mild hepatic or renal impairment; active metabolites can accumulate.
        - Avoid in moderate to severe hepatic impairment or hepatic encephalopathy.
    - Lorazepam: 1 mg orally every 4 to 6 hours as needed (maximum 6 mg daily)
        - Relatively safe in mild to moderate hepatic impairment; use of reduced dose may be needed.
        - Avoid in severe hepatic impairment or hepatic encephalopathy.
        - IV and IM administration available; use with caution in renal impairment due to propylene glycol diluent. Parenteral and oral dosing are the same.
    - Alprazolam: Not suggested due to short half-life and highly reinforcing nature.

- ♦ GI symptoms
    - ◊ Abdominal cramping
        - Dicyclomine, 10 to 20 mg orally every 6 to 8 hours as needed (maximum 160 mg daily); IM administration available (lower doses are used)
        - Use with caution and reduce dose in renal or hepatic impairment
    - ◊ Diarrhea
        - Bismuth, 524 mg orally every 30 to 60 min as needed (up to 4200 mg daily)
            - Monitor for dehydration and maintain fluid levels with oral and/or IV hydration.
        - Loperamide, 4 mg orally followed by 2 mg after each loose stool (maximum 16 mg daily)
    - ◊ Nausea/vomiting
        - Ondansetron, 4 to 8 mg orally or IV every 12 hours as needed (maximum 16 mg/day)
            - Monitor for dehydration and maintain fluid levels with oral and/or IV hydration dose-dependent QT interval prolongation.
            - Use with caution and reduce dose (50%) in severe hepatic impairment.
        - Prochlorperazine, 5 to 10 mg orally three times daily before meals or every 6 hours as needed (maximum 40 mg/day)
            - Monitor for dehydration and maintain fluid levels with oral and/or IV hydration.
            - Use with caution in mild to moderate hepatic impairment; avoid in severe hepatic impairment IV; rectal administration available.

- Promethazine, 25 mg orally every 4 to 6 hours as needed (maximum 50 mg/day)
  - Monitor for dehydration and maintain fluid levels with oral and/or IV hydration.
  - Use with caution in mild to moderate hepatic impairment; avoid in severe hepatic impairment; IM and rectal administration is available.

♦ Insomnia

◊ Trazodone, 25 to 100 mg orally at bedtime; may titrate nightly up to 300 mg at bedtime if needed. Use with caution in severe hepatic or renal impairment.

- Watch with other serotonergic medications. May induce priapism in younger men.

◊ Doxepin, 6 to 50 mg orally at bedtime

- Use with caution and reduce dose in severe hepatic impairment

◊ Mirtazapine, 7.5 to 15 mg orally at bedtime

- May need to use lower dose in moderate to severe hepatic or renal impairment

◊ Quetiapine, 50 to 100 mg orally at bedtime

- Use lower initial dose (25 mg) in hepatic impairment and adjust based on response

◊ Zolpidem, 5 to 10 mg orally at bedtime

- A dose of 5 mg is usually appropriate for female clients and those with mild or moderate hepatic impairment
- Avoid in severe hepatic impairment or hepatic encephalopathy. This is a controlled substance with some addiction risk.

♦ Muscle aches, joint pain, headache

◊ Ibuprofen, 400 mg orally every 4 to 6 hours as needed (maximum 2400 mg daily). Client should be well hydrated and without significant kidney disease. Use with caution in mild to moderate hepatic or renal impairment.

◊ Acetaminophen, 650 to 1000 mg orally every 4 to 6 hours as needed (maximum 4000 mg daily). Appropriate analgesic for most clients.

- Use reduced dose (i.e., 2000 mg daily) or avoid in hepatic impairment or if malnourished.

◊ Naproxen, 500 mg orally twice daily with meals

- Client should be well hydrated and without significant kidney disease. Use with caution in mild to moderate hepatic or renal impairment. Avoid all non-steroidal anti-inflammatory drugs (NSAIDs) in severe renal or hepatic impairment or cirrhosis. May increase gastric irritation.

◊ Avoid all NSAIDs in severe renal or hepatic impairment or cirrhosis. May increase gastric irritation.

- Muscle spasm, restless legs
  - Cyclobenzaprine, 5 to 10 mg orally every 8 hours as needed (maximum 30 mg daily). Use reduced dose in mild hepatic impairment.
    - Avoid in moderate to severe hepatic impairment
  - Diazepam, 5 to 10 mg orally every 6 to 12 hours as needed (maximum 40 mg daily). Use with caution in hepatic or renal impairment
    - Avoid in severe hepatic impairment or hepatic encephalopathy
    - IM and IV administration available; dosing less than oral. This is a long-acting benzodiazepine—controlled substance.
  - Methocarbamol, 750 to 1500 mg orally every 8 hours as needed (maximum 6 g daily) Use with caution in hepatic or renal impairment.
    - IM and IV administration available (lower doses are used); avoid parenteral formulation in renal impairment (propylene glycol additive)

Nonpharmacological Management

- Multimodality treatment needed
- Lifetime treatment is often required.
- Inpatient treatment is usually needed for safe and effective withdrawal from alcohol.
- Indications for inpatient alcohol detoxification include history of severe withdrawal symptoms, seizures, or delirium tremens; multiple past detoxifications; additional medical or psychiatric illness; recent significant alcohol consumption; lack of reliable support system; and pregnancy.
- Reduce central nervous system stimulation by maintaining a quiet environment; put the client in room close to the nurses' station to facilitate frequent observation and monitoring; minimize abrupt changes in environment; decrease bright light and sharp, sudden noises; decrease room clutter; and do not restrain.
- Maintain hydration by monitoring intake and anticholinergic effects of benzodiazepines. Frequently offer fluids.
- Before discharge from acute-care setting, have a definite plan for follow-up treatment.
- Connect client and family with support groups.
  - 12-step groups in community
  - Concrete plan for first week of support group attendance (may need daily)
- Connect client with counseling or psychotherapy.
- Identify a primary health care provider.

- Note medical problems that will require further evaluation and potential treatment:
  - Neurological sequelae of chronic alcohol consumption
  - Nutritional deficiencies
  - Cardiomyopathy, hypertension, arrhythmias, ischemic heart disease
  - Blood dyscrasias
  - Gastrointestinal inflammations
  - Esophageal, liver, nasopharyngeal, and laryngeal cancers
- Client care needs include the following:
  - Substance use education classes
  - Substance use counseling program
  - Continued 12-step program involvement (e.g., Alcoholics Anonymous, Narcotics Anonymous)
  - Halfway housing
  - Cognitive behavioral therapy
- Family care needs include the following:
  - Current and understandable information about condition, progress, and treatment plan
  - Connect family to community support groups such as Al-Anon and Alateen
  - Management of feelings such as guilt and anger
  - Referrals to community resources
  - Specific considerations: Relationship with treatment team; role strain; financial stresses; social isolation and "code of silence"; family support systems; family violence; marital and family strife; family members' work and school functioning; history of mental disorders, including substance-related disorders
  - Assist family in coping with difficulties incorporating drinking member back into routines; encourage further counseling to resolve these difficulties
  - Refer for further treatment if family members report symptom clusters from anxiety and mood disorders, eating disorders, and addiction
- Non-pharmacological care issues in opioid withdrawal management
  - A calm, quiet environment with supportive and reassuring staff can be instrumental in helping clients overcome most symptoms of acute opioid withdrawal and decrease the need for pharmacological interventions.
  - Clients who have diarrhea, vomiting, or sweating should be monitored for dehydration, and fluid levels should be maintained with oral and/or intravenous fluids.

- ◊ Treatment of OUD and other addictions
    - The most effective treatment is medically assisted treatment plus a therapeutic program. Program alone is less likely to keep a person off illicit opioids.
- ◊ Psychotherapeutic treatments
    - Cognitive behavioral therapy (CBT)—including psychoeducation, functional analysis of use, identifying triggers, enhancing overall functioning, building healthy coping skills
    - Contingency management—behavior modification through use of incentives (and less often punishment) to assist client in staying in treatment and progressing through program
    - 12-step facilitation—has the advantage of a group setting and social support
    - Addiction counseling
    - Family therapy
- ◊ Motivational interviewing
    - A method of assessing a person's willingness to engage in treatment and a tool to help the person to make decisions about treatment
    - It is not meant to convince or coerce the person into accepting treatment; the core concept in motivational interviewing is meeting the person where they are.
    - Guiding the person to help them look toward "change thinking" can help to increase motivation and consider positive changes.
- ◊ Relapse prevention (Melemis, 2015)
    - Relapse prevention is key to staying sober and achieving recovery. These concepts can be integrated into group or individual therapy and skill building.
    - There are four key concepts:
        - Relapse is a gradual process with distinct stages; people can learn to recognize the early warning signs.
        - Recovery is a process of personal growth with stages that each have their own risk of relapse.
        - The main tools of relapse prevention are cognitive therapy and mind–body relaxation, which change negative thinking and develop healthy coping skills.
        - Most relapses can be explained in terms of a few basic rules. Educating clients in these few rules can help them focus on what is important.
- ◊ Dual diagnosis
    - There is a strong correlation between addiction and psychiatric illness. Although psychiatric symptoms are often obscured when a person is using, it

is important to treat both psychiatric and addiction simultaneously to obtain the best result.

LIFE SPAN CONSIDERATIONS

- Children and adolescents
    - Most common period for starting drug use
    - Significant impact of peer pressure on substance use patterns
    - 30% to 40% of adolescents report drinking frequently
    - 15% of adolescents report binge-drinking patterns
    - Approximately 50% of high school–age students report at least a one-time use of illicit drugs.
- Older adults
    - Referral to specialized treatment program that emphasizes interventions to deal with losses
    - Large-print psychoeducation materials
    - Transportation to service locations
    - Treatment with same-age peer group
    - Adaptations to home environment to cope with physical disabilities
    - Close collaboration with primary-care physician for follow-up

CASE STUDY

R.J. is a 61-year-old widow who has multiple health problems. The client has been diagnosed with essential hypertension, chronic bronchitis, and non–insulin-dependent diabetes. R.J. has been coming to this clinic for 6 months to receive all care, and before that had been receiving care from multiple other providers in the community. The client receives Social Security Disability Insurance.

The chief complaint for the past few months has been stasis ulcers on the lower left leg, which have not healed well despite multiple approaches to care. R.J. also complains of problems with "nerves." Current medications include the following:

- Multivitamin daily
- Ranitidine, 150 mg q 12 h
- Alprazolam, 1 mg b.i.d.
- Glipizide, 20 mg b.i.d.

The client is in today, and this is the first time you see this client. On initial approach, R.J. is visibly upset, arms are crossed at his chest, sitting forward in his chair with a raised voice and difficult to get information from, stating, "You should know all this; you have my chart right there in your hand." The client requests a refill of all of prescriptions and wants you to write a letter to the landlord to "stop harassing me." Per the client, the landlord is insisting that garbage is placed in the containers in the parking lot of the complex. R.J. feels that is too far for to walk and wants a letter supporting the current practice of leaving garbage bags in the hallway outside the apartment door.

The client also reports "my nerves are worse, and the pain in my legs is worse too." R.J. states "my chronic bronchitis has returned," and is requesting an antibiotic, an increase in the alprazolam and would like you to add codeine or morphine or "any other thing like that" for "constant pain." The client states, "Just do this and get me out of here. I know what I need."

Mental Status Exam

- Appearance: Moderately obese, well-dressed with appropriate hygiene, poor eye contact
- Motor: Mild psychomotor restlessness, slightly ataxic gait, tremulous
- Speech: Loud and pressured
- Affect: Angry
- Mood: Self-described as "cranky"; assessed as irritable
- Thought processes: Goal-directed and organized without evidence of psychotic processing but does show some mild thought-blocking and tangentiality

- Thought content: Thematic for mistrust of health providers and for fear of pain continuing
- Memory: One-third of objects after 15 minutes
- Concentration: Refuses to do numbers testing, stating "I was never good with book work or numbers"
- Abstraction: Is abstract on proverbs; asks, "You got any more dumb questions?"
- Judgment: Intact for self-welfare
- Education: Completed 12th grade and went to 2-year secretarial business school
- Employment history: Was a medical claims clerk for 32 years at the VA Medical Center
- Social history: No children; lives alone; history of 2-pack-a-day smoker and "I drink a six-pack or so at night to relax myself—wouldn't you?"

Physical exam is overall unremarkable. Vital signs are within the documented baseline, with blood pressure 132/88, pulse 96, respiratory rate 26, temp 98.5° F, and weight 209 lbs. Lungs are overall clear. On the left leg there is a stasis ulcer, which is circular and ~6 cm in circumference. It is open and oozing white–yellow liquid drainage, with redness around the borders. The client reports it is painful to touch and increasingly painful when weight-bearing. Silver sulfadiazine treatments with cling wrap and hot soaks q 6 hours was ordered but client refused to cover it because "it hurts when I remove the bandage" and is not very clear about whether the hot soaks are occurring. Recent labs are all within normal limits, including thyroid-stimulating hormone, electrolytes, and CBC.

1. What is the primary health care concern of this client?
2. What method of interviewing would be useful?
3. What further laboratory testing should be considered?
4. If the client is unwilling to participate in further assessment, how will you deal with her health needs?

ANSWERS TO CASE STUDY DISCUSSION QUESTIONS

1. Given that the laboratory values are within normal limits and there are no physical signs of a respiratory infection, the main concern is current or risk for addiction.
2. The method of interviewing this client would be using the Screening, Brief Intervention, and Referral to Treatment (SBIRT) technique.
3. Additional laboratory assessments should be obtained, which include LFTs, including ALT, AST, gamma-glutamyl transferase (GGT), albumin, and possibly uric acid level.
4. If this client is unwilling to engage in a further assessment, the use of motivational interviewing techniques, building rapport, and keeping the client engaged would be indicated.

REFERENCES AND RESOURCES

American College of Obstetricians and Gynecologists Committee on Health Care for Underserved Women. (2012). ACOG Committee Opinion No. 524: Opioid abuse, dependence, and addiction in pregnancy. Obstetrics and Gynecology, 119(5), 1070–1076.

American Psychiatric Association. (2022). Diagnostic and statistical manual of mental disorders (5th ed., Text rev.).

Barbosa, C., Cowell, A., Bray, J., & Aldridge, A. (2015). The cost effectiveness of alcohol screening, brief intervention, and referral to treatment (SBIRT) in emergency and outpatient medical settings. Journal of Substance Abuse Treatment, 53, 1–8.

DiClemente, C., Bellino, L., & Neavins, T. (1999). Motivation for change and alcoholism treatment. Alcohol Research and Health, 23(2), 86–92.

Domino, F. J., Baldor, R. A., Golding, J., & Stephens, M. B. (2015). The 5-minute clinical consult standard (24th ed.). Wolters Kluwer.

Dunn, K., Saulsgiver, K., Miller, M., Nuzzo, P., & Sigmon, S. (2015). Characterizing opioid withdrawal during double blind buprenorphine detoxification. Drug and Alcohol Dependence, 151(1), 47–55.

Farrell, M. (1994). Opioid withdrawal. Addiction, 89(11), 1471–1475. https://onlinelibrary.wiley.com/doi/abs/10.1111/j.1360-0443.1994.tb03745.x

Galanter, M. (1993). Network therapy for alcohol and drug abuse. Basic Books.

Goldberg, J. F., & Stahl, S. (2021). Practical psychopharmacology. Cambridge University Press.

Graham, A. W., & Schultz, T. K. (2007). Principles of addiction medicine (3rd ed.). American Society of Addiction Medicine.

Hanna, J., & Swetter, S. (2018). A case of delirium and rhabdomyolysis in severe iatrogenic opioid withdrawal. Psychosomatics, 59(4), 405–407. https://doi.org/10.1016/j.psym.2017.12.002

Ling, W., Amass, L., Shoptaw, S., Annon, J. J., Hillhouse, M., Babcock, D., . . . Buprenorphine Study Protocol Group. (2005). A multi-center randomized trial of buprenorphine-naloxone versus clonidine for opioid detoxification: Findings from the National Institute on Drug Abuse Clinical Trials Network. Addiction, 100(8), 1090–1100. https://doi.org/10.1111/j.1360-0443.2005.01154.x

Mayfield, D., McLeod, G., & Hall, P. (1974). The CAGE questionnaire: Validation of a new alcoholism instrument. American Journal of Psychiatry, 131, 1121–1123.

Melemis, S. M. (2015). Relapse prevention and the five rules of recovery. The Yale Journal of Biology and Medicine, 88(3), 325–332.

Miller, N., Gold, M., & Smith, D. (1997). Manual of therapeutics for addictions. Wiley-Liss.

National Institute on Alcohol Abuse and Alcoholism. (1997). Alcohol and health. U.S. Department of Health and Human Services. https://files.eric.ed.gov/fulltext/ED418362.pdf

National Institute on Alcohol Abuse and Alcoholism. (2016). Alcohol's effects on the body. U.S. Department of Health and Human Services. http:// www.niaaa.nih.gov/alcohol-health/alcohols-effects-body

National Institute on Drug Abuse. (2012). Medical consequences of drug abuse: Mental health effects. National Institutes of Health. http://www.drugabuse. gov/publications/medical-consequences-drug-abuse/mental-health-effects

Perese, E. F. (2012). Psychiatric advanced practice nursing: A biopsychosocial foundation for practice. F. A. Davis.

Prendergast, M., Podus, D., Finney, J., Greenwell, L., & Roll, J. (2006). Contingency management for treatment of substance use disorders: a meta-analysis. Addiction, 101(11), 1546–1560. https://doi.org/10.1111/j.1360-0443.2006.01581.x

Sadock, B., Sadock, V., & Ruiz, P. (2017). Kaplan and Sadock's comprehensive textbook of psychiatry (10th ed.). Wolters Kluwer.

Scholl, L., Seth, P., Kariisa, M., Wilson, N., Baldwin, G. (2019). Drug and opioid-involved overdose deaths—United States, 2013–2017. Morbidity and Mortality Weekly Report, 67, 1419–1427. http://dx.doi.org/10.15585/mmwr.mm675152e1

Sevarino, K.A. (2019). Medically supervised opioid withdrawal during treatment for addiction. UpToDate. https://medilib.ir/uptodate/show/7808

Skinner, H. (1982). Guide for using the Drug Abuse Screening Test (DAST). York University. https://socwel.ku.edu/sites/socwel/files/documents/Research%20Projects/Family%20First/Survey%20Measures/DAST%20Guide%202019%20-%20Remediated.pdf

Stahl, S. M. (2020). Stahl's essential psychopharmacology: Prescriber's guide (7th ed.). Cambridge University Press.

Substance Abuse and Mental Health Services Administration (SAMHSA). (2016). Screening and assessment. U.S. Department of Health and Human Services. https://www.samhsa.gov/resource/dbhis/screening-assessment

Sullivan J. T., Sykora, K., Schneiderman, J., Naranjo, C. A., & Sellers, E. M. (1989). Assessment of alcohol withdrawal: The revised Clinical Institute Withdrawal Instrument for Alcohol Scale (CIWA-Ar). British Journal of Addiction 84(11), 1353–1357.

The Commonwealth Group. (2023). Overdose deaths decline but remained near record levels during the first nine months of 2022 as states cope with synthetic opioids. www.commonwealthfund.org/blog/2023/overdose-deaths-declined-remained-near-record-levels-during-first-nine-months-2022-states#:~:text=In%202012%2C%20synthetic%20opioids%20were,of%20106%2C699%20deaths%20in%202021

U.S. Food and Drug Administration. (2019). FDA Safety Announcement: FDA identifies harm reported from sudden discontinuation of opioid pain medicines and requires label changes to guide prescribers on gradual, individualized tapering. www.fda.gov/drugs/drug-safety-and-availability/fda-identifies-harm-reported-sudden-discontinuation-opioid-pain-medicines-and-requires-label-change

Wesson, D. R., & Ling, W. (2003). The Clinical Opiate Withdrawal Scale (COWS). Journal of Psychoactive Drugs, 35(2), 253–599.

Wheeler, K. (2022). Psychotherapy for the advanced practice psychiatric nurse: A how-to guide for evidence-based practice (3rd ed.). Springer Publishing.

CHAPTER 14

PERSONALITY DISORDERS

This chapter reviews a category of illnesses called personality disorders, common disorders that can affect the quality of the general health care that a person receives. Although these disorders can create great difficulty for the given person, they remain able to perform routine daily functions. Often the person does not recognize a problem or seek treatment.

This chapter briefly reviews the concept of personality and then its disorders. Assessment and clinical management of features of personality disorders are discussed.

PERSONALITY

DESCRIPTION

- Personality is the sum total of all emotional, cognitive, and behavioral attributes of a person.
- Personality involves an enduring pattern of perceiving, relating to, and thinking about the environment and oneself that is exhibited in a wide array of social and personal contexts.
- When healthy, personality structures allow for realistic, happy, and satisfying self-perceptions and interpersonal interactions.
- Characteristics
    - Personality is organized early in life and is dynamic and deeply ingrained; however, it can be altered.
    - Patterns of behavior based on personality can be perceived by the person as comfortable (ego-syntonic) or uncomfortable (ego-dystonic):
        - Ego-syntonic
            - Behavior consistent with personality
            - Causes little concern to the person
            - Person generally fails to recognize problem
            - Person does not seek treatment
        - Ego-dystonic
            - Behavior inconsistent with personality
            - Causes discomfort and concern to the person

      - Person generally recognizes problem
      - Person often seeks treatment
      - Personality is reflected in behavioral traits habitually displayed by the person

- Coping
  - Interpersonal or interactive style
  - Perceptions
  - Cognitive beliefs about events, people, and situations

PERSONALITY DISORDERS

DESCRIPTION

- Personality disorders are chronically maladaptive patterns of behavior that cause functional impairment in work, school, or relationships.
- These disorders manifest as maladaptive patterns in four areas of functionality:
  - Maladaptive affective traits, such as overly affectual patterns of response
  - Maladaptive behavioral traits, such as poor impulse control patterns of response
  - Maladaptive cognitive traits, such as unrealistic perceptual patterns of response
  - Maladaptive social traits, such as maladaptive unsatisfying interpersonal patterns of response
- These disorders can cause subjective distress.
  - A person is unlikely to recognize the problem or seek help if maladaptive patterns of behavior are ego-syntonic.
  - A person is more likely to recognize a problem and seek help if maladaptive patterns of behavior are ego-dystonic.
  - Maladaptive patterns are inflexible and pervasive across most personal and social situations.
  - These disorders are coded in the Diagnostic and Statistical Manual of Mental Disorders, Fifth Edition, Text Revision (DSM-5-TR; American Psychiatric Association [APA]; see Table 14–1).
  - Clients seldom fit neatly into one personality disorder diagnosis; rather, they often exhibit features of several similar disorders.
  - For this reason, personality disorders often are referred to by the category of commonly manifesting symptom clusters (A, B, or C).

TABLE 14–1.
CATEGORIES OF PERSONALITY DISORDERS

CATEGORY	CHARACTERISTIC BEHAVIOR	DISORDERS
Cluster A	Odd, unusual, eccentric, asocial	Paranoid personality disorder Schizoid personality disorder Schizotypal personality disorder
Cluster B	Dramatic, affective instability	Antisocial personality disorder Borderline personality disorder Histrionic personality disorder Narcissistic personality disorder
Cluster C	Anxious	Avoidant personality disorder Dependent personality disorder Obsessive–compulsive personality disorder

ETIOLOGY

- Multiple theories ranging from psychological to neurobiological
- Probable multifactorial etiological profile
- Less empirical data available on neurobiological etiological factors
- Borderline personality disorder is the most well researched.
- Two common types of theories of personality disorders:
  1. Psychodynamic theory (primarily borderline personality disorder)
     - Based on etiological factors:
       - Early separation problems
         - Object relations theory
         - Internalized intrapsychic experiences of interpersonal relationships
         - Mental representation of the self in relation to others
         - Stability and depth of a person's relationships
         - During development, child must accomplish two tasks: separation and individuation.
           - Separation: Develop intrapsychic self-representation distinct and separate from mother
           - Individuation: Form distinct identity with characteristics unique to the person

- Failure in separation–individuation is etiologically linked to development of personality disorders.
- Different personality disorders linked to problems with different stages of the separation–individuation process.
  - Disturbed parental interaction
  - Family background assumed to be dysfunctional
    - Enmeshed family patterns
    - Role-reversal patterns of child–parent interaction
    - Restricted involvement of family with the rest of the environment
    - Social isolation
    - Confusion of parental authority and nurturing roles
    - Blurred family boundaries
  - Dysfunctional family patterns block separation–individuation processes; family rejection occurs if a person attempts individuation.

2. Biological theory
   - Genetic factors
     - Familial tendency
     - Genetic overlap between loading for some disorders
   - Structural abnormalities
     - Reduced gray matter volume in prefrontal cortex
     - Limbic system deregulation
   - Neurotransmitter dysfunction
     - Decreased levels of serotonin
     - Elevated levels of norepinephrine
     - Dysregulation of dopamine receptors
   - Neurobiological impact of trauma
     - Most studied in borderline personality disorder
     - Assumes early childhood trauma alters basic brain patterns of response
     - In genetically susceptible people, may function as the environmental vulnerability that causes expression of genetic load

INCIDENCE AND DEMOGRAPHICS

- Difficult to estimate because people with personality disorders are rarely hospitalized and often receive no treatment
- Incidence varies with disorder
- Generally assumed to be 0.5% to 5.4% in the general U.S. population

RISK FACTORS

- Genetic loading
- Dysfunctional family of origin

PREVENTION AND SCREENING

- At-risk family education
- Community education
    - Stigma reduction
    - Signs and symptoms of illness
    - Treatment potential for control of symptoms
- Early recognition, intervention, and initiation of treatment
- Preventative work with young children in identified dysfunctional family settings

ASSESSMENT

- Symptoms of personality disorder are enduring maladaptive patterns of behavior, generally seen as problems with living.
- Often several interviews are needed to clarify the diagnostic picture.

Client History

- Assess for the following:
    - Detailed history of present illness, including time frame, progression, and associated symptoms

- ◊ Social history, including present living situation; marital status; occupation; education; and alcohol, tobacco, and illicit drug use
- ◊ Medication use, including prescription, over-the-counter, alternative, supplements, and home remedies
- ◊ Initial and periodic functional history and assessment
- ◊ Validate history with family member

- ♦ Long-term patterns of functioning
  - ◊ Stability of traits over time and across situations
- ♦ Cultural issues versus maladaptive personality traits
  - ◊ Issues of acculturation in new immigrants
  - ◊ Cultural expression of habitual behavior
  - ◊ Custom or religious practices

Assessment for Cluster A Disorders

- ♦ Patterns of pervasive distrust and suspiciousness, with odd and unusual behavior
  - ◊ Present in a variety of contexts, even without supportive evidence
- ♦ Distrust usually not at psychotic level but can display brief psychotic episodes under stress
- ♦ Significant history includes the following:
  - ◊ Limited social network
  - ◊ Poor interpersonal relationships
  - ◊ Limited disclosure or revealing of self to others, often refusing to answer personal questions
  - ◊ Compliments often misinterpreted
  - ◊ Pathological jealousy common
  - ◊ Difficult to get along with
  - ◊ Appearing cold and lacking in feelings
  - ◊ High control needs
  - ◊ Rigid and critical of others
  - ◊ Often highly litigious
  - ◊ Negatively perceive others; often biased and prone to stereotypes
- ♦ Differences in Cluster A disorders are in degree of suspiciousness and mistrust and in behavioral manifestations of those traits (see Table 14–2).

TABLE 14–2.
CHARACTERISTICS OF CLUSTER A PERSONALITY DISORDERS

DISORDER	CHARACTERISTIC
Schizoid personality disorder	Neither desires nor enjoys close relationships Chooses solitary activities Shows little to no interest in sexual activity with another person Derives no pleasure in social activities Lacks close friends or social supports Is indifferent to opinion of others Appears cold and detached Exhibits affective flattening
Schizotypal personality disorder	Ideas of reference Odd beliefs Magical thinking Unusual perceptual experiences Paranoid ideation Inappropriate or constricted affect Behavior overtly odd, eccentric, or peculiar Few or no close friends Excessive social anxiety

Assessment for Cluster B Disorders

- Patterns of pervasive affective and interpersonal disruption
  - Present in a variety of contexts, even without supportive evidence
- Disturbance usually not at psychotic level but can display brief psychotic episodes under stress
- Of all clusters, disorders of Cluster B type may require hospitalization during period of active symptom expression and when client is under significant levels of stress
- Significant history includes the following:
  - Fluctuating emotional states
  - Dramatic qualities to how a person lives their life
- Antisocial personality disorder
  - Usually diagnosed by age 18
  - More common in men

- High substance use comorbidity
- High impulsivity
- Often diagnosed with conduct disorder as children

- Borderline personality disorder
  - Predominantly in women
  - Often with positive history of significant childhood physical abuse, sexual abuse, neglect, or early parental separation or loss
- Differences in Cluster B disorders are in degree of affective instability, type of interpersonal disruption, and behavioral manifestations of those traits (see Table 14–3).

Assessment for Cluster C Disorders

- Patterns of pervasive anxiety and fear
  - Present in a variety of contexts, even without supportive evidence
- Disturbance usually not at psychotic level but can display brief psychotic episodes under stress
- Significant history includes the following:
  - Avoidant behavior
  - Procrastination
  - Difficulty in following through
  - Fearful of rejection and criticism
  - Difficulty relaxing
- Avoidant personality disorder
  - Must consider cultural variable when looking at avoidant behavior
  - Disorder equal for both genders
- Dependent personality disorder
  - Most frequently diagnosed personality disorder
  - Rates higher in women than in men
  - Commonly diagnosed in people with history of chronic physical illnesses
- Obsessive–compulsive personality disorder
  - Predominantly in men
  - Symptoms similar to but less severe than obsessive–compulsive disorder
- Differences in Cluster C disorders are in the degree of anxiety and fear and in behavioral manifestations of those traits (see Table 14–4).

TABLE 14–3.
CHARACTERISTICS OF CLUSTER B PERSONALITY DISORDERS

DISORDER	CHARACTERISTIC
Antisocial personality disorder	Failure to conform to social norms Repeated acts that are grounds for arrest Deceitfulness, lying, and use of aliases for profit or pleasure Impulsivity and failure of future planning Reckless disregard for the welfare of others Consistent irresponsibility Lack of remorse; indifference to the feelings of others
Borderline personality disorder	Frantic efforts to avoid real or imagined abandonment Pattern of unstable, intense interpersonal relationships Identity disturbances Impulsivity, often with self-damaging behavior Recurrent suicidal behavior Chronic feelings of emptiness Inappropriate, intensified affective anger responses Transient psychotic symptoms of paranoia and dissociation
Histrionic personality disorder	Uncomfortable in situations in which they are not center of attention Interactions with others characterized by inappropriate seductive or sexualized or provocative behavior, rapid shifting, and shallow emotional responses Consistent use of physical appearance to draw attention to self Speech is excessively impressionistic and lacking in detail Suggestible and easily influenced Relationships considered more intimate than they are
Narcissistic personality disorder	Grandiose sense of self-importance Preoccupation with fantasies of power, success, brilliance, and beauty Belief of self-importance and being special and unique Excessive admiration required Unreasonable expectations or sense of entitlement Interpersonally exploitative Empathy lacking Envy of others and belief that others envy them Arrogant and haughty behaviors

TABLE 14–4.
CHARACTERISTICS OF CLUSTER C PERSONALITY DISORDERS

DISORDER	CHARACTERISTIC
Avoidant personality disorder	Avoidance of activities involving significant interpersonal contact Fear of criticism, disapproval, or rejection Unwillingness to be involved with people unless sure of being liked Restraint in intimate relationships for fear of being shamed Preoccupation with being criticized or rejected in social settings View of self as socially inept, personally unappealing, or inferior Unusual reluctance to take personal risks or engage in new activities
Dependent personality disorder	Difficulty making everyday decisions without excessive advice Needing others to assume responsibility for most areas of life Difficulty expressing disagreement Difficulty initiating projects by themselves Going to excessive lengths to obtain nurturing and support from others Urgent seeking of another relationship if a close relationship ends Unrealistic preoccupation with fears of being left alone
Obsessive–compulsive personality disorder	Preoccupation with details, rules, order, and organization Perfectionism that interferes with task completion Excessive devotion to work and productivity Overly conscientious, scrupulous, and inflexible on issues of morality Inability to discard worn-out or worthless objects Reluctance to delegate tasks or work with others Adoption of a miserly spending style toward self and others Rigidity and stubbornness

Physical Exam Findings

- No physical exam findings specific to personality disorders

Diagnostic and Laboratory Findings

- Complete blood count (CBC), chemistry profile, and thyroid function tests to rule out metabolic causes or unidentified conditions
- Drug toxicity screening if indicated by history

DIFFERENTIAL DIAGNOSIS

- Comorbidity is common
- Mood disorders (see Chapter 9)
    - Affective instability of borderline personality disorder often mistaken for bipolar affective disorder
- Substance-induced disorders (see Chapter 13)

CLINICAL MANAGEMENT

- Rule out or treat any conditions that may contribute to cognitive impairment.
- Personality disorders are generally managed in a community setting.
- In some cases, hospitalization may be required.

Pharmacological Management

- No specific class of pharmacological agents used to treat personality disorders
- Individualized symptom control
    - Impulsivity
        - Selective serotonin reuptake inhibitors (SSRIs)
        - Anticonvulsant mood stabilizers
    - Affective instability
        - SSRIs
        - Anticonvulsant mood stabilizers
    - Anxiety
        - Non-benzodiazepine anxiolytics
        - SSRIs
        - Benzodiazepines are used with extreme caution

Nonpharmacological Management

- Most common form of treatment for personality disorders
- Focus on issues of limit-setting, protection from self-harm, improved coping, and enhanced interpersonal functioning

- Multiple therapeutic interventions may be used, such as the following:
  - Case management
  - Psychotherapy
- Focus on the person gaining control
- Improvement of interpersonal skill level
- Enhanced coping
- Alteration of problematic patterns of behavior
- Forms of therapy include the following:
  - Dialectical behavioral therapy
  - Psychodynamic therapy
  - Interpersonal therapy
  - Behavioral therapy
  - Cognitive behavioral therapy (CBT)
  - Milieu therapy
- Assist with realistic expectation formation
- Structure environment
- Improve realistic self-appraisal ability

LIFE SPAN CONSIDERATIONS

- Children
  - Before diagnosis is determined, sufficient life experiences must occur so that chronicity of maladaptive patterns can be observed.
  - Features of personality disorder usually become apparent during adolescence to early adulthood.
  - It is unusual for someone to be given personality disorder diagnosis before ages 16 to 18 (an exception is antisocial personality disorder, which often is observable by onset of puberty; however, diagnosis of antisocial personality disorder is not made until age 18).
  - Separation anxiety and chronic physical illness often precede and predict onset of dependent personality disorder.

FOLLOW-UP

- These are chronic disorders, and clients may be resistant to change.
- Relapse is common and frequent.
- How long to treat and success rates vary with client characteristics and motivation.
- Prognosis is poor without treatment.
- Prognosis improves if treatment is started as early in life as possible.

CASE STUDY

T.D. is a 42-year-old new client who seeks health care for a general physical exam. The family nurse practitioner who examines T.D. asks the psychiatric-mental health nurse practitioner (PMHNP) to speak with him because of his odd presentation. The client discusses with the PMHNP an unusual, recurrent experience he has been having.

The client lives in an apartment building downtown, works as a bartender in the late evening, and tells the PMHNP that every night when walking home from work they watch to see if the wind "blows north to south or south to north." The client relates that, on the occasions that wind goes north to south, that is a sign that a woman will visit him. The client tells of a woman who rides a bicycle down the road and she passes a blessing from her that protects him from those who wish him harm. He believes the woman is a "spirit from the other side" and that no one but he can see the woman.

As T.D. tells the story, affect is inappropriate, mood pleasant and happy, and he exhibits some paranoid ideation as he worries that others will try to take away the spirit. The mental status examination (MSE) shows ideas of reference and some magical thinking as he shares his "blessing" with customers in the bar, and describes odd, eccentric, and peculiar behaviors. The client is not at all bothered by his unusual experience and seems to enjoy telling it to others. He considers himself lucky to have "special powers" and to see and understand things that others do not. T.D. denies the presence of any typical manifestations of hallucinations or delusions, any mood disturbance or anxiety, and alcohol or other drug use. Reports having several close friends, a strong support network, and is in general good health but does experience significant social anxiety. He does not believe his unusual experience is a symptom of an illness and wishes no intervention or assistance at this time.

1. What is the most probable diagnosis for this client?
2. What further assessment should occur?
3. If the client desires no treatment, should the PMHNP attempt to follow-up with him?
4. What treatment should be suggested at this time?

ANSWERS TO CASE STUDY DISCUSSION QUESTIONS

1. The most likely diagnosis for this client is schizotypal personality disorder.
2. Medical workup including drug screen is indicated to complete a thorough assessment.
3. If the client is unwilling to engage in treatment, the PMHNP should try to follow-up with the client at regular intervals and continue to build a therapeutic alliance.
4. If the client is willing to engage in treatment, treatment indicated is using a CBT approach would be helpful for the client to find "evidence" for his unusual thoughts and beliefs.

REFERENCES AND RESOURCES

American Psychiatric Association. (2022). Neurodevelopmental disorders. In Diagnostic and statistical manual of mental disorders (5th ed., Text rev.).

American Psychiatric Nurses Association. (2022). The essentials of caring for persons who are diagnosed with personality disorders. www.apna.org/apna-personality-disorders-resource/.

Linehan, M. M., Comtois, K. A., Murray, A. M., Brown, M. Z., Gallop, R. J., Heard, H. L., . . . Lindenboim, N. (2006). Two-year randomized controlled trial and follow-up of dialectical behavior therapy vs therapy by experts for suicidal behaviors and borderline personality disorder. Archives of General Psychiatry, 63(7), 757–766. https://doi.org/10.1001/archpsyc.63.7.757

Neacsiu, A., Lungu, A., Harned, M., Rizvi, S., & Linehan, M. (2014). Impact of dialectical behavioral therapy versus community treatment by experts on emotional experience, expression, and acceptance in borderline personality disorder. Behaviour Research and Therapy, 53, 47–54.

Nelson, K., Zagoloff, A., Quinn, S., Swanson, H., Garber, C., & Schulz, C. (2014). Borderline personality disorder: Treatment approaches and perspectives. Clinical Practice, 11(3), 341–349.

Perese, E. F. (2012). Psychiatric advanced practice nursing: A biopsychosocial foundation for practice. F. A. Davis.

Rees, C., & Prichard, R. (2015). Brief cognitive therapy for avoidant personality disorder. Psychotherapy, 52(1), 45–55.

Reichborn-Kjennerud, T., Czajkowski, N., Ystrom, E., Orstavik, R., Aggen, S., & Kendler, K. (2015) A longitudinal twin study of borderline and antisocial disorder traits in early to middle adulthood. Psychological Medicine, 45(14), 3121–1331.

Sadock, B., Sadock, V., & Ruiz, P. (2017). Kaplan and Sadock's comprehensive textbook of psychiatry (10th ed.). Wolters Kluwer.

Schmahl, C. G., McGlashan, T., & Bremner, J. D. (2002). Neurobiological correlates of borderline personality disorder. Psychopharmacology Bulletin, 36(2), 69–78.

Tusaie, K., & Fitzpatrick, J. (2022). Advanced practice psychiatric nursing integrating psychotherapy, psychopharmacology, and complementary and alternative approaches across the life span (3rd ed.). Springer Publishing Company.

Wheeler, K. (2022). Psychotherapy for the advanced practice psychiatric nurse: A how-to guide for evidence-based practice (3rd ed.). Springer Publishing Company.

CHAPTER 15

DISORDERS OF CHILDHOOD AND ADOLESCENCE

Disorders first diagnosed in infancy, childhood, or adolescence, such as conduct disorder, oppositional defiant disorder, attention-deficit/hyperactivity disorder, Rett syndrome, autism spectrum disorder, eating disorders, and intellectual disabilities, are considered brain-based illnesses and have many similarities to disorders diagnosed more commonly in adulthood. In addition, these disorders often are missed during childhood and adolescent years and are, therefore, not identified until early adulthood.

The disorders diagnosed during childhood or in adolescent differ in presentation based on the developmental context of the person, age at onset, and sex. Assessment, treatment planning, and therapeutic interventions for these disorders must always occur within the context of the family and assume a multimodal, systems-oriented approach to care. In addition, assessment of children is different from assessment of adults. Prior to making a psychiatric diagnosis, all possible medical causes of the symptoms must be ruled out. Therefore, psychiatric-mental health nurse practitioners (PMHNPs) must apply principles of child assessment to care and have a good understanding of normal growth and development to detect what is disordered. Effective assessment, diagnosis, and treatment is completed in the context of the family system; however, family is defined for the client.

ASSESSMENT AND CARE PLANNING FOR CHILDREN AND ADOLESCENTS

- Requires alteration in assessment process
    - Generally takes more time
    - PMHNP must develop trusting relationship with the child to put them at ease
    - Interview the child and parent separately: Child can provide information on internal symptoms and family or care providers on external signs (Hamrin & Gray Deering, 2012)
    - Must attend to developmental needs and interests of the child
    - Must attend to the cognitive and language abilities of the child

- Mental status examination (Sadock et al., 2017)
  - Modified to reflect developmental and other age-related issues in children
  - Often requires establishment of a play environment to open communication with the child
  - Appearance
    - Conclusions must consider age and developmental processes (e.g., physical appearance and dress for weather and age group).
    - Gait and motor skills are assessed according to expected normative behaviors for age.
    - Parent–child interaction
      - Observe interaction in waiting room
      - Examine way parent and child talk with one another and emotional overtones
      - Separation and reunion
      - Examine how child reacts to separation and reunion with parent
  - Social relatedness
    - Child's response to interviewer
  - Motor behavior
    - Coordination, activity level, involuntary movements, tremors, tics, unusual asymmetries
  - Speech and language
    - Assessed on expected normative and appropriate language use for age
    - Comprehension, word selection, and range of vocabulary
    - Rate, rhythm, latency, intonation, spontaneity
  - Mood and affect
    - Mood: Verbal admission of feelings or assessment based on themes, play, and fantasy
    - Affect: Range of emotions expressed; appropriateness of affect to thought content
  - Thought process and content
    - Thought process: Looseness of associations, magical thinking, preservation, echolalia, ability to distinguish fantasy from reality (by age 4 children have some understanding of what is real or made up), flight of ideas
    - Thought content: Suicidal or homicidal ideation, perceptual disturbances (hallucinations)
  - Cognition
    - Intellectual functioning and problem-solving abilities

- ◊ Judgement and insight
    - Child's view of problem
    - Child's understanding of what they can do to help the problem
- ◊ Memory
    - Test recall after 5 minutes (school-age children should be able to remember three objects after 5 minutes)
- ◊ Abstraction
    - Assessed on expected normative behaviors for age
    - Children ages 12 or younger are not expected to have abstractive thought abilities. (Young children have concrete thinking.)
    - Proverb testing and similarity testing require prior exposure to concept, word choices, and ability to think abstractly

- ♦ Therapeutic care planning
    - ◊ Variety of effective treatments commonly used with children and adolescents
        - Play therapy
        - Art therapy
        - Bibliotherapy
        - Orative therapy (such as storytelling, family narrative therapy)
        - Behavioral therapy
        - Interpersonal therapy
        - Cognitive therapy
        - Milieu therapy
        - Pharmacotherapy

OPPOSITIONAL DEFIANT DISORDER

DESCRIPTION

- ♦ Oppositional defiant disorder (ODD) is an enduring pattern of angry or irritable mood and argumentative, defiant, or vindictive behavior lasting at least 6 months with at least four of the associated symptoms:
    - ◊ Loses temper
    - ◊ Touchy or easily annoyed
    - ◊ Angry or resentful

- ◊ Argues with authority
- ◊ Actively defies or refuses to comply with request or rules from authority figures
- ◊ Blames others
- ◊ Deliberately annoys others
- ◊ Spiteful or vindictive

ETIOLOGY

- Temperament
- Parents who model extreme ways of expressing emotions
- Trauma
- Unresolved conflicts

PREVALENCE AND DEMOGRAPHICS

- ODD is more common in children of parents with a history of ODD, conduct disorder, attention-deficit/hyperactivity disorder (ADHD), antisocial personality disorder, mood disorders, or substance use disorder.
- It affects 1% to 11% of the general U.S. population, with an average of 3.3%.
- More common in males (1.4:1)
- About 30% of children with ODD develop conduct disorder.

RISK FACTORS

- Genetic and physiological
- Temperamental
- Environmental

PREVENTION AND SCREENING

- At-risk family education
- Community education

- ◊ Stigma reduction
- ◊ Signs and symptoms of illness
- ◊ Treatment potential for control of symptoms

- ♦ Well-child visit mental health screening
- ♦ Early recognition, intervention, and initiation of treatment
  - ◊ Secondary prevention important in younger clients

ASSESSMENT

Client History

- ♦ Assess for the following:
  - ◊ Detailed history of present illness, including time frame, progression, and associated symptoms
  - ◊ Social history, including present living situation; education; and alcohol, tobacco, or illicit drug use
  - ◊ Medication use, including prescription, over-the-counter, alternative, supplements, and home remedies
  - ◊ Initial and periodic functional history and assessment
  - ◊ Validate history with a family member
  - ◊ Substance or alcohol use

Physical Exam Findings

- ♦ No physical exam findings specific to ODD

Mental Status Exam Findings

- ♦ Mood
  - ◊ Lability: Low frustration tolerance, angry, argues and loses temper
- ♦ Concentration
  - ◊ Impaired
- ♦ Thought content
  - ◊ Often blame others for mistakes

Diagnostic and Laboratory Findings

- No specific laboratory tests
- Complete blood count (CBC), chemistry profile, thyroid function tests, and B_{12} level to rule out metabolic causes or unidentified conditions
- Drug toxicity screening, if indicated by history
    - Lead toxicity
    - Toxicology screen to rule out a substance use disorder

DIFFERENTIAL DIAGNOSIS

- ADHD (see the following sections)
- Mood disorders (see Chapter 9)
- Substance use disorders (see Chapter 13)
- Intellectual disability (see the following sections)
- Conduct disorder (see the following sections)
- Psychotic disorders (see Chapter 11)

CLINICAL MANAGEMENT

- Rule out or treat any conditions that may contribute to current symptom manifestation.

Pharmacological Management

- Nonspecific: Not first-line treatment
- Pharmacological management, if needed, should target symptoms of mood or aggression.

Nonpharmacological Management

- Therapy is mainstay
    - Individual therapy
    - Family therapy, with emphasis on child management skills

- ◊ Evidence-based treatment: Child and parent problem-solving skills training (American Academy of Child and Adolescent Psychiatry [AACAP], 2007b).
- ◊ Incredible Years (group intervention)
- ◊ Parent–child interactional therapy (individual or family intervention)
- ◊ Adolescent Transitions Program (ATP; individual or family and group intervention)

CONDUCT DISORDER

DESCRIPTION

- Conduct disorder is a repetitive and persistent pattern of behavior in which the rights of others or societal norms or rules are violated. The presence of at least three of the following criteria must be present in the past 12 months, with one in the past 6 months:
  - ◊ Aggression toward people or animals—bullies, threatens, intimidates, initiates physical fights, uses a weapon to cause physical harm to others, is physically cruel to people or animals, steals while confronting a victim, forces sexual activity on someone
  - ◊ Destruction of property—engaged in fire-setting, destroyed others' property
  - ◊ Deceit or theft—broke into house, building, or car; lies, steals items
  - ◊ Serious violation of rules—stays out late before age 13, runs away from home, truant before age 13
  - ◊ Child onset at or before age 10 or adolescent onset after the age of 10

ETIOLOGY

- No single factor accounts for presentation.
- Etiology is largely unknown.
- Many biopsychosocial factors contribute to the development.

PREVALENCE

- Conduct disorder is more common in children of parents with antisocial personality disorder, alcohol dependence, mood disorders, or schizophrenia than in the general population.

INCIDENCE AND DEMOGRAPHICS

- Affects 2% to 10% of the general U.S. population, 6% to 16% of boys and 2% to 9% of girls
- Onset is earlier for boys (10 to 12 years) than for girls (16 years)

RISK FACTORS

- Genetic loading
- Temperamental: Lower than average IQ
- Environmental: Family rejection and neglect, unsupervised, physical or sexual abuse, substance use

PREVENTION AND SCREENING

- At-risk family education
- Community education
  - Stigma reduction
  - Signs and symptoms of illness
  - Treatment potential for control of symptoms
- Early recognition, intervention, and initiation of treatment
  - Secondary prevention is important in younger clients

ASSESSMENT

Client History

- Assess for the following:
  - Detailed history of present illness, including time frame, progression, and associated symptoms
  - Social history, including present living situation; education; and alcohol, tobacco, or illicit drug use

    - Medication use, including prescription, over-the-counter, alternative, supplements, and home remedies
    - Initial and periodic functional history and assessment
    - Developmental history
    - Validate history with a family member

Physical Exam Findings

- No physical exam findings specific to conduct disorder

Mental Status Exam Findings

- Affect
    - Irritable
    - Angry
    - Uncooperative
- Mood
    - Anger
- Thought content
    - Lack of empathy or concern for others
- Concentration
    - Distractible
- Insight
    - Poor

Diagnostic and Laboratory Findings

- No specific laboratory tests
- Drug screening to rule out possible substance use
- CBC, chemistry profile, thyroid function tests, and B_{12} level to rule out metabolic causes or unidentified conditions

DIFFERENTIAL DIAGNOSIS

- ADHD (see the following sections)
- ODD (see the following sections)
- Mood disorders (see Chapter 9)
- Posttraumatic stress disorder (see Chapter 10)
- Substance use disorders (see Chapter 11)
- Developmental disorders (see the following sections)

CLINICAL MANAGEMENT

- Rule out or treat any conditions that may contribute to current symptom manifestation.

Pharmacological Management

- No specific pharmacological interventions
- Pharmacological management for symptoms of aggression and agitation have been treated with antipsychotics, mood stabilizers, selective serotonin reuptake inhibitors (SSRIs), and alpha agonists.

Nonpharmacological Management

- Multimodality treatment programs that use all available family and community resources
- Behavioral therapy is mainstay
  - Individual therapy
  - Family therapy

LIFE SPAN CONSIDERATIONS

- May be diagnosed in clients ages 18 years or older if criteria for antisocial personality disorder are not met

ATTENTION-DEFICIT/HYPERACTIVITY DISORDER DESCRIPTION

- Attention-deficit hyperactivity disorder (ADHD) is a persistent pattern of inattention or hyperactivity, impulsivity, or both, that interferes with functioning and development.
  - Inattention, six or more of the following:
    - Fails to give attention to details
    - Difficulty sustaining attention
    - Does not listen when spoken to
    - Does not follow through on instructions
    - Disorganized
    - Avoids or dislikes tasks requiring sustained mental effort
    - Loses things
    - Distracted
    - Forgetful
  - Hyperactive and impulsive, six or more of the following:
    - Fidgets
    - Leaves seat
    - Runs or climbs
    - Unable to engage in quiet activities
    - "On the go"
    - Talks excessively
    - Blurts out information
    - Difficulty waiting turn
    - Interrupts others
    - Several symptoms were present prior to age 12
  - Subtypes:
    - ADHD, inattentive type
      - Inattentive symptoms dominate
      - Lack of criterion symptoms for hyperactivity or impulsivity

- ◊ ADHD, hyperactive type
  - Hyperactivity or impulsivity symptoms dominate
  - Lack of criterion symptoms for inattention
- ◊ ADHD, combined type
  - Criterion symptoms met for inattention and hyperactivity or impulsivity

ETIOLOGY

- ♦ Many biopsychosocial factors contribute to the development of ADHD.
- ♦ Polygenic neurobiological deficits are associated with ADHD.
  - ◊ Problems with executive functioning
  - ◊ Abnormalities of fronto-subcortical pathways
- ♦ Frontal cortex
- ♦ Basal ganglia
  - ◊ Abnormalities of reticular activating system
  - ◊ Structural abnormalities producing neurotransmitter abnormalities
- ♦ Dopamine dysfunction
- ♦ Norepinephrine dysfunction

INCIDENCE AND DEMOGRAPHICS

- ♦ 5% of children and 2.5% of adults in the United States have ADHD.
- ♦ Boys are more likely than girls to be diagnosed—13% vs. 6%, respectively (Centers for Disease Control and Prevention [CDC], 2022b).
- ♦ Average age at onset is 3 years; mean age at diagnosis is 9 years
- ♦ Approximately 60% of clients have symptoms persisting into adulthood.
  - ◊ Inattention symptoms are more persistent than hyperactivity and impulsivity symptoms.

RISK FACTORS

- Genetic loading
  - Pregnancy and perinatal complications
  - Family conflict
- Environmental
  - Low birth weight
  - Neglect, foster placement
  - Alcohol exposure in utero
- Temperamental
  - Reduced behavioral inhibition

PREVENTION AND SCREENING

- At-risk family education
- Community education
  - Stigma reduction
  - Signs and symptoms of illness
  - Treatment potential for control of symptoms
- Early recognition, intervention, and initiation of treatment
  - Secondary prevention is important in young clients.
- Vanderbilt ADHD Diagnostic Rating Scale (VADRS; NovoPsych, 2022)
  - Initial screening: Must be completed in two different setting such as home and school. Teachers who complete the scale must report behaviors in academic classes.
    - Parent/guardian
    - Teacher
  - Follow-up screening: Shorter version that can be compared to the initial screening. Often used to assessment treatment. Also must be completed in two different settings such as home and school.
    - Parent/guardian
    - Teacher

ASSESSMENT

Physical Exam Findings

- No physical exam findings specific to ADHD
- Minor physical anomalies that have been found to occur at higher rates in people with ADHD than in the general population:
  - Hypertelorism
  - Highly arched palate
  - Low-set ears
- Higher-than-average accidental injury rates

Mental Status Exam Findings

- Restlessness
- Inattention
- Distractible speech patterns
- Overproductive speech patterns
- Affective lability
- Poor memory
- Poor concentration

Diagnostic and Laboratory Findings

- No specific diagnostic lab findings exist.

DIFFERENTIAL DIAGNOSIS

- Understimulated home environment
- Substance use disorder
- Major depressive disorder (MDD)
- Bipolar disorder
- Stereotypic movement disorder

CLINICAL MANAGEMENT

Pharmacological Management

- Most commonly used agents (see Table 15–1) are stimulants (Schedule II)—controlled substances that carry risk for misuse.
  - Monitor for side effects and adverse effects of stimulants:
    - Gastrointestinal (GI) upset
    - Cramps
    - Anorexia
    - Weight loss
    - Blood pressure changes
    - Increased pulse rate
    - Growth suppression (rare)
    - Headache, dizziness
    - Irritability
    - Psychosis (rare)

Nonpharmacological Management

- Behavioral therapy
- Client and parent cognitive behavioral training program
- Psychoeducation
- Treatment of learning disorders
- Family therapy and education
  - Parents of children with ADHD have many difficult emotions:
    - Stress
    - Self-blame
    - Social isolation
    - Embarrassment
    - Depressive reaction
    - Marital discord

TABLE 15–1
COMMONLY USED AGENTS FOR ADHD

MEDICATIONS USED TO TREAT ATTENTION-DEFICIT DISORDER AND ATTENTION-DEFICIT/ HYPERACTIVITY DISORDER*	
Stimulants: Methylphenidate	Dexmethylphenidate hydrochloride Methylphenidate Methylphenidate hydrochloride Serdexmethylphenidate/dexmethylphenidate
Stimulants: Amphetamine	Amphetamine Amphetamine sulfate Dextroamphetamine mixed salts/amphetamine Dextroamphetamine sulfate Lisdexamfetamine dimesylate Mixed salts of a single-entity amphetamine Methamphetamine hydrochloride
Non-stimulants	Atomoxetine hydrochloride Bupropion Clonidine Clonidine hydrochloride Desipramine Guanfacine Guanfacine hydrochloride Imipramine hydrochloride (off label) Nortriptyline (off label) Venlafaxine (off label) Viloxazine

*Medications listed in this table are FDA approved for the indicated use unless otherwise indicated as "off label"

- ◊ Typical family concerns include the following:
  - Stigma
  - Anger
  - Concerns over treatment options
- ◊ Presence of controversial information in media
  - Claims of dietary causes of disorder
  - Belief in family etiological factors
- ◊ Family educational needs

- ◊ Environmental structuring
- ◊ Psychiatric comorbidities
- ◊ School issues and concerns
- ◊ Peer relationship-building
- ◊ Smoking and substance use rates
- ◊ Stress management
- ◊ Common comorbidities
    - Major depressive disorder (see Chapter 9)
    - Bipolar disorder (see Chapter 9)
    - Anxiety disorders (see Chapter 10)
    - ODD (see previous section)
    - Substance use disorders (see Chapter 13)
    - Tic disorder
    - Learning disorders

FOLLOW-UP

- ♦ Monitor clinical progress over time.
- ♦ Use standardized rating scales such as the following:
    - ◊ Conners' Parent and Teacher Rating Scales (copyrighted)
    - ◊ Vanderbilt ADHD Diagnostic Parent and Teacher Rating Scales (public domain)
- ♦ Monitor attainment of growth and development milestones.
- ♦ Symptoms may persist into adulthood.
    - ◊ Plan for long-term needs.

AUTISM SPECTRUM DISORDER

DESCRIPTION

- ♦ Persistent deficits in social communication and social interaction across multiple settings associated with deficits in the following:
    - ◊ Social reciprocity
    - ◊ Nonverbal communication
    - ◊ Developing, maintaining, and understanding relationships

- Restricted repetitive behavior
  - Stereotyped or repetitive motor movements
  - Insistence on sameness
  - Highly restricted with fixed interests
  - Hyper- or hyposensory input

ETIOLOGY

- No single factor can account for presentation.
- Etiology is largely unknown.
- Many biopsychosocial factors contribute to the development.

PREVALENCE

- The disorder appears to be more common in families in which other members have autism spectrum disorder (ASD).
- Affects 2.8% of children; 4.3% of boys and 1.1% of girls (National Institute of Mental Health [NIMH], 2023).
- Imbalances of glutamate, serotonin, and γ-aminobutyric acid (GABA) are thought to be implicated in causation.
- Brain imaging studies of children with autism revealed microscopic and macroscopic abnormalities of the amygdala, hippocampus, and cerebellum.
- Decreased numbers of Purkinje cells in the cerebellum are thought to play a role in the development.

INCIDENCE AND DEMOGRAPHICS

- ASD is more common in children with a family history of pervasive developmental disorders.
- The concordant rate for an identical twin with autism is 60%.
- The incidence is 2 to 5 cases per 10,000 in the United States.
- The male-to-female ratio is 4:1.
- Onset of symptoms is before age 3 years.

- About 10% of people with autism also have a genetic or chromosomal condition such as Down syndrome or fragile X syndrome (CDC, 2022a).

RISK FACTORS

- Male
- Intellectual disability
- Genetic loading

PREVENTION AND SCREENING

- At-risk family education
- Community education
  - Stigma reduction
  - Signs and symptoms of illness
  - Treatment potential for control of symptoms
- Early recognition, intervention, and initiation of treatment
  - Secondary prevention is important in young clients.

ASSESSMENT

Client History

- Assess for the following:
  - Impairment with social interaction, communications, and behavior
  - Impaired social interactions such as abnormal gaze, posture, and expression in social interactions
  - Lack of peer relationships, emotional reciprocity, and spontaneous seeking of enjoyment
  - Impaired communication, such as a delay or lack in the development of spoken language, impaired ability to initiate and sustain conversations, repetitive and stereotyped use of language, and inability to play with others
  - Restricted repetitive and stereotyped patterns of behavior, interests, and activities, such as inflexible adherence to specific nonfunctional routines and repetitive, stereotyped motor mannerisms (e.g., hand or finger flapping, rocking, swaying)

- ◇ Parents may report any of the following symptoms:
  - No cooing by age 1 year, no single words by age 16 months, no two-word phrases by age 24 months
  - Loss of language skills at any time
  - No imaginary play
  - Little interest in playing with other children
  - Extremely short attention span
  - No response when called by name
  - Little or no eye contact
  - Intense tantrums
  - Fixations on single objects
  - Unusually strong resistance to changes in routines
  - Oversensitivity to certain sounds, textures, or smells
  - Appetite or sleep–rest disturbance, or both
  - Self-injurious behavior

Physical Exam Findings

- No physical exam findings specific to ASD

Mental Status Exam Findings

- Little or no eye contact
- Flat or blunted affect
- Lack of emotional reciprocity
- Stereotyped or repetitive motor mannerisms
- Expressive and receptive-language impairment

Screening

- Screened for developmental delays at well-child visit (CDC, 2022)
  - ◇ Modified Checklist for Autism in Toddlers (M-CHAT)
  - ◇ Autism Diagnostic Observation Schedule—Generic (ADOS-G)
  - ◇ Ages and Stages Questionnaires (ASQ)

Diagnostic and Laboratory Findings

- No specific laboratory tests

DIFFERENTIAL DIAGNOSIS

- Rett syndrome (see the following sections)
- Childhood disintegrative disorder
- Intellectual disability (see the following sections)
- Hearing impairment
- Developmental language and speech disorders
- Tic disorders
- Stereotypic movement disorder
- Schizophrenia (see Chapter 11)
- Cluster A personality disorders (see Chapter 14)

CLINICAL MANAGEMENT

Pharmacological Management

- No specific pharmacological interventions
- Antipsychotics effective for symptoms such as tantrums; aggressive behavior; self-injurious behavior; hyperactivity; and repetitive, stereotyped behaviors
- Antidepressants, naltrexone, clonidine, and stimulants to diminish self-injurious and hyperactive and obsessive behaviors

Nonpharmacological Management

- Behavioral therapy to improve cognitive functioning and reduce inappropriate behavior
- Occupational therapy to improve sensory integration and motor skills
- Speech therapy to address communication and language barriers
- Pivotal response training
- Appropriate school placement with a highly structured approach

RETT SYNDROME

DESCRIPTION

- A genetic neurological disorder causing a regression in skills following a period of typical development after birth, usually between 6-18 months of age

ETIOLOGY

- Etiology is unknown.
- There is a known, progressive, and deteriorating course after an initial period without apparent disability.
- It is compatible with probable metabolic disorder.
- Genetic mutation is suspected.

INCIDENCE AND DEMOGRAPHICS

- The disorder occurs primarily in girls.
- It is usually associated with an intellectual disability (see the following sections).

RISK FACTORS

- Seizure disorder

PREVENTION AND SCREENING

- At-risk family education
- Community education
  - Stigma reduction
  - Signs and symptoms of illness
  - Treatment potential for control of symptoms
- Early recognition, intervention, and initiation of treatment
  - Secondary prevention is important in young clients

ASSESSMENT

- Detailed history of present illness, including time frame, progression, and associated symptoms
- Social history, including present living situation and education
- Medication use, including prescription, over-the-counter, alternative, supplements, and home remedies
- Initial and periodic functional history and assessment
- Validate all physical health findings with a family member.

Client History

- Assess for the following:
    - Normal prenatal and perinatal development
    - Normal psychomotor development through the first 5 months after birth
    - Normal head circumference at birth
    - Onset of all of the following after the period of normal development:
        - Deceleration of head growth between the ages of 5 and 48 months
        - Loss of previously acquired purposeful hand skills between the ages of 5 and 30 months, with the subsequent development of stereotyped hand movements
        - Early loss of social engagement
        - Appearance of poorly coordinated gait or trunk movements
        - Severely impaired expressive and receptive-language development with severe psychomotor retardation

Physical Exam Findings

- Associated features
    - Seizures
    - Irregular respirations
    - Scoliosis
    - Loss of purposeful hand skills
    - Stereotypic hand movements

Mental Status Exam Findings

- Appearance
  - Stereotypic hand movements
- Speech
  - Expressive and receptive-language impairment
- Affect
  - Flat or blunted affect
  - Diagnostic and laboratory findings
  - No specific laboratory or diagnostic findings
  - CBC, chemistry profile, thyroid function tests, and B_{12} level to rule out metabolic causes or unidentified conditions
  - Drug toxicity screening, if indicated by history
  - Electroencephalogram (EEG) and nonspecific abnormalities on brain imaging

DIFFERENTIAL DIAGNOSIS

- Intellectual disability (see the following sections)
- ASD (see the preceding sections)

CLINICAL MANAGEMENT

- Rule out or treat any conditions that may contribute to current symptom manifestation.

Pharmacological Management

- Nonspecific

Nonpharmacological Management

- Multimodality treatment
- Treatment aimed at symptomatic intervention

EATING DISORDERS

DESCRIPTION

- Eating disorders: Characterized in the Diagnostic and Statistical Manual of Mental Disorders (DSM-5-TR) as "persistent disturbance of eating or eating-related behavior that results in the altered consumption or absorption of food and that significantly impairs physical health or psychosocial functioning" (American Psychiatric Association [APA], 2022, p. 372).
- Common forms of eating disorders include the following:
  - Anorexia nervosa
    - Clients refuse to maintain a normal body weight.
    - Involves restricted caloric intake
    - Clients have an intense fear of gaining weight because of a distorted body image.
  - Bulimia nervosa
    - Clients engage in binge eating, combined with inappropriate ways of stopping weight gain.
    - Associated with efforts made to lose weight
    - Usually normal or slightly overweight
  - Binge eating disorder
    - Recurrent episodes of binge eating with lack of control
    - Bingeing occurs at least 2 days weekly for 6 months
    - Not regularly associated with compensatory behaviors

ETIOLOGY

- Etiology is multifactorial, with biological, social, and psychological factors implicated in causation.
- Neurobiological factors include decreased hypothalamic norepinephrine activation, dysfunction of lateral hypothalamus, and decreased serotonin.

INCIDENCE AND DEMOGRAPHICS

- Incidence is more common in women and girls, with 85% to 95% of occurrences.
- Anorexia nervosa affects approximately 0.28% of the U.S. population.
- Bulimia nervosa affects approximately 1.0% of the general U.S. population.

- Binge eating disorder affects approximately 1.2% of U.S. population.
- Onset is typically between ages 14 and 18 years.

RISK FACTORS

- Genetic loading
- Increased risk of eating disorders among first-degree biological relatives of people with certain other psychiatric disorders including the following:
  - Eating disorders
  - Mood disorders
  - Substance use disorders

PREVENTION AND SCREENING

- At-risk family education
- Community education
  - Stigma reduction
  - Signs and symptoms of illness
  - Treatment potential for control of symptoms
- Early recognition, intervention, and initiation of treatment
  - Secondary prevention is important in young clients.

ASSESSMENT

- Detailed history of present illness, including time frame, progression, and associated symptoms
- Social history, including present living situation; marital status; occupation; education; and alcohol, tobacco, or illicit drug use
- Medication use, including prescription, over-the-counter, alternative, supplements, and home remedies
- Initial and periodic functional history and assessment
- Validate history with a family member.

Client History

- Assess for the following:
  - Anorexia nervosa
    - Refusal to maintain a minimally normal body weight
    - Weight less than 85% of expected weight
    - Fear of gaining weight or becoming fat
    - Distorted body image
    - Restricting type: During the current episode, the person has not regularly engaged in binge eating or purging behavior.
    - Binge eating or purging type: During the current episode, the person has regularly engaged in binge eating or purging behavior.
  - Bulimia nervosa
    - Recurrent, episodic binge eating
    - Both binge eating and inappropriate compensatory behaviors occur at least twice weekly for 3 months
    - Recurrent, inappropriate compensatory behaviors to prevent weight gain including the following:
      - Self-induced vomiting
      - Laxatives
      - Enemas
      - Diuretics
      - Stimulants
      - Misuse of diet pills
      - Fasting
      - Excessive exercise
    - Self-evaluation unduly influenced by body shape and weight
    - Purging type: During the current episode, the person has engaged regularly in purging or the misuse of laxatives, enemas, or diuretics.
    - Nonpurging type: During the current episode, the person has used other inappropriate compensatory behaviors, such as fasting or excessive exercise, but has not engaged regularly in purging or misuse of laxatives, enemas, or diuretics.
  - Binge eating disorder
    - Recurrent, episodic binge eating which occur at least once a week for 3 months
    - Marked distress about binge eating
    - Absence of inappropriate compensatory behaviors associated with bulimia nervosa

Physical Exam Findings

- Anorexia nervosa
    - Low body mass index
    - Amenorrhea
    - Emaciation
    - Bradycardia
    - Hypotension
    - ECG changes
        - Inversion of T waves
        - ST segment depression
        - Prolonged QT interval
    - Hypothermia
    - Yellow skin secondary to carotenemia
    - Dry skin
    - Brittle hair and nails
    - Lanugo growth on face, extremities, and trunk
    - Peripheral edema
    - Hypertrophy of the salivary glands
    - Erosion of dental enamel
    - Russell's sign—scarring or calluses on the dorsum of the hand, secondary to self-induced vomiting
- Bulimia nervosa
    - Weight usually within normal range
    - Erosion of dental enamel
    - Russell's sign
    - Hypertrophy of salivary glands
    - Rectal prolapse
- Binge eating disorder
    - No physical exam findings specific to binge eating disorder

Mental Status Exam Findings

- Appearance
  - Emaciated appearance with anorexia nervosa
- Affect
  - Lability
  - Anxiety
  - Constricted and sad
- Mood
  - Dysphoric mood
- Thought content
  - Preoccupation with food and body weight
  - Suicidal ideation
  - Low self-esteem
- Concentration
  - Decreased concentration
- Judgment
  - Impaired for self-welfare
- Insight
  - Impaired

Diagnostic and Laboratory Findings

- CBC, chemistry profile, thyroid function tests, and B_{12} level to rule out metabolic causes or unidentified conditions
- Drug toxicity screening, if indicated by history
- Anorexia nervosa
  - No definitive laboratory test for diagnosis
  - Laboratory changes
    - Normochromic, normocytic anemia
    - Leukopenia
    - Neutropenia
    - Anemia

- Thrombocytopenia
- Hypokalemia
- Hypomagnesemia
- Hypoglycemia
- Decreased luteinizing hormone (LH) and follicle-stimulating hormone (FSH)

♦ Bulimia nervosa

◊ No definitive laboratory tests

◊ Laboratory changes:

- Hypotension
- Bradycardia
- Hypokalemia
- Hyponatremia
- Hypochloremia
- Hypomagnesemia
- Metabolic acidosis or alkalosis
- Elevated serum amylase

♦ Binge eating disorder

◊ No lab findings specific to binge eating disorder

DIFFERENTIAL DIAGNOSIS

♦ General medical condition

♦ Mood disorders (see Chapter 9)

♦ Cluster B personality disorders (see Chapter 14)

♦ Obsessive–compulsive disorder (OCD; see Chapter 10)

♦ Schizophrenia (see Chapter 11)

CLINICAL MANAGEMENT

♦ Rule out or treat any conditions that may contribute to current symptom manifestation.

Pharmacological Management

- Medication management as adjunctive therapy to psychotherapy
- No specific medication therapy for anorexia nervosa
- Fluoxetine is approved by the U.S. Food and Drug Administration (FDA) for bulimia nervosa.
- SSRIs and tricyclic antidepressants (TCAs) are effective in reducing the frequency of bingeing and purging.
- Treat associated symptoms, such as depression and anxiety, with appropriate pharmacological therapy.

Nonpharmacological Management

- Multimodal treatment
  - Medical and nutritional stabilization
    - Weight restoration
    - Correction of electrolyte disturbance
    - Vitamin supplementation
    - Nutrition counseling
    - Dental care
- Psychotherapeutic interventions
  - Individual psychotherapy
  - Behavioral therapy
  - Cognitive behavioral therapy
  - Family therapy
  - Group therapy
- Community resources
  - Eating disorder support groups
  - 12-step programs

FOLLOW-UP

- Regular follow-up with a multidisciplinary team is necessary.

INTELLECTUAL DISABILITY

DESCRIPTION

- Intellectual disability has an onset during the developmental period and includes low intellect and adaptive functioning.
- Onset must occur before age 18.
- Mild, moderate, severe, or profound
  - Based on adaptive functioning and not IQ scores
  - IQ scores are less valid on the lower end of IQ range

ETIOLOGY

- Heredity accounts for 5% of cases
  - Inborn errors of metabolism (e.g., Tay-Sachs disease)
  - Single-gene abnormalities (e.g., tuberous sclerosis)
  - Chromosomal aberrations (e.g., translocation of chromosome 21 [Down syndrome] and X-linked gene of FMR-1 [fragile X syndrome]).
- Early alterations of embryonic development account for 30% of cases.
  - Prenatal exposure to toxins (e.g., maternal alcohol consumption, infections)
- Pregnancy and perinatal problems account for 10% of cases.
  - Fetal malnutrition
  - Premature birth
  - Fetal hypoxia
  - Birth trauma
- General medical conditions acquired during infancy or childhood contribute to approximately 5% of cases.
  - Infections
  - Brain trauma
  - Exposure to toxins (e.g., lead poisoning)
- No clear etiology can be found in 30% to 50% of cases.

- The most preventable cause of intellectual disability is fetal alcohol syndrome.
    - Characteristics of fetal alcohol syndrome include the following
        - Epicanthal skin folds
        - Low nasal bridge
        - Short nose
        - Indistinct philtrum
        - Small head circumference
        - Small eye openings
        - Wide-set eyes
        - Thin upper lip

PREVALENCE

- 1% of the general population

DEMOGRAPHICS

- Highest rates are reported in school-age children (10–14 years of age).
- 1.5% more males than females

RISK FACTORS

- Genetic loading
- Adverse birth events

PREVENTION AND SCREENING

- At well-baby examinations
- School screenings

ASSESSMENT

Physical Exam Findings

- Oblique eye folds
- Small, flattened skull
- Large tongue
- Broad hands with stumpy fingers
- Single transverse palm crease
- High cheekbones
- Short height
- Brushfield spots on iris
- Abnormal finger and toe prints
- Cryptorchidism
- Congenital cardiac defects
- Early dementia
- Hypothyroidism

Mental Status Exam Findings

- Communication deficits
- Dependency
- Passivity
- Poor self-esteem
- Low frustration tolerance
- Aggressiveness
- Stereotyped, repetitive motor movement
- Self-injurious behavior

Diagnostic and Laboratory Findings

- No specific laboratory findings

- Some laboratory findings associated with a variety of causes of intellectual disability (e.g., metabolic disturbances)

DIFFERENTIAL DIAGNOSIS

- Borderline intellectual functioning
- Learning and communication disorders
- Pervasive developmental disorder (PDD)
  - 75% of people with a PDD have comorbid intellectual disability.
- ADHD (see previous sections)
- Stereotypic movement disorder
- General medical condition

CLINICAL MANAGEMENT

Pharmacological Management

- Pharmacological treatment is symptom-specific.
  - Treat concomitant psychopathology (e.g., ADHD, depressive disorder, anxiety disorder, schizophrenia).
  - Aggressive or self-injurious behavior may be controlled with antipsychotics and mood stabilizers.

Nonpharmacological Management

- Therapy
  - Behavioral therapy
  - Group therapy
  - Family therapy
- Community resources
  - Day care settings
  - Sheltered workshops
  - Group homes

DISRUPTIVE MOOD DYSREGULATION DISORDER

DESCRIPTION

- Childhood depressive disorder that is diagnosed in children older than age 6 but younger than age 18.
- The features of this disorder are
  - chronic dysregulated mood,
  - frequent temper outbursts, and
  - severe irritability.

ETIOLOGY

- Cause is unknown

PREVALENCE AND DEMOGRAPHICS

- Affects about 2% to 5% of children and adolescents
- Higher incidence in boys than girls and in school-aged children than adolescents

RISK FACTORS

- Complicated psychiatric history including comorbid attention deficit disorder (ADD) and ADHD

PREVENTION AND SCREENING

- Children and adolescents should be screened for a personal and family history of bipolar disorder as symptoms of disruptive mood dysregulation disorder can be similar to those of bipolar disorder using an evidence-based screener.

ASSESSMENT

- Assess for comorbid conditions such as the following:

- ◊ Bipolar disorder
- ◊ ODD
- ◊ ADHD
- ◊ Depressive and anxiety disorders
- ◊ ASD

CLINICAL MANAGEMENT

Pharmacologic Management

- ♦ Medications can be used to treat the target symptoms of the disorder.
- ♦ SSRIs, mood stabilizers, and atypical antipsychotics can be helpful.

Nonpharmacologic Management

- ♦ Individual, group, and family therapy are helpful.

FOLLOW-UP

- ♦ Regular follow-up is necessary, as is ongoing assessment for comorbid conditions.

CASE STUDY

The parents of a 14-year-old with ADHD ask to speak to you privately after you complete your assessment of their child. They tell you they have several questions that they want answered, and they want to ask you to keep the answers to yourself and not tell their son what they ask. Their first question is about diet. They have read that ADHD can be managed by dietary therapy instead of medications, and they want your opinion about trying this strategy with their child. They also want to know how likely it is that he will "outgrow" the disorder. You have many issues to consider before answering the parents' questions.

1. What is the most accepted theory of etiology regarding ADHD?
2. What is the empirical database for dietary treatment in ADHD clients?
3. What is the natural course of this illness? Is it likely that the son's symptoms will improve as he ages?
4. What are the other issues to consider regarding the parents' request to keep confidential the concerns that they are expressing?

ANSWERS TO CASE STUDY DISCUSSION QUESTIONS

1. The accepted theory is that ADHD is a neurobiological disorder
2. The best-studied treatment for ADHD is stimulant medication. Elimination of food allergens, sugar, and aspartame can be helpful to decrease hyperactivity. Limited evidence exists about the use of herbal remedies; however, it is always best to meet the client and parents where they are and if nonpharmacological treatments or dietary alterations are requested, the PMHNP should provide evidence for treatment of ADHD so the family can make an informed decision.
3. ADHD is a life span disorder; however, as children progress into adulthood, symptoms of inattention usually remain, with a decrease in impulsive and hyperactive symptoms.
4. Other issues of concern in a child with ADHD include that a lack of involvement of the child in treatment might lead to nonadherence by the child. Working in family therapy would be beneficial.

REFERENCES AND RESOURCES

American Academy of Child and Adolescent Psychiatry. (1997). Practice parameters for the treatment of children and adolescents with conduct disorder. Journal of the American Academy of Child and Adolescent Psychiatry, 36(10), 122S–139S.

American Academy of Child and Adolescent Psychiatry. (2001). Practice parameters for the assessment and treatment of children and adolescents with suicidal behavior. Journal of the American Academy of Child and Adolescent Psychiatry, 4(Suppl. 7), 245–478.

American Academy of Child and Adolescent Psychiatry. (2007a). Practice parameter for the assessment and treatment of children and adolescents with attention-deficit/hyperactivity disorder. Journal of the American Academy of Child and Adolescent Psychiatry, 46(7), 894–921.

American Academy of Child and Adolescent Psychiatry. (2007b). Practice parameter for the assessment and treatment of children and adolescents with oppositional defiant disorder. Journal of the American Academy of Child and Adolescent Psychiatry, 46(1), 126–141.

American Psychiatric Association. (2009). Practice parameters on the use of psychotropic medication in children and adolescents. Journal of the American Academy of Child and Adolescent Psychiatry, 48(9), 961–973.

American Psychiatric Association. (2022). Diagnostic and statistical manual of mental disorders (5th ed., Text rev.).

Centers for Disease Control and Prevention. (2010). Increasing prevalence of parent reported attention-deficit/hyperactivity disorder among children—United States, 2003 and 2007. Morbidity and Mortality Weekly Report, 59(44), 1439–1443.

Centers for Disease Control and Prevention. (2022a). Facts about ASD. Retrieved from https://www.cdc.gov/ncbddd/autism/facts.html

Centers for Disease Control and Prevention. (2022b). Attention-deficit/hyperactivity disorder. www.cdc.gov/ncbddd/adhd/data.html

Hamrin, V., & Gray Deering, C. (2012). Mental health assessment of children and adolescents. In M. Boyd (Ed.), Psychiatric nursing contemporary practice (5th ed., pp. 661–678). Lippincott Williams & Wilkins.

Lock, J., LaVia, M., & The American Academy of Child and Adolescent Psychiatry Committee on Quality Issues. (2015). Practice parameter for the assessment and treatment of children and adolescents with eating disorders. Journal of the American Academy of Child and Adolescent Psychiatry, 54(5), 412–425.

Murphy, T., Lewin, A., Storch, E., Stock, S., & The American Academy of Child and Adolescent Psychiatry Committee on Quality Issues. (2013). Practice parameter for the assessment and treatment of children and adolescents with tic disorders. Journal of the American Academy of Child and Adolescent Psychiatry, 52(12), 1341–1359.

National Institute of Mental Health. (2023). Autism spectrum disorder. www.nimh.nih.gov/health/statistics/autism-spectrum-disorder-asd

Nolan, E., Gadow, K., & Sprafkin, J. (2001). Teacher reports of DSM-IV ADHD, ODD, and CD symptoms in school children. Journal of the American Academy of Child and Adolescent Psychiatry, 40, 241–249.

NovoPsych. (2022). Vanderbilt ADHD diagnostic rating scale. https://novopsych.com.au/assessments/

Sadock, B. J., Sadock, A. V., & Ruiz, P. (2017). Kaplan & Sadock's comprehensive textbook of psychiatry (10th ed.). Wolters Kluwer.

U. S. Department of Health and Human Services. (2000). Mental health: A report of the Surgeon General. https://profiles.nlm.nih.gov/spotlight/nn/catalog/nlm:nlmuid-101584932X120-doc

Volkmar, F., Siegel, M., Woodbury-Smith, M., King, B., McCracken, J., & The American Academy of Child and Adolescent Psychiatry Committee on Quality Issues. (2014). Practice parameter for the assessment and treatment of children and adolescents with autism spectrum disorder. Journal of the American Academy of Child and Adolescent Psychiatry, 53(2), 237–257.

CHAPTER 16

SLEEP

This chapter addresses sleep issues and disorders commonly encountered by the psychiatric-mental health nurse practitioner (PMHNP). These conditions and clinical problems may co-occur with the disorders already discussed or may present in clients with no other identifiable psychiatric or mental health problems. They also may be frequent findings in primary care settings while working with clients with general medical conditions.

GENERAL CONSIDERATIONS

- Must be systematically assessed
- Comparison of present level of sleep to historical baseline
- Can be measured by polysomnography
- Rapid eye movement (REM) alternating with four distinct non–rapid eye movement stages (NREM)
  - Stage I NREM
    - Transitional stage from wakefulness to sleep
    - 5% of total normal sleep cycle
  - Stage II NREM
    - Specific electroencephalogram (EEG) waveforms
    - 50% of total sleep cycle
  - Stages III and IV NREM
    - Slow-wave sleep period
    - Deepest level of sleep
    - 20% to 25% of total sleep cycle
  - Sleep stages are organized and sequential during sleep period.
  - Stages III and IV tend to occur in first one-third to one-half of sleep period.
- REM occurs cyclically throughout the night, alternating with NREM on average every 80 to 100 minutes.

- REM increases in duration toward morning.
- Sleep patterns vary with age.
  - Children and adolescents have large amounts of slow-wave sleep.
  - Sleep continuity and depth decrease with age.
  - Consider age when assessing for sleep–rest problems.
- Sleep patterns vary with medication use.
  - Many medications and substances of use affect sleep cycle.
  - Assess recent changes in medication or substance use in a person presenting with sleep pattern disturbances.

SLEEP DISORDERS

INSOMNIA

Description

- Insomnia is the inability to get the amount of sleep needed to function efficiently during the day.
- Situational or acute insomnia lasts from days to weeks.
- Insomnia disorder is characterized by a significant inability to initiate or maintain sleep, or early morning awakening with inability to return to sleep and occurs at least 3 nights per week and is present for at least 1 month (episodic insomnia disorder) and may persist for greater than 3 months (persistent insomnia disorder).
- Insomnia disorder is associated with increased mortality, poor career performance, overeating, and increased hospitalization.
- Insomnia disorder is not better explained by or occurring exclusively during the course of another sleep disorder and is not attributable to the effects of a substance.

Etiology

- Dysfunction in sleep–wake circuits of the brainstem
- Neurochemical imbalances impinging on these circuits
- May be stress-related in brief episodic insomnia

Incidence and Demographics

- 33% of Americans have difficulty sleeping.
- Up to 10% meet criteria for insomnia disorder.
- Insomnia is highly comorbid with other psychiatric disorders.

Risk Factors

- Female sex and advancing age
- Past history of insomnia
- Significant stress
- Forced pattern changes
    - Working alternating shifts
    - Swing-shift work patterns
    - Travel across time zones
- Genetic (obstructive sleep apnea)
- High-use patterns of medications or substances known to affect sleep cycles
    - Caffeine, other stimulants
    - Alcohol
    - Benzodiazepines

Prevention and Screening

- At-risk family education for children and adolescents
- Limits on shift work
- Avoidance of medications known to affect sleep patterns
- Good sleep hygiene patterns
- Avoidance of stimulants late in the day
- Early recognition, intervention, and initiation of treatment
    - Routine screening at all health care settings

HYPERSOMNOLENCE DISORDER

Description

- Self-reported excessive sleepiness despite adequate main sleep period
- Difficulty being fully awake—"groggy" after abrupt awakening
- Occurs at least 3 times per week and lasts for several months
- Causes significant distress or impairment
- Not better explained by another sleep disorder, viral infection, or physiologic effect of a substance
- May occur within 18 months of experiencing a head trauma
- Comorbidity includes various depressive disorders (e.g., major depression with atypical features, seasonal affective disorder [SAD], bipolar disorder depressed state)

Etiology

- 10% of cases are preceeded or accompanied by viral infection.
- Common after traumatic brain injury
- Genetic

Incidence and Demographics

- In the United States, approximately 5%–10% of clients who consult in sleep disorder clinics about complaints of daytime sleepiness are diagnosed with hypersomnolence disorder (American Psychiatric Association [APA], 2022).
- Onset usually late adolescence or early adulthood

OBSTRUCTIVE SLEEP APNEA (OSA)

Description

- Breathing-related sleep disorder characterized by repeated episodes of upper airway obstruction during sleep called apneas and hypoapneas:

  - ◇ Apneas: total absence of airflow
  - ◇ Hypoapnea: reduction of airflow
- Hallmark of disorder is snoring and repeated apnea during sleep
- Daytime sleepiness or sense of feeling unrefreshed despite adequate sleep period is prominent.
- Headache upon awakening is common.
- Consequences include panic attacks (waking up "gasping"), attention-deficit/hyperactivity disorder (ADHD), depression, hypertension, and motor vehicle and workplace accidents.

Etiology

- Abnormally small nasopharynx, tonsillar tissue in children; obesity

Incidence and Demographics

- Affects up to 2% of children, up to 15% to 20% of adults

ASSESSMENT

- Detailed history of present insomnia, including time frame, progression, and associated symptoms
- Social history, including present living situation; marital status; occupation; education; and alcohol, tobacco, or illicit drug use
- Medication use, including prescription, over-the-counter, alternative, supplements, and home remedies
- Initial and periodic functional history and assessment
- Number of hours in usual sleep pattern
- Initial or middle-phase insomnia; early morning awakening
- Use of sleep aids
- Bed position, use of pillows
- Environment: Temperature, sound, light

Physical Exam Findings

- No physical exam findings specific to sleep disorders
- Clients in whom a sleep disorder is suspected should have full exam.

Mental Status Exam Findings

- May have preoccupation or excessive worry about "not getting enough sleep"
- Depending on duration of sleep deprivation, many areas of mental status exam (MSE) may be affected

Diagnostic and Laboratory Findings

- Complete blood count (CBC), chemistry profile, thyroid function tests, ferritin level (if restless legs), and B_{12} level to rule out metabolic causes or unidentified conditions
- Drug toxicity screening, if indicated by history
- Polysomnography needed to make the definitive diagnosis
    - Sleep disturbance is often a manifestation of an underlying disorder.

DIFFERENTIAL DIAGNOSIS

- More than 50% of insomnia cases are related to a primary psychiatric disorder.
    - Mood disorders (see Chapter 9)
    - Anxiety disorders (see Chapter 10)
    - Substance-related disorders (see Chapter 13)
    - ADHD (see Chapter 15)
    - Early-morning wakefulness is a possible sign of depression.
    - Sudden, dramatic decrease in sleep is a sign of possible mania or schizophrenia.
    - Poor sleep is a sign of possible obsessive–compulsive disorder (OCD; see Chapter 10).
    - Panic and anxiety episodes during sleep are signs of possible panic disorder.
    - Alcohol may cause numerous awakenings during the night.
- Cardiac illnesses
- Parasomnias
- Gastrointestinal (GI) disorders

- Chronic obstructive pulmonary disease
- Medication side effects
- Sleep apnea
- Restless leg syndrome
- Chronic pain
- Stress reaction
- Active substance use
- Drug use
    - Caffeine
    - Stimulants

CLINICAL MANAGEMENT

- Rule out or treat any conditions that may contribute to current symptom manifestation.
- Weight loss and avoiding supine sleep position may alleviate sleep apnea.
- Positive airway pressure: continuous (CPAP) or bilevel (BPAP) for OSA

Pharmacological Management (Stahl, 2020)

- Melatonin is particularly useful to correct sleep-onset issues and may be helpful for the person with ADHD.
- Benzodiazepine or hypnotics (should not be used in OSA)
- Flurazepam
    - Long-lasting agent
    - May cause excess drowsiness
    - Avoid in older adults
- Temazepam
    - Intermediate acting agent
- Triazolam
    - Short-acting agent
    - Little to no excess sedation

- ◊ Common side effects:
  - Impaired memory
- ◊ Efficacy decreases over time
- ◊ Should not be used on a long-term basis

- ♦ Nonbenzodiazepine hypnotics
  - ◊ Zaleplon
    - Ultra-short half-life makes this drug particularly useful for initial or middle phase insomnia
  - ◊ Zolpidem
    - Short half-life drugs, but may affect person the next morning; must allow for 8 hours before planned awakening
    - Give on empty stomach
  - ◊ Eszopiclone
    - Intermediate-acting agent
  - ◊ Ramelteon
    - melatonin receptor agonist
  - ◊ Suvorexant
    - Orexin antagonist, suppresses wakefulness
    - Must consider long half-life
- ♦ Antidepressants
  - ◊ Used for sedating properties
  - ◊ Amitriptyline doxepin—generally avoid use in older adults
  - ◊ Mirtazapine
  - ◊ Trazadone
- ♦ Wake-promoting drugs
  - ◊ Armodafinil indicated for daytime sleepiness associated with OSA

Nonpharmacological Management

- ♦ Sleep hygiene practices
  - ◊ Establish a bedtime routine.
  - ◊ Have a regular time to sleep and wake.
  - ◊ Avoid computer and other electronic device use 1 hour before bedtime.

  - Never lie in bed for more than 15 minutes if not able to sleep.
  - Reduce stress.
  - Do stress reduction activities before bedtime.
  - Avoid late-in-the-day exercise intensive.
  - Avoid late-in-the-day stimulant use, such as caffeine.
  - Use bed/bedroom for sleep or sex only.
  - Consider moving phone and other devices away from sleeping area; restrict phone and computer use to 1 or more hours before bedtime.
  - Psychotherapy
  - Cognitive therapy for insomnia
- Relaxation and other therapies
  - Abdominal breathing
  - Progressive muscle relaxation
  - Meditation
  - Imaging
  - Hypnosis
  - Biofeedback
  - Stimulus control
  - Sleep curtailment
  - Light therapy
- Somatic and other therapies
- Exercise (during the day)
- Warm bath
- Warm milk
- Change bedroom environment

LIFE SPAN CONSIDERATIONS

Insomnia in children

- Most commonly related to stress
- Children with insomnia often have been poor sleepers since birth.
- Pharmacological treatment is not recommended for most children.

Insomnia in older adults

- If the first presentation is in older years, insomnia often is the result of changes in chronobiological rhythms. Older adults often become sleepier early in the evening and wake up early.
- Sleep latency, decreased REM sleep, and increased sleep fragmentation are common.
- Insomnia may be related to underlying psychiatric disorders:
    - Mood disorders
    - Anxiety disorders
    - ADHD
    - Alzheimer's disease
- Older adults often manifest confusion and restlessness as aspects of insomnia.
- A careful, complete assessment is necessary when pharmacological interventions are planned.

CASE STUDY 1

M.K., a 43-year-old receptionist, presents at the PMHNP's clinic with a primary complaint of insomnia. The client reports lifelong problem with sleeping that "comes and goes" depending on her stress level and general health and recently has been experiencing a 4- to 5-day period of poor sleeping, reporting only 3 to 4 hours of sleep and early morning awakening. M.K. has tried over-the-counter medication and has received no relief. Also reports health is generally good but says is a 2-pack-a-day smoker and has increased the recreational use of alcohol to 1 to 2 drinks a night in the past few weeks in order to get to sleep. The insomnia is now beginning to impair daily functioning and interest in social activities. M.K. reports an irritable mood since sleep has been difficult and problems with memory and concentration in the morning after poor sleep has been experienced. The client denies depression or any other mood problem and currently is taking no routine medication. The physical exam is unremarkable, and routine lab studies, including thyroid-stimulating hormone (TSH), CBC, and electrolytes, are all normal.

1. What is the most likely diagnosis for this client at this time?
2. What further assessment should the PMHNP make?
3. What treatment should the PMHNP consider?
4. Is medication warranted at this time to induce sleep?

CASE STUDY 2

B.C., a 40-year-old, presents to the PMHNP with a chief complaint of "I can't fall asleep. I've tried everything. Nothing works! That medicine the doctor gave me made me feel worse. It made me feel really anxious. I'm exhausted! I can't function. I'm going to lose my job." States the primary care provider has prescribed various sleeping medications, "Ambien, Lunesta, and Ativan," which have all caused a worsening of the insomnia. The physical exam and routine labs performed by the primary care provider have all been within normal limits.

1. What further assessment should the PMHNP make at this time?
2. What treatment should the PMHNP consider?
3. Why might a person report feeling more anxious and have more trouble sleeping in response to a hypnotic or anxiolytic medication?
4. The client begins psychotherapy with the PMHNP and starts to discuss growing up in a family with excessive alcohol use, and parents fighting at night after the children went to bed. In addition to continuing psychotherapy, should medication be considered?

CASE STUDY 3

G.L., 39-year-old, single, obese client is self-referred to the PMHNP for assessment and treatment of a chief complaint of "depression and exhaustion." The client states "I sleep just fine, but I'm always tired. My doctor did some blood work and said that everything was normal. I can't concentrate. I'm dragging at work. The other day I had to go out to my car and take a nap. I can't take this anymore! This is really getting me down. Do you think an antidepressant would help?" G.L. has had a CBC, comprehensive metabolic panel, serum iron, B_{12}, folate levels, and thyroid function tests which were all within normal limits.

1. What further assessment should be completed?
2. Should the client be started on medication?

ANSWERS TO CASE STUDY DISCUSSION QUESTIONS

CASE STUDY 1

1. The client has transient insomnia.
2. The PMHNP should identify life stressors, complete a full psychiatric assessment, and identify any other mental health needs.
3. The PMHNP should assist the client in managing sleep by using effective sleep hygiene strategies, encouraging diet changes, reducing smoking, and omitting the use of alcohol for sleep induction.
4. Short-term use of sleep induction medications such as a low-dose sedating antidepressant would provide relief with little risk to this client and may help reduce the current reliance on alcohol.

CASE STUDY 2

1. The PMHNP should complete a comprehensive psychiatric evaluation exploring for signs and symptoms of a mood or anxiety disorder. The history should include a thorough evaluation of past sleep patterns and issues with insomnia. The PMHNP should carefully assess for issues such as childhood or more recent trauma, alcohol, or other related violence exposure. Clients who have experienced significant trauma directed at them, or who have been raised in an environment of violence, may have fear related to falling asleep.
2. The PMHNP should consider psychotherapy, which should include psychoeducation about insomnia, the impact of anxiety on sleep, and sleep hygiene measures.
3. Children raised in traumatic environments commonly have difficulty falling and staying asleep. Many children become hypervigilant. These patterns can persist into adulthood. Adults may not be cognizant of the connection between current sleep issues and childhood trauma. Any medication that prevents a person from being hypervigilant could be experienced as a lack of control, thus causing an increase in anxiety and insomnia.
4. The PMHNP should discuss the possibility of using a selective serotonin reuptake inhibitor (SSRI) or perhaps another sedating antidepressant to address the heightened arousal and insomnia.

CASE STUDY 3

1. The PMHNP should complete a comprehensive psychiatric evaluation to rule out a mood, anxiety, or substance use disorder. A careful sleep and energy history should be taken and the PMHNP should screen for evidence of snoring or apnea. Further assessment should be done by a sleep specialist to rule out OSA or other sleep disorder.
2. The PMHNP should consider that medications may be indicated. If the client does have OSA, will be treated with a continuous or bilevel airway pressure device (CPAP or BPAP). Wake-promoting medication such as armodafinil may also be helpful in reducing excessive daytime sleepiness.

REFERENCES AND RESOURCES

American Psychiatric Association. (2022). Diagnostic and statistical manual of mental disorders (5th ed., Text rev.).

Buysse, D. (2013). Insomnia. JAMA, 309(7), 706–716. https://doi.org/10.1001/jama.2013.193

Rajput, V., & Johnson, R. (1999). Chronic insomnia: A practical review. American Family Practice, 11, 1–6.

Redeker, N., & McEnany, G.P. (2011). Sleep disorders and sleep promotion in nursing practice. Springer Publishing Company.

Stahl, S. M. (2020). Stahl's essential psychopharmacology: Prescriber's guide (7th ed.). Cambridge University Press.

CHAPTER 17

VIOLENCE

This chapter deals with the psychiatric-mental health nurse practitioner's (PMHNP's) role in identifying and treating clients who are impacted by intimate partner violence (IPV), sexual assault, homicide, and suicide. Assessment of lethality will also be reviewed. These issues may co-occur with the disorders already discussed or may present in clients with no other identifiable psychiatric or mental health problems. They also may be frequent findings in primary care settings while working with clients with general medical conditions.

INTIMATE PARTNER VIOLENCE

DESCRIPTION

- IPV is physical, emotional, economic, or sexual pain and injury that is intentionally inflicted by a person's intimate partner.
- The goal of the abuser is to
  - Establish power,
  - Manipulate the other person,
  - Intimidate the other person, and
  - Control the other person.

ETIOLOGY

- Characteristics of abusers
  - Personality disorders
    - Antisocial personality disorder
    - Narcissistic personality disorder
    - Borderline personality disorder

- ◇ Environmental stressors
    - Financial difficulties
    - Ending of a relationship
    - Unemployment

INCIDENCE AND DEMOGRAPHICS (NATIONAL COALITION AGAINST DOMESTIC VIOLENCE, 2023)

- IPV occurs among heterosexual and homosexual couples.
- IPV is the leading cause of injury to women ages 15–44.
- It is the leading cause of death among African American women between the ages of 15 and 24.
- 1 in 10 female high school students in the United States have reported violence from their dating partners.
- 15% to 25% of pregnant women are physically abused.
- 22% to 35% of all women seen in emergency rooms have experienced injuries as a result of IPV.
- 1 in 3 women and 1 in 4 men are victims of IPV.
- 50% of women who are unhoused experience IPV.
- 63% of men incarcerated for murder between the ages of 11 and 20 have murdered their mother's abuser.
- The presence of a gun in a domestic violence situation increases the risk of homicide by 500%.
- Only 34% of people who are injured by intimate partners receive medical care for their injuries.

RISK FACTORS

- For abusers
    - ◇ Exposure to violence at an early developmental age
    - ◇ Low self-esteem
    - ◇ Social isolation

- ◊ Lack of support
- ◊ Cognitive impairment
- ◊ Physical or financial dependency

PREVENTION AND SCREENING

- ♦ Public education and awareness beginning in high school
- ♦ Social programs
- ♦ At-risk family education
- ♦ Community education
    - ◊ Stigma reduction to allow victims to come forward
    - ◊ Signs and symptoms of being the victim of abuse
    - ◊ Prevention programs
    - ◊ Early recognition, intervention, and initiation of treatment for victims
    - ◊ Routine screening for victimization in all health care settings

ASSESSMENT

- ♦ Interview the person who has experienced the violence alone.
- ♦ Determine primary caregivers, living arrangements, and legal custodian.

Client History

- ♦ Assess for the following:
    - ◊ Determine recurrent history of medical treatment consistent with abuse:
        - Accidents
        - Suspicious or repeated fractures
        - Physical injuries
        - Traumas
        - Refusal of ongoing treatment or follow-up
        - Missed medical appointments
    - ◊ Determine environmental, psychosocial, and financial stressors.

Physical Exam Findings

- Monitor nutritional status for dehydration and malnutrition.
- Look for lacerations, bruises, wounds, burns, or fractures.
- Look for poor skin and personal hygiene.

Mental Status Exam Findings

- Findings of traits and behaviors suggestive of experiencing abuse include the following:
    - Fearful
    - Evasive
    - Guarded
    - Depressed
    - Passive
    - Dependent

Diagnostic and Laboratory Findings

- None specific to abuse
- Determine general health and nutritional status.

DIFFERENTIAL DIAGNOSIS

- Accidental injuries
- Mood disorders (see Chapter 9)
- Anxiety disorders (see Chapter 10)
- Substance use disorders (see Chapter 13)

CLINICAL MANAGEMENT

- Most state laws mandate reporting of suspected abuse and neglect of vulnerable populations:
    - Older adults

- ◇ People with disabilities
- ◇ Children

Pharmacological Management

- None specific to condition

Nonpharmacological Management

- The safety and medical well-being of the person experiencing the abuse is most important.
- Refer the person to a domestic abuse shelter when feasible.
- Help the person develop a safety plan.
  - Assist client in developing a "code word" for family or other support system as an attempt to inform them that the person needs help.
  - Advise client to tell one person in their support system about the situation.
  - Advise client to pack an "emergency bag" and hide it in case of need to leave quickly.
  - Advise client to keep the IPV hotline and other telephone numbers (e.g., police department, counselor, shelter) in a secure place.
  - Monitor medical status as symptomology presents.
  - Monitor nutritional status and vital signs.
  - Suggest psychotherapy to assist in gaining insight and in developing new coping skills.
  - Suggest hospitalization when in the best interest of the client.

SEXUAL ASSAULT AND ABUSE

DESCRIPTION

- Sexual assault or abuse is any sexual act or penetration committed through coercion or physical force.
  - This includes rape, incest, sodomy, oral and anal acts, and use of a foreign object.
  - It is an act of violence and humiliation expressed through sexual means.
  - It is used to express power or anger.

ETIOLOGY

- For abusers
  - Behavioral disorders, also called personality disorders
  - Behavioral act of violence is reinforcing
  - Once done, likely to repeat
  - Social exposure to violence in culture, media, and home

INCIDENCE AND DEMOGRAPHICS

- Women have a greater incidence of being assaulted than men.
- Sexual assault is the most common form of abuse.
- Perpetrators are more frequently men than women.
  - Sexual assaults are often committed by fathers and stepfathers, uncles, older siblings, other family members, and men that women are dating.
- Alcohol is involved in 34% of all rapes.
- Only 1 in 3 rapes is reported.

FACTORS THAT INCREASE INCIDENTS OF ABUSE

- Substance use disorders
- Psychiatric disorders
- Divorce
- Family or personal history of physical or sexual abuse
- Long-term exposure to violence
- Social isolation and lack of support systems
- Environmental stressors such as unwanted pregnancy in an intimate partner, unemployment, or financial difficulty

PREVENTION AND SCREENING OF VICTIMS

- Public education and awareness campaigns
- Community resources and support

- Community emergency shelters, help lines, and safe houses
- Assertiveness training and self-defense
- Early recognition, intervention, and initiation of treatment
  - Routine screening in all health care settings

ASSESSMENT

- Interview persons who have experienced the assault alone, when possible.
- Establish a safe, trusting relationship to promote sharing.
  - Routine inclusion of questions concerning sexual assault in medical history.
  - Interview alone and not in presence of family, friend, or partner.
  - Interview for social history, including history of living arrangements and relationships.

Physical Exam Findings

- No physical exam findings specific to sexual assault and abuse
- Presentation of traits and behaviors consistent with potential for having experienced sexual assault or other abuse:
  - Withdrawn
  - Frightened appearance
  - Hyperreactive to touch
- Associated findings include the following:
  - Unexplained bruises, abrasions, cuts, laceration, burns, soft-tissue swellings, and hematomas
  - Sexually transmitted diseases
  - Genital rash or discharge
  - Rectal tissue swelling or discharge
- Physical signs that are strongly suggestive of sexual abuse in children include the following:
  - Lacerations, ecchymosis, and newly healed scars of the hymen or posterior fourchette
  - No hymenal tissue in 3- to 9-o'clock area
  - Healed hymenal transactions, especially in the aforementioned area

- ◊ Perianal lacerations

Remember that any child presenting with concerning physical signs should be evaluated by a sexual abuse expert. A complete history and a sexual abuse examination need to take place.

Mental Status Exam Findings

- Withdrawn
- Frightened
- Anxious
- Scattered appearance
- Hyperreactive to touch
- Dissociative

Diagnostic and Laboratory Findings

- No specific diagnostic lab findings exist.
- Assessment and documentation labs
- Forensic specimens
- Pregnancy tests
- Rectal, throat, and vaginal cultures
- Screening for sexually transmitted diseases: Syphilis, HIV, hepatitis B, herpes simplex, human papillomavirus, trichomonas vaginalis

DIFFERENTIAL DIAGNOSIS

- Accidental injuries
- Consensual sexual activity
- Lichen sclerosis
- Posttraumatic stress disorder
- Anxiety disorder (see Chapter 10)

CLINICAL MANAGEMENT

- Use sensitivity and respectful care.
- Be aware of legal reporting requirements.
- Use available community resources.

Nonpharmacological Management

- Ensure safety and well-being.
- Ensure confidentiality.
- Complete accurate documentation.
- Assess for potential suicidal ideation if the person is showing any depressive symptoms.
- Suggest cognitive behavioral therapy (CBT).
- Offer support groups and community resources.
- Assist with access to criminal and legal supports.

LETHALITY ASSESSMENT

- Lethality assessment: Evaluation, screening, or testing
- Lethality refers to the likelihood that a person will end their own life or commit homicide—focused violence at the extreme.
- Violence: The behavioral expression of anger, rage, and hostility that is demonstrated by the use of physical force directed toward persons (in case of suicide, toward self) or property

VIOLENCE IN SCHOOL

- Serious physical fighting with peers or family members
- Severe destruction of property
- Severe rage for seemingly minor reasons
- Detailed threats of lethal violence

- Possession, use, or both of firearms or other weapons
- Self-injurious behaviors or threats of suicide
- Bullying or being bullied
- When warning signs indicate that danger is imminent, safety must always be the primary consideration. Action must be taken immediately. Immediate intervention by school authorities and possibly law enforcement officers is needed when a child
    - Has presented a detailed plan (time, place, method) to harm or kill others, particularly if the child has a history of aggression or has attempted to carry out threats in the past; or
    - Is carrying a weapon, particularly a firearm, and has threatened to use it.

SUICIDE ASSESSMENT

RISK FACTORS

- Depression
- All antidepressants have U.S. Food and Drug Administration (FDA) box warnings about an increased risk of suicide in children, adolescents, and young adults under the age of 24.
- Prior attempt to end their own life
- Family history of mental disorder or substance use
- Family history of death by suicide
- Family violence
- Firearms in the home
- Incarceration
- Males are 5 times more likely than females to die by suicide.
- White males over age 85 have the highest rate of death by suicide.

SIGNS OF IMMINENT DANGER

- Threatening to hurt or kill oneself
- Looking for ways to kill oneself (weapons, pills, or other means)
- Talking or writing about death, dying, or suicide
- Plans or preparations for a potentially serious attempt
- Alcohol use increases the risk of a person attempting to end their own life in persons with ideation.

HOMICIDE: EARLY WARNING SIGNS

- Prior history of threatening or violent behavior
- Paranoia or easily panicked behavior
- A fascination or preoccupation with weapons, particularly weapons or explosives that could be used for mass destruction, such as semi-automatic guns
- Extreme stress from personal problems or a life crisis
- Identifying with incidents of workplace violence reported in the media and either condoning or sympathizing with the actions of the persons committing violence
- Being a loner with little or no involvement with other employees
- Engaging in frequent disputes with supervisors or coworkers
- Persistent violation of company policy
- Obsessive involvement with one's job, particularly where it occurs with no apparent outside interests
- Volatile or violent home or other personal situation that has the potential to bring violence into the workplace

THREATS OF VIOLENCE

- Throwing objects
- Making a verbal threat to harm another person or destroy property
- Making menacing gestures or physical posturing without actually touching the person
- Displaying an intense or obsessive romantic interest that exceeds the normal bounds of interpersonal interest
- Attempting to intimidate or harass other persons
- Behavior indicating that the person is significantly out of touch with reality and that they may pose a danger to themselves or to others
- Volatile or violent personal situations such as found in some custody battles
- Alcohol use increases the risk for violence

Safety is the number one priority and any threatening behavior must be taken seriously.

CASE STUDY

T.R. is 24 years old, single, and is referred to the PMHNP for persistent insomnia and depression after being treated in the emergency department of the local hospital for headaches, stomach pain, and various other physical complaints five times in the past 6 months. The PMHNP suspects the client is a victim of IPV.

1. What should the PMHNP's assessment include?
2. How should the PMHNP approach suspicions of IPV?
3. Should anyone besides T.R. be interviewed?
4. If the PMHNP concludes that the client meets criteria for major depression, should medication be included as part of the treatment plan?

Assume T.R. is an immigrant.

5. What other considerations must be included in the assessment?
6. How should the PMHNP approach the client with her suspicions of IPV?
7. What other considerations must be included in the treatment plan?

Assume the client is 80 years old and widowed.

8. What other considerations must be included in the assessment?
9. Who should be included in the assessment findings?
10. What other considerations must be included in the treatment plan for any person suspected of being the victim of IPV?

ANSWERS TO CASE STUDY DISCUSSION QUESTIONS

1. The client should undergo a complete physical assessment, labs as indicated (likely working in conjunction with primary care providers), and a comprehensive psychiatric evaluation. The PMHNP should also inquire about sexual partner(s), sexual behaviors, birth control, and possibility of sexually transmitted infection.
2. The PMHNP should approach the client privately (1:1). Questions should be posed in a matter-of-fact manner, using language that is not stigmatizing, such as "Has ________________________ ever threatened you or made you feel afraid?" or "Does _____'s temper ever make you feel scared?"
3. Generally no one else besides the victim should be interviewed. Clients often feel reluctant to discuss being abused because they think if their partner finds out, things will get worse. They may feel embarrassed or judged if anyone else were to know what is going on.
4. Possibly, treating significant depression will allow the client to be in a better position to make decisions and take action.
5. The PMHNP must make sure the interview is done in the client's native language. Interpreters must not be a family member or friend.
6. The PMHNP must consider that different cultures may have different perceptions of IPV. The PMHNP must use culturally sensitive language. The PMHNP will need to consider the woman's concerns about legal issues related to immigration status.
7. Culturally sensitive and relevant resources for therapy and medication management should be available.
8. The client's living situation and ability to care for their own needs, whether or not the client has caregivers, and whether or not family member or other caregivers are possibly abusing the client should be considered.
9. All states have mandatory reporting for suspected elder abuse.
10. A safety plan should be first and foremost. The victim should know where and how to get help. Resources should include 24-hour hotlines, shelters, support groups, and the like. The victim should have an escape plan that includes having some clothing and money packed and ready in case they decide to leave.

REFERENCES AND RESOURCES

American Nurses Association, American Psychiatric Nurses Association, & International Society of Psychiatric-Mental Health Nursing. (2022). Psychiatric-mental health nursing: Scope and standards of practice (3rd ed.). American Nurses Association.

Blunt, E., & Reinisch, C. (2013) The family nurse practitioner review manual (4th ed). American Nurses Credentialing Center.

Davidson, J. R. (2000). Trauma: The impact of post-traumatic stress disorder. Journal of Psychopharmacology, 14(Suppl. 1), 5–12.

National Coalition Against Domestic Violence. (2023). National statistics. https://www.ncadv.org/learn/statistics

Sadock, B., Sadock, V., & Ruiz, P. (2017). Kaplan and Sadock's comprehensive textbook of psychiatry (10th ed.). Wolters Kluwer.

Tusaie, K., & Fitzpatrick, J. (2022). Advanced practice psychiatric nursing: Integrating psychotherapy, psychopharmacology and complementary and alternative approaches (3rd ed.). Springer Publishing Company.

U. S. Department of Health and Human Services. (1999). Mental health: A report of the Surgeon General. https://profiles.nlm.nih.gov/spotlight/nn/catalog/nlm:nlmuid-101584932X120-doc

APPENDIX A

REVIEW QUESTIONS

1. What is the purpose of the Psychiatric-Mental Health Nursing: Scope and Standards of Practice?

   a. Define the roles and actions of psychiatric-mental health nurses at registered nurse (RN) and advanced practice registered nurse (APRN) levels

   b. Establish the legal authority for the prescription of psychotropic medications

   c. Define the legal statutes of the role of the psychiatric mental health nurse practitioner (PMHNP)

   d. Define the differences between the physician role and the NP role

2. Primary prevention care practices are an essential aspect of the PMHNP role. Which of the following is the best example of a primary prevention care strategy for community behavioral health?

   a. Aftercare program for chronically mentally ill clients recently discharged from the hospital

   b. Court-ordered counseling for abusive parents

   c. 24-hour crisis hotlines

   d. Parenting skills classes for pregnant adolescents

3. Which of the following has been the trend in legal rulings on cases involving mental illness over the past 25 years?

   a. Encourage juries to find defendants not guilty by reason of insanity

   b. Protect the person's freedoms or rights when they are committed to a mental hospital

   c. Place increasing trust in mental health professionals to make good and ethical decisions

   d. Decrease the "red tape" associated with commitments so that commitments are faster and easier

4. An involuntarily hospitalized client experiencing symptoms of hearing voices and seeing people who are not present refuses to take any of the ordered medication. The client states, "Jesus Christ told me I am the prophet and must fast for a year." Your actions should be based on your knowledge of which of the following?

   a. Psychiatric clients cannot refuse treatment.

   b. Psychiatric clients do not always know what is good for them.

   c. Psychiatric clients can refuse treatment.

   d. Psychiatric clients cannot be trusted to make good health care decisions and, therefore, the nurse's best clinical judgment should guide actions.

5. Which of the following statements best reflects the difference between the nurse–client (N–C) relationship and a social relationship?

    a. In the N–C relationship, the primary focus is on the client and the client's needs.
    b. Goals in the N–C relationship are deliberately left vague and unspoken so that the client can work on any issue.
    c. In the N–C relationship, the nurse is solely responsible for making the relationship work.
    d. In the N–C relationship, there is no place for social interaction.

6. A community has an unusually high incidence of depression and drug use in the teenage population. The public health nurses decide to address this problem, in part, by modifying the environment and strengthening the capacities of families to prevent the development of new cases of depression and drug use. What is this is an example of?

    a. Primary prevention
    b. Secondary prevention
    c. Tertiary prevention
    d. Protective factorial prevention

7. K.C. is voluntarily admitted to the hospital. After 24 hours, the client wishes to leave because "this place can't help me." Which of the following is the best nursing action that reflects the legal right of this client?

    a. Discharge the client.
    b. Explain that the client cannot leave until you can complete further assessment.
    c. Allow the client to leave but have her sign forms stating she is leaving against medical advice.
    d. Immediately start the paperwork to commit the client and to allow you to treat her against her wishes.

8. In forming a therapeutic relationship with clients, the PMHNP must consider developing many characteristics that are known to be helpful in relationship building. Which of the following is an essential part of building a therapeutic relationship?

    a. Collecting a family history
    b. Like-mindedness
    c. Authenticity
    d. Accuracy in assessment

9. According to the Diagnostic and Statistical Manual of Mental Disorders, Fifth Edition, Text Revision (DSM-5-TR), which of the following is true?

    a. A mental disorder is equivalent to the need for treatment.
    b. Diagnostic criteria are used to inform clinical judgment.
    c. Socially deviant behavior is considered a mental disorder.
    d. A culturally expected response to a stressor is not a mental disorder.

10. Your client has been in individual therapy with you for the past 3 months and has shown much growth and improvement in functioning and insight and is to discontinue services within the next few weeks. In the next session, after you discuss service termination, the client suddenly begins to demonstrate the original symptoms that had brought them to treatment initially. Now the client is hesitant to discharge, wants to continue services, and is displaying an increase in regressive defense mechanisms. What is the best explanation for this behavior?

    a. An exacerbation of her symptoms related to stress
    b. The normal cyclic nature of chronic mental health symptoms
    c. A sign of normal resistance to termination seen in the termination phase of therapy
    d. A sign of pathological attachment to the therapist that must be addressed

11. A client is displaying low self-esteem, poor self-control, self-doubt, and a high level of dependency. These behaviors indicate developmental failure of which of the following stages of development?

    a. Infancy
    b. Early childhood
    c. Late childhood
    d. School age

12. W.P. reports being forgetful lately, for example, forgetting where the keys are placed or what time appointments are scheduled, and states "these are just random behaviors that have no particular meaning." Which Freudian-based psychodynamic principle assumes that all behavior and actions are purposeful?

    a. Pleasure principle
    b. Psychic determinism principle
    c. Reality principle
    d. Unconsciousness principle

13. Which of the following is an example of a mature, healthy defense mechanism?

    a. Denial
    b. Rationalization
    c. Repression
    d. Suppression

14. H.D. is a 54-year-old client you have been seeing for several weeks in therapy. While discussing the current concerns of marital stress, the client lies on the floor and assumes the fetal position. This is most likely an example of which of the following?

    a. Immature regressive defense mechanism
    b. Denial of reality
    c. Immature fantasy defense mechanism
    d. Repressive behavior

15. Which of the following defense mechanisms are best viewed as a function of the ego?

    a. To alert us to harm and danger
    b. To alert us to problems
    c. Used to resolve a conflict
    d. Used to protect the id

16. One of the health care changes that has occurred as a result of the Patient Protection and Affordable Care Act (ACA) is that providers/hospitals/clinic groups or health systems are coming together and assuming the responsibility for quality care to large groups of individuals insured by Medicare. The health care clinics/systems providers or hospitals that join together are called which of the following?

    a. Health Maintenance Organization (HMO)
    b. Preferred Provider Network (PPO)
    c. Accountable Care Organization (ACO)
    d. Individual Health Plan (IHP)

17. Health care economics is concerned with making decisions so that the benefits outweigh the cost of resource utilization. What are two concepts that health care economics is concerned with in regard to fair distribution of resources and allocation?

    a. Equity and efficiency
    b. Cost and benefits
    c. Opportunity and waste
    d. Affordability and quality

18. What four elements need to be present for a malpractice lawsuit to be filed?

    a. Beneficence, non-maleficence, truthfulness, and justice

    b. Professional standard of care, breach of standard of care, injury caused by the breach, and resulting damage.

    c. Abandonment, breach of care, violation of ethics, and reimbursement for poor care

    d. Breach of standard of care, injury, deceit, and malpractice

19. A PMHNP who is working in a hospitalist role has encountered over five incidents in which attending psychiatrists and medical residents have been demeaning to nursing staff and not answering calls in the middle of the night or telling the nursing staff to write orders and the medical doctor (MD) would sign off in the a.m. The PMHNP is concerned about errors and wants to improve quality and reduce errors to promote safety. What concept is being employed?

    a. Bullying

    b. Abuse

    c. Civil disobedience

    d. Just culture

20. The role of neurotransmitters in the central nervous system is to function as which of the following?

    a. A communication medium

    b. A gatekeeper for transmissions

    c. A building block for amino acids

    d. An agent to break down enzymes

21. Serotonin is produced in which of the following locations?

    a. Locus ceruleus

    b. Nucleus basalis

    c. Raphe nuclei

    d. Substantia nigra

22. Dopamine is produced in which of the following locations?

    a. Locus ceruleus

    b. Nucleus basalis

    c. Raphe nuclei

    d. Substantia nigra

23. A client presents with complaints of changes in appetite, feeling fatigued, problems with sleep–rest cycle, and changes in libido. What is the neuroanatomical area of the brain that is responsible for the normal regulation of these functions?

    a. Thalamus
    b. Hypothalamus
    c. Limbic system
    d. Hippocampus

24. In considering whether to order a magnetic resonance imaging (MRI) of the brain for a client, which of the following would be a contraindication to this diagnostic test?

    a. Prosthetic limb
    b. History of head trauma
    c. Pacemaker
    d. Pregnancy

25. What is the primary excitatory neurotransmitter?

    a. gamma-aminobutyric acid (GABA)
    b. Serotonin
    c. Dopamine
    d. Glutamate

26. A client who is experiencing difficulties with working memory, planning and prioritizing, insight into his problems, and impulse control presents for assessment. In planning his care, the PMHNP should apply the knowledge that these symptoms represent problems with which of the following?

    a. Frontal lobe
    b. Temporal lobe
    c. Parietal lobe
    d. Occipital lobe

27. Which of the following best explains the concept of target symptom identification?

    a. Identification of the major clinical presentation of the client
    b. Identification of specific, precise, and individualized symptoms reasonably expected to improve with medication
    c. Identification of the secondary messenger system syndrome
    d. Intentional modulation of synaptic pathways

28. Which of the following is the goal of the psychiatric assessment process performed by the PMHNP?

    a. Gain an understanding of the life experiences of the client

    b. Correctly diagnose the client

    c. Identify the mental health needs of the client

    d. Be able to communicate with other staff about the client's health needs

29. S.W. is a client newly admitted to an inpatient psychiatric hospital. The PMHNP on call at the facility plans to perform the initial intake assessment and diagnostic process. The client asks to please talk in the room because, "people make me nervous." S.W.'s room is at the end of the hallway and is the farthest from the nursing station. The PMHNP's action should be based on awareness that the best location to do the assessment is which of the following?

    a. In the client's room, because it is least noisy and most comfortable for him, thus facilitating data collection

    b. In the dayroom, which is full of people, to observe his interactions with other people

    c. In a quiet place, but public enough to get assistance with client care should it be required during the assessment

    d. In the treatment room with the door closed, a neutral location

30. Which communication technique is the PMHNP using in the following situation? Client: "Sorry I was late. I did not realize what time it was." PMHNP: "This is the third time now that you have been late for our sessions. I am wondering how committed you are to our working on your problems."

    a. Theming

    b. Recognizing

    c. Validating

    d. Sequencing

31. In assessing a client, you ask him the meaning of the proverb "People who live in glass houses shouldn't throw stones." The client replies, "Because it will break the windows." Which of the following is the correct interpretation of this findings?

    a. Client has a probable mood disorder

    b. Client has a probable anxiety disorder

    c. Client has limited intellectual ability

    d. Unable to interpret the finding without knowing the client's age

32. The PMHNP is planning to work with a client using an individual therapy model of care. During the first session, the client makes the following statement: "This is the third time my son has run away. I've grounded him, taken away his bike, even tried cutting off his allowance and confining him to his room. What should I do now?" Which of the following is the most therapeutic response for the PMHNP to make?

    a. "I wonder if confining him to his room was abusive?"
    b. "Maybe that depends on what you are trying to accomplish."
    c. "Perhaps talking to his friends and teachers would help."
    d. Remain silent

33. A client says to the PMHNP, "Some days life is just not worth it. All my spouse and I ever do is fight and scream. Things at home would be calmer and simpler if I just wasn't there anymore." Which of the following is the most therapeutic response for the PMHNP to make?

    a. "Do you mean that you are thinking about leaving your wife and moving out?"
    b. "Tell me what you mean by 'it would be simpler if you just weren't there anymore.'"
    c. "So you are thinking suicide might be an option for you?"
    d. Remain silent

34. F.L. has come to the mental health center seeking treatment for depression and has a history of attempting to end their own life by overdose 1 month ago. The client was started on imipramine, a tricyclic antidepressant (TCA), after that event but stopped taking the medication 1 week later because it "did no good." The PMHNP meets with the client to establish a plan of care. Which of the following is the most appropriate initial action?

    a. Asking the client how to help
    b. Providing client teaching about the long timeframe for TCAs to work
    c. Contracting with the client for 6 sessions of individual therapy
    d. Providing the client with feedback about how suicide might affect the family

35. In completing the PMHNP assessment for F.L., what is the most appropriate lab test for the PMHNP to order at this time?

    a. complete blood count (CBC)
    b. thyroid stimulating hormone (TSH)
    c. Liver function tests
    d. Electrolyte panel

36. A client comes into the clinic with a longstanding history of depression and chronic renal failure and is on an antidepressant and a diuretic and complains of increased depression, mild confusion, irritability, and overall apathy from being too tired to do anything. Which of the following is the best initial PMHNP action to take at this time?

    a. Increase his dose of antidepressant medication to better capture symptoms
    b. Change him to another antidepressant for better symptom control
    c. Augment his antidepressant with an atypical antipsychotic medication
    d. Order a comprehensive metabolic panel

37. S.F. presents for her initial intake appointment with complaints of depression and is being treated for hypertension and asthma by her primary care provider. Knowing that certain medications can cause or exacerbate depression, you obtain a complete medication history. Which of the following medications is known to exacerbate or cause depression?

    a. Omeprazole
    b. Propranolol
    c. Levothyroxine
    d. Clarithromycin

38. When treating older adults, you should keep in mind that they are more sensitive to issues of drug toxicity because of which of the following reasons?

    a. Decreased body fat
    b. Increased liver capacity
    c. Decreased protein binding
    d. Increased muscle concentration

39. Which known teratogenic effects can be caused by the common psychotropic medications divalproex and lithium?

    a. Divalproex—Ebstein's anomaly; lithium—cleft palate
    b. Divalproex—spina bifida; lithium—Ebstein's anomaly
    c. Divalproex—limb malformations; lithium—seizure disorder
    d. Divalproex—mental retardation; lithium—spina bifida

40. What is the study of what the body does to drugs called?

    a. Pharmacodynamics
    b. Pharmacology
    c. Pharmacokinetics
    d. Distribution

41. Your client S.A. is being treated for panic disorder with agoraphobia and is currently being prescribed paroxetine ER, 37.5 mg q.d., and clonazepam, 0.5 mg q.d., p.r.n. S.A. has been taking clonazepam for 2 years and admits to needing four pills to achieve the same effect that one pill initially produced. This is possibly an example of which process?

    a. Kindling
    b. Addiction
    c. Tolerance
    d. Potency

42. Why is group therapy beneficial?

    a. It assists the client to focus on self
    b. It lacks theoretical frameworks
    c. It enables participants to acquire therapeutic factors
    d. It is always time limited

43. Which of the following is the best rationale for using cognitive behavioral therapy (CBT)?

    a. Recognize and change client's automatic thoughts
    b. Convince the client to see reality as you see it
    c. Change client's reality by changing their environment
    d. Recognize and accept that automatic thoughts suggest delusional thinking

44. When working with a family that is struggling conflict, roles, and boundaries, you find that the father, Jim, worries excessively and is resistant to change. You give Jim a paradoxical directive to worry extremely well for 1 hour per day, knowing that he will likely be noncompliant, and thus change will occur. With this technique, you are using which type of therapy?

    a. Experiential therapy
    b. Structural therapy
    c. Strategic therapy
    d. Solution-focused therapy

45. Which of the following best describes homeostasis in a family system?

 a. Choices a family makes to keep the peace
 b. Balance or stability that the family returns to despite its dysfunction
 c. Need for change and balance in a family
 d. Calm in a family that returns after a crisis

46. In an attempt to bring the client toward the goal they are working on, you ask the client, "If a miracle were to happen tonight while you slept, and you awoke in the morning and the problem no longer existed, how would you know, and what would be different?" This technique is used in which type of therapy?

 a. Behavioral therapy
 b. Solution-focused therapy
 c. Adlerian therapy
 d. Existential therapy

47. T.R. has been diagnosed with major depressive disorder (MDD) and is placed on fluoxetine, 20 mg q.d., for her depression. For the PMHNP to effectively monitor her use of the medication, which of the following actions should be part of ongoing care?

 a. Use of a standardized rating scale of depression
 b. Monitoring for potential abuse of the medication
 c. Monitoring of labs for renal functioning
 d. Monitoring for potential cardiac side effects

48. Which of the following is the best reason for considering selective serotonin reuptake inhibitors (SSRIs) among the first-line drug choices for treating symptoms of major depression?

 a. Need to stair-step initial dosages
 b. Sedating and calming effect of the medication
 c. Safe use in suicidal overdose clients
 d. Ability to obtain therapeutic serum drug levels

49. A 23-year-old is brought to the emergency department after attempting end their own life by cutting their wrists. Which nursing action by the PMHNP would be of highest priority initially?

 a. Assess coping behaviors
 b. Assess current level of suicidality
 c. Take vital signs
 d. Assess health history

50. Which of the following interventions by the PMHNP for a person experiencing ataque de nervios demonstrates culturally informed care?

    a. Offering brief supportive psychotherapy

    b. Offering a brief hospitalization

    c. Requesting a family member act as an interpreter

    d. Offering low-dose, short-term anxiolytic medication

51. The PMHNP working at a student mental health clinic has now been working with a first-year student for several weeks. The PMHNP learns that the student considers themselves shy and tells the PMHNP they have always felt uncomfortable in social situations or when they have had to do oral presentations in class. The client has had few friends up until the senior year of high school when it was discovered the client could enjoy themselves if "I had a couple of drinks before going out." The client has continued this pattern in college and now occasionally drinks "2 to 3 beers" on weekends as well. According to the DSM-5-TR, does the student have a mental disorder?

    a. Yes, alcohol use disorder, mild

    b. Yes, generalized anxiety disorder

    c. No, at this point, the student does not meet criteria for a mental disorder.

    d. Yes, adjustment disorder with mixed features

52. J.K. misses several appointments. The PMHNP recognizes feeling resentful toward the client and is struggling with how to respond to J.K. when they finally come in for the appointment. Which of the following demonstrates a therapeutic response?

    a. "J.K., since you have missed several appointments, we are closing your case."

    b. "J.K., it's pretty clear to me that you don't want to be here."

    c. "J.K., you are ambivalent about seeking treatment."

    d. "J.K., help me understand what's going on so we can figure out how to proceed."

53. Which is true about pharmacologic treatment of anxiety in older adults?

    a. The course of treatment is generally shorter than for younger adults.

    b. Older adults may have a decreased sensitivity to the effects of medications.

    c. The therapeutic dose of SSRIs is generally lower than for young adults.

    d. Highly lipophilic drugs have a more linear elimination in older adults.

54. A client returns for a follow-up appointment 3 weeks after starting on fluoxetine, 20 mg q.d. During this appointment you notice that speech is a little rapid, in marked contrast to the psychomotor retardation and paucity of spontaneous speech that was displayed on the first visit. Instead of looking at the floor, the client now makes normal eye contact, the affect has gone from constricted to expansive. The client continues to have difficulty sleeping, but the energy has improved and the client states, "I feel so much better!" What should you conclude about the shift in the client's presentation?

    a. The client is experiencing the activating side effects of fluoxetine.

    b. The client is becoming euthymic.

    c. The client is becoming hypomanic.

    d. The client is in a mixed state.

55. D.S. is a 35-year-old, married, high-tech industry executive who is referred to the PMHNP for "insomnia." D.S. reports falling asleep quickly, but has difficulty staying asleep, wakes up several times during the night, and believes they "toss and turn" even when sleeping. The client wakes up feeling exhausted and drinks "a pot of coffee" to stay awake and concentrate during the long workday. D.S. reports drinking one glass of wine most evenings and denies any illicit substance use. The client denies any symptoms of a mood or anxiety disorder but is feeling increasingly frustrated and concerned about the sleep issues. Which of the following is the most likely contributing factor to D.S.'s ongoing middle insomnia?

    a. Obstructive sleep apnea (OSA)

    b. Caffeine dependence

    c. Alcohol withdrawal

    d. Attention-deficit/hyperactivity disorder (ADHD)

56. A PMHNP who has been practicing for over 20 years is considering making application to a Doctor of Nursing Practice (DNP) program but states "if a DNP is required to practice I'll get grandfathered in, no need for me to go back to school." Following the 2008 License, Accreditation, Certification, and Education (LACE) Consensus Model for Advanced Practice Registered Nurse Regulation, which statement is correct?

    a. The PMHNP is correct: If the DNP becomes a requirement, they will be grandfathered in and obtain a DNP degree.

    b. The DNP is an academic terminal degree and there will not be an opportunity for the PMHNP to be grandfathered into a DNP.

    c. The PMHNP will be grandfathered in and obtain a DNP only if her state requires a DNP to practice as an APRN.

    d. The DNP is a certification and the PMHNP will have to take an examination to be grandfathered in to obtain a DNP.

57. A board-certified PMHNP working in a busy community mental health center (CMHC) is currently seeing a client diagnosed with bipolar I disorder who has comorbid hypertension and diabetes. During the visit, the client's blood pressure is 160/94 mm Hg, and they deny headaches, nausea, chest pain, or shortness of breath. The client states "I can't afford all these medications so I haven't seen my doctor in 7 months and I am out of all my blood pressure and sugar medications. Can you give me some?" What is the PMHNP's most appropriate action?

   a. Call the pharmacy to find out what medications the client is taking and refill for 1 month to cover until she can get in to see his primary care provider.

   b. Tell the client he cannot refill her medications and direct her to go to the emergency room should she develop any signs or symptoms of elevated blood pressure or hyperglycemia.

   c. Call the client's primary care provider, explain the situation, and coordinate the client getting an appointment and medication refills.

   d. Send the client to an urgent care clinic to get refills today.

58. The chief nursing officer of a large behavioral health system approached the PMHNP to discuss the new Healthcare Effectiveness Data and Information Set (HEDIS) behavioral health measures and specifications. The PMHNP is asked to do a retrospective chart review of all hospital discharge clients who received a follow-up visit within 7 days of discharge and within 30 days of discharge. The PMHNP has been asked to engage in which of the following?

   a. Needs assessment project

   b. Plan, do, study, act project

   c. A task that is outside of the PMHNP's scope of practice

   d. Quality improvement initiative

59. A PMHNP who is working on the consult liaison service is referred to a client in the medical intensive care unit by the attending hospitalist. The consult note read "Evaluate the client for competency to make independent medical decisions and consent for a surgical procedure." Based on the scope of practice of a PMHNP, which response would be most appropriate?

   a. Complete the client assessment and write up the findings in the client's medical record.

   b. Complete a client assessment, including the Mini-Mental Status Exam and obtaining family collateral data to determine competency.

   c. Call the hospitalist and provide education that competency is a legal concept and explain that you can assess the client for the capacity to make medical decisions.

   d. Refuse the consult and inform the hospitalist that this is outside your scope of practice.

60. You are asked by a church organization to work with members within your health system to develop a flu vaccination program. According to public health principles, this is an example of what level of prevention?

    a. Secondary

    b. Preventative

    c. Tertiary

    d. Primary

61. A client with a diagnosis of bipolar I disorder presents to your PMHNP office for a follow-up visit. During the visit, the client informs you that they no longer want to be treated with medication, and "do not have bipolar disorder; that was a misdiagnosis." The client further informs you they stopped all medication 2 months ago and is here to thank you for your care and tell you they no longer need follow-up appointments. Understanding the ethical conflict, you use which of the following ethical principles in working with this client?

    a. Autonomy

    b. Nonmaleficence

    c. Justice

    d. Beneficence

62. A new client reveals to the PMHNP that their boyfriend screams and has repeatedly slapped and pushed them in front of her 3-year-old son. The client goes on to say that the boyfriend has thrown things and on one occasion threw a glass of water that hit her son in the back. Should the PMHNP report this to child protective services (CPS)?

    a. Yes, the client is issuing a cry for help for the son.

    b. Yes, the PMHNP has a duty to report.

    c. No, this does not constitute a reportable offense.

    d. No, a report to CPS will escalate the violence.

63. Which of the following is a function of the psychiatric interview?

    a. Understand the client's psychosocial needs and communicate them to the treatment team.

    b. Identify the mental health needs of the client.

    c. Review previous medical records.

    d. Evaluate a treatment plan.

64. A 74-year-old, married female was referred to you by her primary care provider for a psychiatric evaluation. She had a normal medical and neurological examination within the last 2 months. The client presents with her husband of 45 years who states, "My wife is just not the same anymore; she is irritable and asks the same question several times, even though I've answered it many times." The client responds, "Oh, Henry, you do the same thing; it's just a normal part of getting older, and the kids think everything is fine." During the assessment you compete the Mini-Mental Status Exam (MMSE) and the client scores 18. As the PMHNP treating the client, you know the results of her MMSE indicate which level of cognitive impairment?

   a. No cognitive impairment
   b. Mild cognitive impairment
   c. Moderate cognitive impairment
   d. Severe cognitive impairment

65. You are the PMHNP treating a 10-year-old boy for ADHD and social anxiety disorder. His mother presents with him for the scheduled individual therapy session. At the end of the session his mother says, "I need to take him to see his pediatrician and at the last visit I was told he needed some HPV shot. I don't know, he's a boy, why would he need that? What do you think?" What is the PMHNP's best response to her question?

   a. "The CDC recommends the human papillomavirus (HPV) vaccine for all boys and girls at age 10. HPV can cause cancer in both men and women, and the vaccine is effective in protecting against the virus. Can you tell me your concerns about this vaccine?"
   b. "While the Centers for Disease Control and Prevention (CDC) recommends the vaccine, every parent has the right to choose and if you do not think he needs this vaccine, as his parent you have the right to refuse."
   c. "The CDC recommends the human papillomavirus (HPV) vaccine for older teenagers, starting at age 18, so you have time to research and think about your decision."
   d. "My daughters received the vaccine, and I'm like you, I did not let my sons receive the vaccine. They don't need it. I agree, vaccines can be scary. Can you tell me your concerns?"

66. As a PMHNP working in a crisis evaluation center, you are aware that the initial focus of a crisis assessment is on which of the following?

   a. Client's past diagnosis and medication trials
   b. Psychosocial history and supports
   c. Safety of the client and others
   d. Current living situation and coping skills

67. When conducting a neurological examination on a client, the PMHNP asks the client to hold out her arms and stick out her tongue while assessing for tremors. Which cranial nerve is being assessed?

    a. Glossopharyngeal
    b. Vagus
    c. Trigeminal
    d. Hypoglossal

68. A 20-year-old client who was recently diagnosed with schizophrenia comes to your office for a follow-up appointment. During the assessment, the client talks about experiences in the group home, saying that the television is sending messages through news anchors during the 10 p.m. evening news. What symptom is the client describing?

    a. Paranoia
    b. Illusions
    c. Ideas of reference
    d. Neologisms

69. You are working with a family: mother, father, and two biological children. The father is very rigid and controlling, which seems to be out of fear that something might happen to his family. He worries daily and it affects his family relationships. You give the father a paradoxical directive and instruct him to intensely worry about everything he can think of for 1 hour a day. Using a paradoxical directive is part of which therapy?

    a. Experimental
    b. Structural
    c. Strategic
    d. Cognitive

70. As a PMHNP working in an outpatient addiction clinic, you often refer your clients to community Alcoholics Anonymous (AA) and Narcotics Anonymous (NA) meetings. Using Yalom's therapeutic factors, you are aware that peer-led groups can inspire and encourage other group participants. Which therapeutic factor is instilled in AA and NA group members?

    a. Hope
    b. Altruism
    c. Catharsis
    d. Existential factors

71. Which of the following client statements best describes imitative behavior as a therapeutic factor in group therapy?

    a. Group members talk over one another so the loudest person is heard.
    b. Group members begin to model aspects of other members of the group and group leaders.
    c. Group members discuss past situations when they were bullied and felt ashamed.
    d. Group leaders take charge of the group and redirect members when they monopolize the group.

72. Dialectical behavioral therapy (DBT) draws on cognitive theory and behavioral theory, along with other theories. Elements of behavioral theory in DBT include which of the following?

    a. Skills training and exposure
    b. Examination of feelings and relating feelings to visceral sensations
    c. Working through the transference with the therapist
    d. Cognitive interpretation of past traumatic experiences

73. DBT affirms dialectical thinking, which involves examining and discussing opposing ideas to find the truth. This philosophy is a supportive principle of DBT training. The central dialectical pattern emphasized in DBT involves the tension between which of the following?

    a. Radical acceptance and change
    b. Cue exposure and block avoidance
    c. Problem avoidance and problem-solving
    d. Crisis survival and acceptance

74. S.P. is a 26-year-old partnered female who works full time as a teacher. S.P. is in a long-term relationship, they are getting along well, and doing well financially. They have two children, ages 2 and 6. S.P. is seeing the PMHNP to address concerns about feeling down and sad for no reason and states, "I know my life is going well but I just don't feel happy. I have always worried a lot and have been sad most of my life." As a PMHNP trained in transactional analysis (TA), you understand that personality is multifaceted and wonder if which of the following is affecting her ability to experience happiness:

    a. Experienced long periods of separation from the primary caregiver as a child and now has a difficult time accepting and receiving love and experiencing happiness
    b. The possibility of a traumatic event in childhood and thoughts and feelings related to the event are locked together in the brain and cannot be accessed
    c. Unhappiness is likely related to distorted thoughts and feelings about the relationship
    d. As an adolescent experienced an event that was processed in an ego state as an older sibling

75. You have been working with a 54-year-old client who has been treated for schizophrenia since age 19. The client has limited social interactions, likes to be alone, and has never dated or had a desire to date. The symptoms are best explained by which of the following?

   a. Antisocial personality disorder
   b. Lack of personal hygiene
   c. Negative symptoms
   d. Positive symptoms

76. Following evidence-based practice (EBP), which laboratory screening tests and assessments should be completed prior to placing a person on a second-generation ("atypical") antipsychotic medication?

   a. Serum glucose, lipid profile, weight, blood pressure, waist circumference, and family history of cardiovascular disease
   b. Comprehensive metabolic panel, body mass index, complete blood count, and thyroid panel
   c. Serum glucose or hemoglobin A1c, lipid profile, weight, body mass index, blood pressure, waist circumference, and family history of cardiovascular disease
   d. Serum glucose, complete blood count, assessment of family history of cardiovascular disease and cancer

77. Which type of hallucination is rare in persons with psychotic illnesses and is often associated with an organic etiology?

   a. Auditory hallucinations
   b. Gustatory hallucinations
   c. Visual hallucinations
   d. Combination hallucinations

78. What differentiates atypical antipsychotic medications from first-generation or typical antipsychotic medications?

   a. 5-HT2A receptor antagonist properties
   b. 5-HT2A receptor agonist properties
   c. Specific dopamine receptor 3 and 5-HT2A blockade
   d. Dopamine receptor 2 antagonist properties

79. You are treating a client with a diagnosis of schizophrenia who takes clozapine. What laboratory values will indicate that the client needs to discontinue treatment?

    a. White blood cell count of less than 1,800/mm^3 and absolute neutrophil count of less than 1,200/mm^3
    b. Absolute neutrophil count of less than 1,000/uL
    c. White blood cell count of less than 1,200/mm^3
    d. Absolute neutrophil count of less than 2,000/uL

80. C.Z. is a 47-year-old Gulf War veteran who was in combat during Operation Desert Storm and has been treated by the PMHNP for symptoms of major depressive disorder and associated anxiety symptoms. During the most recent visit, the PMHNP learns that C.Z. sustained a traumatic brain injury (TBI) during service, which was recently diagnosed at the TBI clinic at the Veterans Affairs (VA) clinic. What is the rationale for the PMHNP to taper C.Z. off clonazepam?

    a. Benzodiazepines cause memory problems and confusion in clients with a history of a TBI.
    b. Benzodiazepines lower the seizure threshold in clients with a history of a TBI.
    c. The VA has banned benzodiazepines from the medication formulary.
    d. Benzodiazepines place clients with a TBI at risk for a second head injury.

81. A.C. is a 68-year-old client who presents to you with concerns about memory. The client explains that memory issues run in the family; their mother and grandmother both experienced dementia and A.C. wants to be able to prevent this terrible disease. The client is treated for hypertension, which is well controlled; other than that, they are in good health. A.C. is socially and physically active and participates in a monthly cooking class, volunteers at church, and plays bridge twice a week at the senior center. A.C. states, "I understand that I am losing brain cells at my age, but I would still like to keep my mind and body active." Which is the best response to A.C.?

    a. "You are correct that you cannot form new brain cells at your age but you should continue with your activities because they offer excellent physical and mental health benefits and in turn will lower your risk for dementia."
    b. "Although most brain development occurs early in life, we still form some new brain cells in a couple of areas of the brain during adulthood. You should continue with your activities because they offer excellent physical and mental health benefits and are neuroprotective."
    c. "Scientists now know that we do continue to form new brain cells throughout the entire brain during adulthood. Continue with your activities because you are producing new brain cells in the frontal lobe and this will decrease your risk of dementia."
    d. "You should continue the social activities such as bridge, volunteering, and the book club but should consider the risks and benefits of physical activities such as dancing. If you were to fall and break a hip, this could lead to prolonged hospitalization, loss of independence, and ultimately increase your risk of dementia."

82. What is the best treatment for AIDS dementia complex?

    a. Acetylcholinesterase inhibitors

    b. Symptom-targeted pharmacologic treatments

    c. Nonpharmacologic supportive care

    d. Antiretroviral therapy

83. As a PMHNP working on the consult liaison team, you know the importance of preventing delirium due to which of the following?

    a. Risk of 1-year mortality rate

    b. Risk of harm to the client and staff

    c. Risk of unremitting psychosis

    d. Risk of aspiration

84. When working with a 26-year-old who presents for treatment of cannabis use and gambling, you use motivational interviewing techniques. As a PMHNP, you are familiar with the core counseling skills used in motivational interviewing. The client made the following statement: "I don't know why I came here in the first place but I thought maybe some medication would help me." You respond by saying, "You're feeling confused about the process" and the client replies, "I never thought I'd need to come to a place like this." You respond, "You kept your appointment today and I appreciate the courage it took for you to come here." What two motivational interviewing techniques are used in this interaction?

    a. Interrupting and reassurance

    b. Affirming and reflecting

    c. Open-ended questions and summarizing

    d. Clarification and data collection

85. You are a PMHNP working in a hospitalist role on an acute inpatient psychiatric unit at a local hospital. As you make rounds, the registered nurse informs you that a 32-year-old client who was admitted for alcohol detox has a score of 17 on the Clinical Institute Withdrawal Assessment for Alcohol (CIWA). What phase of withdrawal is this client in?

    a. Mild withdrawal

    b. Moderate withdrawal

    c. Severe withdrawal

    d. Delirium tremens

86. A client who has been addicted to opioids has not used in 15 days. During your medication management visit, the client states, "I'm going to die from not having my Opana. You need to give me something now." What is the PMHNP's best response?

    a. "I know you are feeling very uncomfortable and we need to get you to the emergency room immediately to prevent a seizure."

    b. "I know you are feeling very uncomfortable; let's take your vital signs and talk about a trial on clonidine to treat your withdrawal symptoms."

    c. "You have been using Opana for a long time and it is going to take several months for the withdrawal to end. In the meantime, I will see you weekly."

    d. "There is no treatment for opioid withdrawal; you will have to wait it out."

87. Signs and symptoms of cannabis intoxication include: which of the following?

    a. Increased sensitivity to external stimuli

    b. Enhanced motor skills

    c. Fast passage of time

    d. Lower heart rate

88. Which defense mechanisms are commonly used by persons with a diagnosis of obsessive–compulsive personality disorder?

    a. Rationalization, isolation, and intellectualization

    b. Projection, distortion, and hypochondriasis

    c. Regression, somatization, and dissociation

    d. Sexualization, displacement, and reaction formation

89. You have been working with D.J., a 30-year-old single client, in weekly individual psychotherapy for 3 weeks. At the start of session 4, D.J. says, "I noticed when I came in that your usual parking spot has a new car in it with temporary tags, and it's a BMW. Nice car." What is the best response from the PMHNP psychotherapist to D.J.?

    a. "Thanks for noticing, it is a nice car."

    b. "How do you know what spot I park in?"

    c. "I noticed you drive a BMW as well; how do you like your car?"

    d. "Sounds like having expensive things is important to you."

90. When working in individual psychotherapy with a client who has a personality disorder, what are the primary treatment goals?

    a. Change the client's personality structure and make them more adaptable in everyday life.

    b. Re-parent the client, following Bowlby's theoretical framework.

    c. Allow the client to reprocess their childhood trauma because all clients with personality disorders have a history of severe abuse.

    d. Assist the client in changing dysfunctional interpersonal relationships and use of immature defense mechanisms.

91. For a client who has a diagnosis of paranoid personality disorder, what are the best treatment strategies?

    a. Confront negative and misinterpreted thoughts and feelings.

    b. Deflate grandiose thoughts.

    c. Engage the client in detailed and emotional responses and dialog.

    d. Do not challenge negative views or recollections of events.

92. G.L., a client with a diagnosis of paranoid personality disorder, states the following: "I noticed there is a red light in the upper corner of your door and it has been going on and off during our sessions. Are you recording me?" What is the PMHNP best response?

    a. "No, it would be illegal for me to record you, and that is not a camera; it's just a red light."

    b. "G.L., thank you for asking the question. The light you see in the upper corner of my door tells me when a client has arrived and is in the waiting room. The client turns on the light, as you do, when they arrive in the waiting room, alerting me to their arrival, and I turn off the light when we get into the office using the switch by my desk."

    c. "Come on G.L., do you think I would record your sessions? You are not that interesting. I'm just kidding. No G.L., it is not a recorder or camera."

    d. "G.L., it takes courage to ask me the question. Tell me a time in your life when you had a similar experience."

93. As a PMHNP, you understand the genetic factors that contribute to psychiatric and personality disorders. Persons who develop antisocial personality disorder often are raised in families with high rates of which of the following?

    a. Psychotic disorders
    b. Alcohol use disorders
    c. Anxiety disorders
    d. Mood disorders

94. Persons with a diagnosis of obsessive–compulsive personality disorder often use isolation as a defense mechanism. Which of the following examples best describes isolation as a defense mechanism?

    a. Staying in the house for days or weeks to clean
    b. Declining invites by friends or family to attend social gatherings
    c. Describing information with very little affect variation
    d. Being an introvert in the work setting to prevent talking with coworkers

95. In the DSM-5-TR, how should a personality disorder be coded?

    a. Coded as the personality disorder
    b. Coded on Axis II
    c. Coded with the major psychiatric disorder
    d. Coded on Axis IV

96. When prescribing a selective SSRI for a child or young adult up to age 24, what education must be included?

    a. Food and Drug Administration (FDA) box warning about increased suicidality in this population
    b. FDA box warning about increased risk of mania in this population
    c. Risk of sexual side effects associated with this class of medication
    d. Risk of stomach upset and headaches, to prevent unnecessary primary care visits

97. K.T. is an 8-year-old who presents to the PMHNP for evaluation of attention-deficit/hyperactivity disorder. The client's mother completed the Vanderbilt ADHD rating scale and brought in the Vanderbilt teaching rating scale. Both your clinical interview and the rating scales indicate that K.T. has met the criteria for ADHD. What assessment indicator(s) need to be completed prior to starting a stimulant mediation?

    a. Get a copy of the rating scale completed by his grandparents.
    b. Assess for family history of cardiovascular disease and, if positive for conduction problems, and order an electrocardiogram before prescribing medication.
    c. Obtain blood pressure and pulse, and begin the stimulant medication.
    d. Assess for a family history of bipolar disorder.

98. A mother brings in her 7-year-old son for a psychiatric follow-up visit with the PMHNP. This is the fourth visit the PMHNP has had with the client, his mother, and his younger sister, Renee, now 7-months-old. You notice that she has a decrease in head growth, along with stereotypic motions of the hands, often licking and slapping. Renee has also lost her language skills. What medical condition do you suspect Renee has developed?

    a. Autism spectrum disorder
    b. Rett syndrome
    c. Selective mutism
    d. Childhood-onset diabetes

99. You are treating a 16-year-old for symptoms of an eating disorder. The client is of normal weight and socially extroverted, at times appearing to seek attention when in a peer group or class. The symptoms are most consistent with which eating disorder?

    a. Anorexia nervosa
    b. Bulimia nervosa
    c. Binge eating disorder
    d. Anxiety-induced eating disorder

100. You are treating a 14-year-old for symptoms of ADHD who has a family history of bipolar disorder. As a PMHNP familiar with symptoms of both ADHD and pediatric bipolar disorder, which of the following are overlapping symptoms of both disorders?

    a. Excessive talking, increased activity, and distractibility
    b. Irritability, sleep problems, and mood swings
    c. Excessive talking, irritability, and sleep problems
    d. Sleep problems, mood swings, and distractibility

APPENDIX B

REVIEW QUESTION ANSWERS

1. Correct Answer: A. The Psychiatric-Mental Health Nursing: Scope and Standards of Practice defines the role and actions of psychiatric-mental health nurses at RN and APRN levels.

2. Correct Answer: D. Information reduces incidence of disease.

3. Correct Answer: B. Identifies the trend of ensuring the protection of individual civil liberties for psychiatric clients.

4. Correct Answer: C. As with any client, psychiatric clients can refuse treatment unless a legal process resulting in involuntary commitment or mandatory court order for treatment has been obtained.

5. Correct Answer: A. Social relationships are mutual interpersonal relationships in which the needs of both parties are addressed. The N–C relationship is most concerned with meeting the needs of the client.

6. Correct Answer: A. This action focuses on interventions designed to reduce the incidence of new cases of disease.

7. Correct Answer: B. Almost every state allows for a brief period of detainment to assess a client for dangerousness to self or others before allowing the client to leave a hospital setting, even if the admission was voluntary.

8. Correct Answer: C. Authenticity. Being genuine, honest, and respectful are essential elements in establishing a working relationship with any client. Like-mindedness is not a part of the therapeutic relationship. Although an important aspect of the PMHNP role, collecting a family history and accuracy in assessment does not in and of itself facilitate relationship-building.

9. Correct Answer: D. All DSM-5-TR disorders need to be made taking a person's culture into account. A cultural expression of a response to grief, loss, or stress is not considered a DSM-5-TR diagnosis.

10. Correct Answer: C. Clients frequently display resistance and regression at the termination of a meaningful therapeutic process. The PMHNP is responsible for planning an effective termination and monitoring clients during the termination period.

11. Correct Answer: B. These signs indicate developmental failure of early childhood.

12. Correct Answer: B. The psychic determinism principle states that all behavior has purpose and meaning, often unconscious in nature, and that no behaviors occur randomly or by coincidence.

13. Correct Answer: D. Suppression is the only defense mechanism listed in which the client channels conflicting energies into growth-promoting activities.

14. Correct Answer: A. Immature regressive defense mechanism is a return to a behavior common to an earlier stage of development.

15. Correct Answer: C. Defense mechanisms are a function of the ego used to resolve a conflict.

16. Correct Answer: C. ACOs are groups of doctors or other health care providers who voluntarily come together and assume the care provided to Medicare clients.

17. Correct Answer: A. Health efficiency evaluates the risk and benefit and decides how health care resources are allocated; health equity requires a fair distribution of resources.

18. Correct Answer: B. The four elements that must be satisfied for malpractice to have occurred are a duty of care between clinician and client, breach of duty which is a breach of standard of care, an injury to the client, and the client's injury must be related to the clinician's breach of care.

19. Correct Answer: D. The ANA position statement on "Just Culture" recognizes individuals should not be held accountable for system failings for which they have no control and also recognizes many errors represent predictable interactions between humans and the system where they work. The model creates an open, fair, and just culture with baseline competencies for accountability and creates opportunities to improve.

20. Correct Answer: A. Neurotransmitters in the central nervous system function as a communication medium.

21. Correct Answer: C. Serotonin is produced in the raphe nuclei.

22. Correct Answer: D. Dopamine is produced in the substantia nigra.

23. Correct Answer: B. Appetite, sleep, and libido are regulated by the hypothalamus.

24. Correct Answer: C. A client with a pacemaker should not receive an MRI of the brain.

25. Correct Answer: D. Glutamate is the primary excitatory neurotransmitter.

26. Correct Answer: A. Problems with working memory, planning and prioritizing, insight into problems, and impulse control indicate a problem in the frontal lobe.

27. Correct Answer: B. Target symptom identification is the identification of specific, precise, and individualized symptoms reasonably expected to improve with a given medication.

28. Correct Answer: C. Although diagnosis is an important aspect of the assessment process, the assessment ultimately should identify the needs of the client.

29. Correct Answer: C. One PMHNP role is to control the milieu as an aspect of assessment, so the PMHNP should choose a quiet place that is immediately accessible to get assistance with client care should it be required during the assessment.

30. Correct Answer: B. This exchange is an illustration of the technique of recognizing.

31. Correct Answer: D. The answer demonstrates concrete thought processes, which are normal in persons 12 years of age or older. To interpret the finding, the PMHNP must know the age of the client.

32. Correct Answer: B. This response will be the most therapeutic in moving forward with the client.

33. Correct Answer: B. This response is the most therapeutic, allowing the client to further clarify and express feelings.

34. Correct Answer: A. Asking the client how to help is an aspect of assessment. All other answers are aspects of interventions, which are not initial actions of the PMHNP.

35. Correct Answer: C. Client overdosed and then was placed on a medication that affects the liver. The PMHNP needs to assess the client's liver function as an aspect of care planning.

36. Correct Answer: D. Client symptoms are consistent with electrolyte imbalance and a physical cause of his symptoms must be ruled out first.

37. Correct Answer: B. Beta blockers can cause or exacerbate depression.

38. Correct Answer: C. Older adults usually have decreased protein levels. Most psychotropic medications are highly protein-bound. It is the unbound (free) concentration of the drug that is active; the bound concentration of the drug is inert. Thus, with decreased protein available for binding, more, free (active) drug remains in the body, which then predisposes older adults to toxicity.

39. Correct Answer: B. Divalproex can cause spina bifida and lithium can cause Ebstein's anomaly.

40. Correct Answer: C. Pharmacokinetics is the study of what the body does to drugs.

41. Correct Answer: C. Tolerance means needing more to achieve the same effect.

42. Correct Answer: D. Group therapy is beneficial because it increases social skills, is cost-effective, and enables participants to acquire the therapeutic factors which can be curative.

43. Correct Answer: A. Cognitive behavioral therapy helps clients recognize and change their automatic thoughts.

44. Correct Answer: C. Paradoxical directives are used in strategic therapy.

45. Correct Answer: B. Homeostasis is balance or stability to which the family returns despite its dysfunction.

46. Correct Answer: B. Miracle questions are used in solution-focused therapy.

47. Correct Answer: A. The use of a standardized rating scale will allow the PMHNP to monitor the level of client symptoms and to evaluate the efficacy of the medication.

48. Correct Answer: C. SSRIs are considered among the first-line medications used to treat depression because of safety in suicidal overdose clients.

49. Correct Answer: C. The PMHNP needs to ensure that their attempt to end her life has not led to medical instability.

50. Correct Answer: A. The literature suggests that although short-term anxiolytic medication may be offered in an emergency room setting, ataque de nervios is best treated by brief supportive therapy by a Spanish-speaking Latino therapist.

51. Correct Answer: C. The student does not meet criteria for alcohol use or other disorder at this point, but if he does not learn alternative coping skills to deal with his shyness, he is at risk of developing an alcohol use disorder.

52. Correct Answer: D. Although the PMHNP's resentment is in response to actual behavior by the client (missing several appointments), clarifying what is going on for him, his expectations for treatment, and the PMHNP's (and the clinic's) expectations in a non-judgmental manner will help to develop a therapeutic alliance.

53. Correct Answer: C. The therapeutic dose of SSRIs is generally lower than for young adults.

54. Correct Answer: C. In this case, you see a shifting set of symptoms, the most important being her expansive mood and statement "so much better" that indicates she has gone beyond euthymia.

55. Correct Answer: A. OSA is the only plausible possibility if the rest of the information given by the client is accurate. OSA causes clients to have frequent awakenings and a sense that they are not sleeping deeply ("tossing and turning") that is caused by apnea. The client should be assessed further for snoring and awareness of apnea. Although the client states he drinks a lot of coffee, this is driven by his sleep issues. Drinking 1 glass of wine in the evening would not cause the degree of sleep pathology he is exhibiting. Other than diminishing concentration that is consistent with sleep deprivation, there are no other signs and symptoms of ADHD.

56. Correct Answer: B. APRNs are not grandfathered into an academic degree; degrees must be earned from accredited academic institutions.

57. Correct Answer: C. It is not within the scope of practice of a PMHNP to treat hypertension. Coordination of care to ensure that the client does not run out of medication is the appropriate course of action.

58. Correct Answer: D. Engaging in a project to assess whether a standard of care was met is a quality improvement project.

59. Correct Answer: C. The legal system makes the determination about whether a person is competent; practitioners can assess and make a determination about a person's capacity to make medical decisions.

60. Correct Answer: D. Prevention of illness is primary prevention and administration of flu vaccinations in a community is intended to prevent a flu outbreak.

61. Correct Answer: A. Clients who are legally competent have the ability to make medical decisions and maintain individual autonomy.

62. Correct Answer: B. PMHNPs are mandated reporters of child abuse. The 3-year-old is being exposed to violence and, although not the target, could have been injured when the boyfriend threw the glass of water.

63. Correct Answer: B. During a psychiatric interview, the PMHNP is responsible for identifying symptoms and needs of a client to develop an appropriate treatment plan.

64. Correct Answer: C. Cut points on the MMSE are as follows: total score 30, 25–30 questionable significance, 20–25 mild impairment, 10–20 moderate impairment, and 10 or lower severe impairment.

65. Correct Answer: A. When family members or clients ask questions about illnesses and treatment, it is the PMHNP's responsibility to provide data and then assess understanding and meaning.

66. Correct Answer: C. In a crisis, the first assessment should be the safety of the client and those near the client.

67. Correct Answer: D. The tongue is controlled by the hypoglossal cranial nerve.

68. Correct Answer: C. Ideas of reference are misinterpretations of incidents and events that one believes have a direct personal reference to oneself.

69. Correct Answer: C. Paradoxical directives may be used in strategic family therapy.

70. Correct Answer: A. Working in support groups such as AA and NA, hearing stories of others who had similar struggles, instills hope.

71. Correct Answer: B. As the group progresses, the leader is less active and the members of the group take over and begin to model other members and the leaders.

72. Correct Answer: A. DBT focuses on cognitive and behavioral techniques, mindfulness including meditation, and emotional regulation.

73. Correct Answer: A. DBT emphasis acceptance of the current reality of what is and the ability to engage in personal change.

74. Correct Answer: B. According to TA, when a person is traumatized the thoughts and feelings get tied together and the process of therapy is to unlock the two.

75. Correct Answer: C. Negative symptoms include flat affect, alogia, avolition, poor attention, and anhedonia. In the case study, the symptoms are avolition and anhedonia.

76. Correct Answer: C. EBP guidelines indicate that all clients should have the following prior to starting antipsychotic medication: fasting glucose or hemoglobin A1c, lipid profile, weight, body mass index, blood pressure, waist circumference, and family history of cardiovascular disease.

77. Correct Answer: B. The most common type of hallucinations in persons with psychotic illnesses are auditory and visual. Tactile and gustatory hallucinations are less common and more likely related to an organic illness.

78. Correct Answer: A. Typical antipsychotic medications block D2 receptors; atypical antipsychotic medications block D2 receptors and have 5HT2A antagonist properties.

79. Correct Answer: B. The recent change in monitoring clozapine clients using the risk evaluation and mitigation strategy (REMS) indicates persons treated on clozapine need to have absolute neutrophil count monitored and, if level drops below 1,000/uL, treatment must be interrupted and can be resumed once the absolute neutrophil count normalizes to 1,000/uL or above.

80. Correct Answer: A. Benzodiazepines are contraindicated in clients with TBI due to increased rates of confusion and memory problems.

81. Correct Answer: B. Although it was once thought that brain neurons did not regenerate, we now know that while most brain development occurs early in life, we continue to form some new brain cells throughout life. As we age, we need to engage in activities that keep our brains healthy by encouraging this growth. Examples are healthy diet, exercise, socialization, and cognitive stimulation.

82. Correct Answer: D. All persons with AIDS should be treated with antiretroviral therapy. Those who develop dementia complex should have those symptoms treated with appropriate pharmacological or nonpharmacological interventions.

83. Correct Answer: A. Studies have identified high rates of mortality post hospitalization for delirium, so the best treatment is prevention.

84. Correct Answer: B. When a person is in the contemplation stage, interventions should be affirming and reflecting.

85. Correct Answer: B. CIWA cutoff scores are as follows: 0–9, absent or very mild withdrawal; 10–15, mild withdrawal; 16–20, moderate withdrawal; and 21–67, severe withdrawal.

86. Correct Answer: B. Opioid withdrawal symptoms can be treated with central alpha agonists.

87. Correct Answer: A. Persons intoxicated on cannabis exhibit distorted perceptions, increased relaxation and sensitivity, and loss of coordination.

88. Correct Answer: A. Persons with obsessive–compulsive personality disorder use defense mechanisms of rationalization, isolation of affect, and intellectualization to make sense of their behavior.

89. Correct Answer: D. In a therapy relationship, the therapist should try to understand the meaning of a client's statement rather than engage in social conversations.

90. Correct Answer: D. Persons with personality disorders have a pervasive maladaptive pattern of behavior and the goal of therapy is to slowly shift how they relate in the world and begin to use higher-order defenses.

91. Correct Answer: D. Persons with fixed false beliefs should not be challenged.

92. Correct Answer: B. When working with a paranoid client, help the person find proof of meaning and explain any questions in a matter-of-fact manner.

93. Correct Answer: B. Being raised in a family with alcohol use disorder increases the likelihood of chaos, unpredictability, and lack of rules and order, leading to higher rates of developing antisocial personality disorder.

94. Correct Answer: C. Isolation is a defense mechanism often used by people with obsessive–compulsive personality disorder and has to do with affect and emotion rather than getting out and being social.

95. Correct Answer: A. Axial system is no longer used and the personality disorder is coded as its own diagnosis.

96. Correct Answer: A. The SSRIs all carry a FDA box warning for increased suicidal ideation for this age group.

97. Correct Answer: B. American Academy of Child and Adolescent Psychiatry practice parameters require physical exam, pulse, weight, height, and blood pressure workup prior to the start of stimulant medication. Because his grandfather had a cardiac conduction problem, an electrocardiogram (ECG) should also be obtained prior to the start of medication.

98. Correct Answer: B. Girls with Rett's syndrome develop normally and around the seventh month regress, with a decrease in the mean head circumference to 2 standard deviations below the normal at 4 years of age and language loss.

99. Correct Answer: B. Clients with bulimia are often of normal weight or overweight and are outgoing.

100. Correct Answer: A. Clients with ADHD and bipolar disorder often have excessive talking, increased activity, and distractibility.

INDEX

Printed and bound by CPI Group (UK) Ltd, Croydon, CR0 4YY

02/06/2026

14891421-0001